Atrial Fibrillation

Guest Editors

RANJAN K. THAKUR, MD, MPH

ANDREA NATALE, MD, FACC, FHRS

CARDIOLOGY CLINICS

www.cardiology.theclinics.com

Consulting Editor
MICHAEL H. CRAWFORD, MD

February 2009 • Volume 27 • Number 1

SAUNDERS an imprint of ELSEVIER, Inc.

W.B. SAUNDERS COMPANY
A Division of Elsevier Inc.

Elsevier, Inc. • 1600 John F. Kennedy Blvd. • Suite 1800 • Philadelphia, Pennsylvania 19103-2899

http://www.theclinics.com

CARDIOLOGY CLINICS Volume 27, Number 1
February 2009 ISSN 0733-8651, ISBN-13: 978-1-4377-0456-3, ISBN-10: 1-4377-0456-5

Editor: Barbara Cohen-Kligerman

Cardiology Clinics (ISSN 0733-8651) is published quarterly by Elsevier Inc., 360 Park Avenue South, New York, NY 10010-1710. Months of issue are February, May, August, and November. Business and editorial Offices: 1600 John F. Kennedy Blvd., Suite 1800, Philadelphia, PA 19103-2899. Customer Service Office: 11830 Westline Industrial Drive, St. Louis, MO 63146. Periodicals postage paid at New York, NY, and additional mailing offices. Subscription prices are $244.00 per year for US individuals, $378.00 per year for US institutions, $122.00 per year for US students and residents, $298.00 per year for Canadian individuals, $470.00 per year for Canadian institutions, $346.00 per year for international individuals, $470.00 per year for international institutions and $173.00 per year for Canadian and foreign students/residents. To receive student/resident rate, orders must be accompanied by name of affiliated institution, data of term, and the *signature* of program/residency coordinator on institution letterhead. Orders will be billed at individual rate until proof of status is received. Foreign air speed delivery is included in all *Clinics* subscription prices. All prices are subject to change without notice. **POSTMASTER:** Send address changes to *Cardiology Clinics*, Elsevier Periodicals Customer Service, 11830 Westline Industrial Drive, St. Louis, MO 63146. **Customer Service: 1-800-654-2452 (US). From outside of the US, call 314-453-7041. Fax: 314-453-5170. E-mail: JournalsCustomer Service-usa@elsevier.com (for print support); JournalsOnlineSupport-usa@elsevier.com (for online support).**

Reprints. For copies of 100 or more, of articles in this publication, please contact the Commercial Reprints Department, Elsevier Inc., 360 Park Avenue South, New York, NY 10010-1710. Tel.: 212-633-3812; Fax: 212-462-1935; Email: reprints@elsevier.com.

Cardiology Clinics is also published in Spanish by McGraw-Hill Interamericana Editores S. A., P.O. Box 5-237, 06500, Mexico D. F., Mexico; in Portuguese by Reichmann and Alfonso Editores Rio de Janeiro, Brazil; and in Greek by Dimitrios P. Lagos, 8 Pondon Street, GR115-28 Ilissia, Greece.

Cardiology Clinics is covered in *MEDLINE/PubMed (Index Medicus)*, *Excerpta Medica*, *The Cumulative Index to Nursing and Allied Health Literature* (CINAHL).

Contributors

CONSULTING EDITOR

MICHAEL H. CRAWFORD, MD
Professor of Medicine, University of California
San Francisco; Lucie Stern Chair in Cardiology,
and Interim Chief of Cardiology, University of
California San Francisco Medical Center, San
Francisco, California

GUEST EDITORS

ANDREA NATALE, MD, FACC, FHRS
Executive Medical Director, Texas Cardiac
Arrhythmia Institute at St. David's Medical
Center, Austin, Texas; Consulting Professor,
Division of Cardiology, Stanford University,
Palo Alto, California; Clinical Associate
Professor of Medicine, Case Western Reserve
University, Cleveland, Ohio; Senior Medical
Director, California Pacific Medical Center
Atrial Fibrillation and Arrhythmia Program, San
Francisco, California

RANJAN K. THAKUR, MD, MPH
Thoracic and Cardiovascular Institute, Sparrow
Health System, Michigan State University,
Lansing, Michigan

AUTHORS

RAMTIN ANOUSHEH, MD, MPH
Loma Linda University Medical Center, Loma
Linda, California

EMELIA J. BENJAMIN, MD, ScM
Professor of Medicine and Epidemiology,
Schools of Medicine and Public Health, Boston
University, Boston; and Framingham Heart
Study, Framingham, Massachusetts

NOEL G. BOYLE, MD, PhD
Professor of Medicine, UCLA Cardiac
Arrhythmia Center, Division of Cardiology,
Department of Medicine, David Geffen School
of Medicine at UCLA, Los Angeles, California

THOMAS D. CALLAHAN IV, MD
Cardiac Pacing and Electrophysiology,
Cleveland Clinic, Cleveland, Ohio

PENG-SHENG CHEN, MD
Professor of Medicine, Medtronic-Zipes Chair
in Cardiology, Director, Krannert Institute of
Cardiology and the Division of Cardiology,
Department of Medicine, Indiana University
School of Medicine, Indianapolis, Indiana

WEI-CHUNG CHEN, MPH
University of California San Diego Medical
Center, San Diego, California

CHUNG-CHUAN CHOU, MD
Assistant Professor of Medicine, Chang Gung
Memorial Hospital and Chang Gung University
College of Medicine, Taiwan, China

EMILY L. CONWAY, MD
Lankenau Hospital, Division of Cardiovascular
Diseases, Wynnewood, Pennsylvania

LUIGI DI BIASE, MD
Cardiac Pacing and Electrophysiology,
Cleveland Clinic, Cleveland, Ohio; Texas
Cardiac Arrhythmia Institute at St. David's
Medical Center, Austin; Department of
Cardiology, University of Foggia, Foggia, Italy

J. KEVIN DONAHUE, MD
Associate Professor, The Heart and Vascular
Research Center, Case Western Reserve
University, MetroHealth Campus, Cleveland,
Ohio

KENNETH ELLENBOGEN, MD
Kontos Professor of Medicine, Vice Chair,
Division of Cardiology, Department of Internal
Medicine, Virginia Commonwealth University,
Richmond; Director, Cardiac
Electrophysiology, Department of Internal
Medicine, Virginia Commonwealth University,
Richmond, Virginia

PATRICK T. ELLINOR, MD, PhD
Assistant Professor, Harvard Medical School,
Boston; Assistant Physician, Cardiac
Arrhythmia Service, and Cardiovascular
Research Center, Massachusetts General
Hospital, Boston, Massachusetts

GREGORY K. FELD, MD
Professor of Medicine, Director,
Electrophysiology Laboratory, Cardiac
Electrophysiology Program, Division of
Cardiology, University of California San Diego
Medical Center, San Diego, California

J. EMANUEL FINET, MD
Resident in Medicine, The Heart and Vascular
Research Center, Case Western Reserve
University, MetroHealth Campus, Cleveland,
Ohio

JOSEPH G. GALLINGHOUSE, MD
Texas Cardiac Arrhythmia Institute at
St. David's Medical Center, Austin, Texas

A. MARC GILLINOV, MD
Associate Professor of Surgery, Lerner School
of Medicine; Surgical Director, Atrial Fibrillation
Center, Cleveland Clinic Foundation
Cleveland, Ohio

RODNEY HORTON, MD
Texas Cardiac Arrhythmia Institute at
St. David's Medical Center, Austin, Texas

KRIT JONGNARANGSIN, MD
Assistant Professor, Division of Cardiovascular
Medicine, Cardiovascular Center, University of
Michigan, Ann Arbor, Michigan

GAUTHAM KALAHASTY, MD
Assistant Professor of Medicine, Division of
Cardiology, Department of Internal Medicine,
Virginia Commonwealth University, Richmond,
Virginia

WILLIAM B. KANNEL, MD, MPH, FACC
Professor of Medicine and Public Health,
National Heart Lung and Blood Institute's
Framingham Heart Study, Framingham;
Boston University School of Medicine's
Framingham Heart Study, Framingham,
Massachusetts

MARY KEEBLER, MD
Massachusetts General Hospital, Harvard
Medical School, Boston, Massachusetts

ATUL KHASNIS, MD
Department of Rheumatic and Immunologic
Diseases, Cleveland Clinic, Cleveland, Ohio

SUSAN S. KIM, MD
Assistant Professor of Medicine, Section of
Cardiology, Department of Medicine, University
of Chicago Medical Center, Chicago, Illinois

BRADLEY P. KNIGHT, MD
Professor of Medicine, Section of Cardiology,
Department of Medicine, University of Chicago
Medical Center, Chicago, Illinois

PETER R. KOWEY, MD
Lankenau Hospital and Institute for Medical
Research, Division of Cardiovascular Diseases,
Main Line Heart Center, Wynnewood; and
Thomas Jefferson University, Philadelphia,
Pennsylvania

STEVEN A. LUBITZ, MD
Clinical Fellow, Cardiovascular Institute, Mount
Sinai School of Medicine, New York, New York;
Research Fellow, Division of Preventive
Medicine, Brigham and Women's Hospital,
Boston, Massachusetts

SIMONE MUSCO, MD
Lankenau Hospital, Division of Cardiovascular
Diseases, Wynnewood, Pennsylvania

ANDREA NATALE, MD, FACC, FHRS
Executive Medical Director, Texas Cardiac
Arrhythmia Institute at St. David's Medical
Center, Austin, Texas; Consulting Professor,
Division of Cardiology, Stanford University,
Palo Alto, California; Clinical Associate
Professor of Medicine, Case Western Reserve
University, Cleveland, Ohio; Senior Medical
Director, California Pacific Medical Center
Atrial Fibrillation and Arrhythmia Program,
San Francisco, California

HAKAN ORAL, MD
Associate Professor, Division of Cardiovascular
Medicine, Cardiovascular Center, University of
Michigan, Ann Arbor, Michigan

BENZY J. PADANILAM, MD
The Care Group, LLC, Indianapolis, Indiana

ERIC N. PRYSTOWSKY, MD
The Care Group, LLC, Indianapolis, Indiana

VIVEK Y. REDDY, MD
Associate Professor of Medicine, Director of
Electrophysiology, University of Miami Hospital
Cardiovascular Clinic, Miami, Florida

DAVID S. ROSENBAUM, MD
Professor and Chairman, The Heart and
Vascular Research Center, Case Western
Reserve University, MetroHealth Campus,
Cleveland, Ohio

RAHUL SAKHUJA, MD, MPP
Massachusetts General Hospital, Harvard
Medical School, Boston, Massachusetts

ADAM E. SALTMAN, MD, PhD
Associate Professor of Surgery, SUNY
Downstate, Director of Cardiothoracic Surgery
Research, Maimonides Medical Center,
Brooklyn, New York

JAVIER SANCHEZ, MD
Texas Cardiac Arrhythmia Institute at
St. David's Medical Center, Austin, Texas

NAVINDER S. SAWHNEY, MD
Assistant Professor of Medicine, Cardiac
Electrophysiology Program, Division of
Cardiology, University of California
San Diego Medical Center, San Diego,
California

ASHOK J. SHAH, MD
Thoracic Cardiovascular Institute, Sparrow
Health System, Michigan State University,
Lansing, Michigan

KALYANAM SHIVKUMAR, MD, PhD
Professor of Medicine, UCLA Cardiac
Arrhythmia Center, Division of Cardiology,
Department of Medicine, David Geffen
School of Medicine at UCLA, Los Angeles,
California

RANJAN K. THAKUR, MD, MPH
Thoracic and Cardiovascular Institute, Sparrow
Health System, Michigan State University,
Lansing, Michigan

ALBERT L. WALDO, MD
The Walter H. Pritchard Professor of
Cardiology, Professor of Medicine, and
Professor of Biomedical Engineering, Division
of Cardiovascular Medicine, Department of
Medicine, Case Western Reserve University/
University Hospitals of Cleveland Case Medical
Center, Cleveland, Ohio

B. ALEXANDER YI, MD, PhD
Clinical and Research Fellow, Cardiology
Division, Massachusetts General Hospital and
Harvard Medical School, Boston,
Massachusetts

Contents

Foreword   xiii

Michael H. Crawford

Preface   xv

Ranjan K. Thakur and Andrea Natale

Dedication   xvii

Atrial Fibrillation: A Historical Perspective   1

Atul Khasnis and Ranjan K. Thakur

> Atrial fibrillation (AF) has undoubtedly become one of the most well-studied arrhythmias today in terms of pathophysiology and diagnostic and therapeutic (interventional) electrophysiology. Although it lends itself to an apparently easy diagnosis on the surface electrocardiography, myriad electromechanical mechanisms underlie its origin. We have now reached an era of technology that makes AF not only "treatable" but potentially "curable." This article aims at walking through the historical "corridors" and "mazes" that led to the present day understanding of this common yet complex arrhythmia.

Current Perceptions of the Epidemiology of Atrial Fibrillation   13

William B. Kannel and Emelia J. Benjamin

> Atrial fibrillation (AF), an escalating dysrhythmia, is accountable for extensive population morbidity and mortality. In the United States, approximately 2.3 million people are presently diagnosed with AF and it is estimated that this prevalence may increase to 5.6 million by 2050. Foremost predisposing risk factors for this dysrhythmia include advanced age and cardiovascular disease and its risk factors. The chief hazard of AF is embolic stroke, which is increased four- to fivefold, and in advanced age, it becomes a dominant stroke risk factor. AF also carries a doubled mortality rate.

Genetics of Atrial Fibrillation   25

Steven A. Lubitz, B. Alexander Yi, and Patrick T. Ellinor

> Recent studies of AF have identified mutations in a series of ion channels; however, these mutations appear to be relatively rare causes of AF. A genome-wide association study has identified novel variants on chromosome 4 associated with AF, although the mechanism of action for these variants remains unknown. Ultimately, a greater understanding of the genetics of AF should yield insights into novel pathways, therapeutic targets, and diagnostic testing for this common arrhythmia.

New Concepts in Atrial Fibrillation: Neural Mechanisms and Calcium Dynamics   35

Chung-Chuan Chou and Peng-Sheng Chen

Atrial fibrillation (AF) is a complex arrhythmia with multiple possible mechanisms. It requires a trigger for initiation and a favorable substrate for maintenance. Pulmonary vein myocardial sleeves have the potential to generate spontaneous activity, and this arrhythmogenic activity is surfaced by modulation of intracellular calcium dynamics. Direct autonomic nerve recordings in canine models show that simultaneous sympathovagal discharges are the most common triggers of paroxysmal atrial tachycardia and paroxysmal AF. Autonomic modulation as a potential therapeutic strategy has been targeted clinically and experimentally, but its effectiveness as an adjunctive therapeutic modality to catheter ablation of AF has been inconsistent. Further studies are warranted before application can be widely implied for therapies of clinical AF.

Information Learned from Animal Models of Atrial Fibrillation   45

J. Emanuel Finet, David S. Rosenbaum, and J. Kevin Donahue

Animal models of atrial fibrillation have taught us about mechanisms of this common disease. A variety of animal models exist, including models of lone atrial fibrillation and models of atrial fibrillation in the setting of heart failure, aging, or pericardial inflammation. This article reviews these various models.

Diagnosis and Management of Typical Atrial Flutter   55

Navinder S. Sawhney, Ramtin Anousheh, Wei-Chung Chen, and Gregory K. Feld

Typical atrial flutter (AFL) is a common atrial arrhythmia that may cause significant symptoms and serious adverse effects including embolic stroke, myocardial ischemia and infarction, and rarely a tachycardia-induced cardiomyopathy as a result of rapid atrioventricular conduction. As a result of the well-defined anatomic and electrophysiological substrate, and the relative pharmacologic resistance of typical AFL, radiofrequency catheter ablation has emerged in the past decade as a safe and effective first-line treatment. This article reviews the electrophysiology of typical AFL and the techniques currently used for its diagnosis and management.

Postoperative Atrial Fibrillation   69

Krit Jongnarangsin and Hakan Oral

Atrial fibrillation is a common arrhythmia that occurs after cardiac surgery. It is associated with an increase in morbidity, length of hospital stay and mortality. Patients who are at higher risk of postoperative atrial fibrillation should receive prophylactic treatment. Atrial fibrillation usually resolves spontaneously after heart rate is controlled; however, if patients are highly symptomatic or hemodynamically unstable, sinus rhythm should be restored by electrical or pharmacologic cardioversion.

Atrial Fibrillation in Congestive Heart Failure: Current Management   79

Noel G. Boyle and Kalyanam Shivkumar

Atrial fibrillation (AF) and congestive heart failure are common conditions and each predisposes to the development of the other. Basic research using animal models of the two conditions continues to yield insights that may improve therapies. The role of medical therapies aimed at the underlying structural changes in AF continues to be a subject of ongoing studies. Cardiac resynchronization therapy is effective in appropriately selected patients with both sinus rhythm and AF. Catheter ablation is emerging as a potential alternative to antiarrhythmic drug therapy, but large randomized trials will be needed to assess its role.

Electrical and Pharmacologic Cardioversion for Atrial Fibrillation   95

Susan S. Kim and Bradley P. Knight

This article describes electrical and pharmacologic cardioversion for atrial fibrillation and discusses indications for cardioversion and management of pericardioversion anticoagulation. Finally, management strategies are offered for immediate recurrence of atrial fibrillation and cardioversion failure.

Drug Therapy for Atrial Fibrillation   109

Emily L. Conway, Simone Musco, and Peter R. Kowey

Atrial fibrillation is the most frequently diagnosed arrhythmia. Prevalence increases with age, and the overall incidence is expected to increase as the population continues to age. Choice of pharmacologic therapy for atrial fibrillation depends on whether or not the goal of treatment is maintaining sinus rhythm or tolerating atrial fibrillation with adequate control of ventricular rates. Many new antiarrhythmic drugs are currently being tested in clinical trials. Drugs that target remodeling and inflammation have shown potential in prevention of atrial fibrillation, or as adjunctive therapy.

Anticoagulation: Stroke Prevention in Patients with Atrial Fibrillation   125

Albert L. Waldo

It is well recognized that during atrial fibrillation (AF), clots may form in the left atrium, which may embolize and cause ischemic stroke or systemic embolism. The presence of AF confers a fivefold increased risk for stroke. AF is the most common and important cause of stroke. This article considers the risks for and anticoagulation prophylaxis against embolic stroke in patients who have AF.

The Role of Pacemakers in the Management of Patients with Atrial Fibrillation   137

Gautham Kalahasty and Kenneth Ellenbogen

This article reviews the wide range of implantable device–based therapies (mainly pacemakers) that are being used in the management of atrial fibrillation (AF), atrial flutter, and atrial tachycardia. The role of pacemakers in the management of patients with AF and in the prevention of AF has been extensively studied. Based on well-designed prospective clinical trials, only a few of these strategies can be recommended for routine clinical use in related subpopulations.

Atrial Fibrillation in Patients with Implantable Defibrillators   151

Rahul Sakhuja, Ashok J. Shah, Mary Keebler, and Ranjan K. Thakur

Atrial fibrillation (AF) is common in patients who have implantable defibrillators and presents some unique challenges and opportunities. AF burden can be assessed more accurately, allowing for evaluation of therapy efficacy (drugs or ablation). It remains to be shown whether home monitoring of defibrillators to detect and treat AF more quickly can reduce cardiovascular and stroke end points. One major goal will be to reduce inappropriate shocks from atrial fibrillation. Otherwise, the goals of therapy remain the same—reduction of symptoms (including heart failure exacerbation and inappropriate implantable cardioverter defibrillator therapies) by controlling rate or rhythm and anticoagulation for stroke prophylaxis.

Catheter Ablation of Atrial Fibrillation   163

Thomas D. Callahan IV, Luigi Di Biase, Rodney Horton, Javier Sanchez, Joseph G. Gallinghouse, and Andrea Natale

Atrial fibrillation is a common arrhythmia associated with significant morbidity, including angina, heart failure, and stroke. Medical therapy remains suboptimal, with significant side effects and toxicities, and a high recurrence rate. Catheter ablation or modification of the atrioventricular node with pacemaker implantation provides rate-control but exposes patients to the hazards associated with implantable devices and does nothing to reduce the risk for stroke. Pulmonary vein antrum isolation offers a nonpharmacologic means of restoring sinus rhythm, thereby eliminating the morbidity of atrial fibrillation and the need for antiarrhythmic drugs.

Surgical Approaches for Atrial Fibrillation   179

Adam E. Saltman and A. Marc Gillinov

For cardiac surgery patients presenting with atrial fibrillation (AF), surgeons offer an operation that corrects the structural heart disease and the AF. With this approach, it is estimated that surgeons will perform more than 10,000 ablation procedures in 2008. Surgeons are developing minimally invasive techniques for stand-alone, epicardial ablation of AF. This article reviews the rationale for surgical ablation of AF, describes the classic maze procedure and its results, details new approaches to surgical ablation of AF, emphasizes the importance of management of the left atrial appendage, and considers challenges and future directions in the ablation of AF.

Atrial Fibrillation: Goals of Therapy and Management Strategies to Achieve the Goals   189

Benzy J. Padanilam and Eric N. Prystowsky

The primary goals in the management of patients who have atrial fibrillation are prevention of stroke and tachycardia-induced cardiomyopathy and amelioration of symptoms. Each patient presents to a physician with a specific constellation of symptoms and signs, but, fortunately, most patients can be assigned to broad categories for therapy. For some, anticoagulation and rate control suffice, whereas others require attempts to restore and maintain sinus rhythm. Physicians and patients should be willing to alter therapeutic plans if an initial strategy of rate or rhythm control is unsuccessful.

Atrial Fibrillation: Unanswered Questions and Future Directions   201

Vivek Y. Reddy

The seminal demonstration of the role of pulmonary vein triggers in the pathogenesis of atrial fibrillation (AF) and the potential therapeutic role of catheter ablation to treat patients who have paroxysmal AF was provided just over a decade ago. This initial observation ushered in the modern era of catheter ablation to treat patients who have AF, and tremendous progress has been made in understanding its pathogenesis and the catheter approaches to treating this rhythm. This article reflects on some of the major unanswered questions about AF management, and the future technologic and investigational directions being explored in the nonpharmacologic management of AF.

Index   **217**

Cardiology Clinics

FORTHCOMING ISSUES

May 2009

Nuclear Cardiology—From Perfusion to Tissue Biology
Frank Bengel, MD, *Guest Editor*

August 2009

Advances in Coronary Angiography
John D. Carroll, MD, and S. James Chen, PhD, *Guest Editors*

November 2009

Advances in Cardiac Computed Tomography
Mario J. Garcia, MD, FACC, *Guest Editor*

RECENT ISSUES

November 2008

Cardiology Drug Update
JoAnne M. Foody, MD, *Guest Editor*

August 2008

Ventricular Arrhythmias
John M. Miller, MD, *Guest Editor*

May 2008

Thromboembolic Disease and Antithrombotic Agents in the Elderly
Laurie G. Jacobs, MD, *Guest Editor*

ISSUES OF RELATED INTEREST

Heart Failure Clinics January 2009 (Vol. 5, No. 1)
Management of Heart Failure in the Emergency Department
James F. Neuenschwander II, MD, FACEP, and W. Frank Peacock, MD, FACEP, *Guest Editors*
Available at http://www.heartfailure.theclinics.com/

Anesthesiology Clinics September 2008 (Vol. 26, No. 3)
Cardiac Anesthesia: Today and Tomorrow
Davy C.H. Cheng, MD, MSc, FRCPC, FCAHS, *Guest Editor*
Available at http://www.anesthesiology.theclinics.com/

Sleep Medicine Clinics December 2007 (Vol. 2, No. 4)
Sleep and Cardiovascular Disease
Shahrokh Javaheri, MD, *Guest Editor*
Available at http://www.sleep.theclinics.com/

THE CLINICS ARE NOW AVAILABLE ONLINE!

Access your subscription at:
www.theclinics.com

Foreword

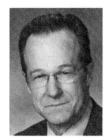

Michael H. Crawford, MD
Consulting Editor

Atrial fibrillation is rapidly becoming the "low back pain" of cardiology. It becomes more common with age, cardiac disease, and certain systemic diseases such as thyrotoxicosis. Hypertension, which affects one third of Americans—two thirds of those over 65 years old—is a harbinger of atrial fibrillation. It is frequent in post-surgical patients and can be precipitated by hyper- or hypovolemia. Sometimes it is the first manifestation of unrecognized underlying cardiac diseases such as mitral stenosis and atrial septal defect. Unfortunately, it is sometimes discovered only after a stroke in which it plays a causal role. Almost all areas of cardiology are touched by atrial fibrillation.

When I saw this excellent issue of *Medical Clinics of North America* volume 92, issue 1, on atrial fibrillation, edited by Drs. Thakur and Natale, I knew it would make a great issue of *Cardiology Clinics*. Fortunately, they agreed to update and modify the issue to make it more relevant to cardiologists. It is now the most current and comprehensive review of atrial fibrillation I know of. There is something for everyone in this issue, from the general cardiologist to the electrophysiology specialist. I found it highly informative and useful, and know you will as well.

Michael H. Crawford, MD
Division of Cardiology
Department of Medicine
University of California
San Francisco Medical Center
505 Parnassus Avenue, Box 0124
San Francisco, CA 94143-0124, USA

E-mail address:
crawfordm@medicine.ucsf.edu

Cardiol Clin 27 (2009) xiii
doi:10.1016/j.ccl.2008.10.005
0733-8651/08/$ – see front matter © 2009 Elsevier Inc. All rights reserved.

cardiology.theclinics.com

Preface

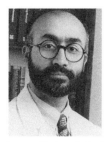 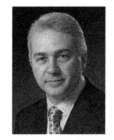

Ranjan K. Thakur, MD, MPH   Andrea Natale, MD, FACC, FHRS
Guest Editors

Atrial fibrillation is the most commonly sustained arrhythmia in man. While it affects millions of people around the globe already, its incidence will reach epidemic proportions as people live longer and we become even more successful in treating other cardiovascular diseases. Until recently, atrial fibrillation did not receive the attention it deserved, in part because we did not have much of a therapeutic armamentarium that could be brought to bear. A new wave of enthusiasm appeared about a decade ago after Haissaguerre and colleagues showed that atrial fibrillation could be initiated by ectopic beats originating in the pulmonary veins and that ablation of these sites can be curative.

An incredible effort by physicians, scientists and the medical industry over the last decade has brought forth new insights and therapeutic tools, and we have reached a level of maturity to indeed cure many patients with atrial fibrillation. We were privileged to take pause and summarize how much we have learned and reflect on what lies ahead in *Medical Clinics of North America* in January 2008. We are pleased that Dr. Michael Crawford, Consulting Editor for *Cardiology Clinics*, felt that its readership would benefit from an updated issue.

Our initial panel of authors has updated their contributions in this issue of *Cardiology Clinics*. We have added three new articles that the readers of the *Clinics* may also find interesting.

We are grateful to our friends and colleagues who have contributed their time and energy in writing these reviews. All of the contributors are busy investigators and well-known experts in the field. We have enjoyed reading their perspectives, and we hope that readers will also find these reviews helpful in obtaining an up-to-date understanding of this ever more important disease.

In addition, we owe special gratitude to Dr. Michael Crawford for this opportunity, and to our wonderful colleagues at Elsevier who worked very hard and made this project possible: Barbara Cohen-Kligerman, Jeannette Forcina and Rachel Glover.

Ranjan K. Thakur, MD, MPH
Thoracic and Cardiovascular Institute
Michigan State University
405 West Greenlawn, Suite 400
Lansing, MI 48910, USA

Andrea Natale, MD, FACC, FHRS
St. David's Medical Center
1015 East 32nd Street, Suite 516
Austin, TX 78705, USA

E-mail addresses:
thakur@msu.edu (R.K. Thakur)
dr.natale@gmail.com (A. Natale)

Cardiol Clin 27 (2009) xv
doi:10.1016/j.ccl.2008.10.001

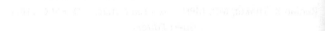

Dedication

To my wife, Niti for her love and support;
Our son Jay and my mother;
Also, to my patients, but especially, Louvenia.

Ranjan K. Thakur

To Marina

Andrea Natale

Cardiol Clin 27 (2009) xvii
doi:10.1016/j.ccl.2008.10.004

cardiology.theclinics.com

Atrial Fibrillation: A Historical Perspective

Atul Khasnis, MD, Ranjan K. Thakur, MD, MPH*

KEYWORDS

- Atrial fibrillation • Historical • Clinical
- Pathophysiology • Drugs • Ablation

We shall not cease from exploring and the end of all our exploring will be to arrive where we started and know the place for the first time.

—*T.S. Eliot*

The foregoing quotation is particularly a propos as we review the historical developments in atrial fibrillation (AF). This is exemplified by the fact that one of the first mechanisms proposed for initiation of AF invoked a focal trigger. For much of the twentieth century, a focal trigger was discounted until the landmark observation by Haissaguerre described pulmonary vein (PV) foci, and thus ushered in the ablation era. Although we engage in this "circus movement" in an attempt to understand AF better, we someday hope to eliminate the "excitable gap" in our knowledge, leading to the "cure" of AF.

AF has undoubtedly become one of the most well-studied arrhythmias today in terms of pathophysiology and diagnostic and therapeutic (interventional) electrophysiology. Although it lends itself to an apparently easy diagnosis on the surface electrocardiography (ECG), myriad electromechanical mechanisms underlie its origin. We have now reached an era of technology that makes AF not only "treatable" but potentially "curable." This article aims at walking through the historical "corridors" and "mazes" that led to the present day understanding of this common yet complex arrhythmia.

EARLIEST CLINICAL SIGHTINGS

The earliest record of AF seems to be in the Yellow Emperor's Classic of Internal Medicine in the seventeenth century.[1] William Harvey is credited with the first description of "auricular fibrillation" in animals, however, in 1628. After Harvey's description, the misunderstanding that the pulse was independent of the heartbeat continued to prevail, likely because of the dissociation that frequently exists between the irregular heart contractions and the palpable radial pulse in AF. This is now well recognized as the "pulse deficit," which can be a valuable clue to the bedside diagnosis of AF. In 1863, Chauveau and Marey[2] conducted various studies on cardiac physiology utilizing the "sphygmograph," an instrument used to record the pulse graphically, and thereby described a pulse tracing from a patient with AF.[1] Various descriptions of the irregular pulse as "intermission of the pulsation of the heart" (Laennec), "ataxia of the pulse" (Bouilland), delirium cordis (Nothnagel), and, finally, "pulsus irregularis perpetuus" (Hering) later ensued.[3] In 1907, Arthur Cushny at University College of London published the first case report of AF in his patient after surgery for an "ovarian fibroid" recorded with a "Jacques sphygmochronograph."[4] This was the first correlative clinical report on the electrical record and palpated irregularity of the pulse in AF. The development of the string galvanometer in 1909 opened the door on the electrical nature of AF, allowing further correlation with the physical examination.

AF is most commonly associated with mitral valve disease. Jean Baptiste Senac connected AF (which he called "rebellious palpitation") and mitral stenosis (MS) in 1783.[5] Robert Adams[6] reported irregular pulses associated with MS in 1827. In 1897, James Mackenzie[7] first noted that the jugular "A wave" was lost in a patient who

A version of this article originally appeared in *Medical Clinics of North America*, volume 92, issue 1.

Thoracic and Cardiovascular Institute, Sparrow Health System, Michigan State University, 405 West Greenlawn, Suite 400, Lansing, MI 48910, USA

* Corresponding author.

E-mail address: thakur@msu.edu (R.K. Thakur).

doi:10.1016/j.ccl.2008.09.013

cardiology.theclinics.com

had MS and that the presystolic murmur of MS disappeared in a patient who went from a normal to irregular rhythm. In more recent literature, AF has been reported to occur in 29% of patients who had isolated MS, in 16% who had isolated mitral regurgitation, and in 52% who had combined MS and regurgitation of rheumatic etiology.[8]

In the years that followed, the pure clinical face of AF was accompanied by further electromechanical insight facilitated by ECG and, over the years, newer recording and imaging modalities.

ELECTROCARDIOGRAPHY: REVEALING THE ELECTRICAL FACE OF ATRIAL FIBRILLATION

The development of ECG by Willem Einthoven (**Fig. 1**)[9] in 1902 provided a simple means for recording the electrical events that represent AF. His device consisted of a string galvanometer (with various complex attachments) and required transmission of electrical signals over telephone wires to his laboratory (**Fig. 2**). He recorded 26 single-lead ECG strips of various cardiac rhythm disturbances, one of which depicted AF (he called this electrical pattern pulsus inequalis and irregularis). In 1909, Thomas Lewis[10] described the classic "absence of P waves" and "irregularity of the

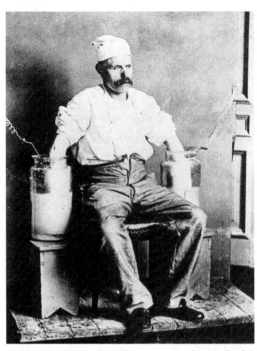

Fig. 2. Patient sitting in the university hospital while his telecardiogram is recorded in the physiology laboratory. His hands are immersed in strong salt (NaCl) solution. (*Courtesy of* The Einthoven Foundation, Leiden, The Netherlands; with permission.)

F waves" that define AF (**Fig. 3**). In 1928, technical advances were made to amplify ECG recordings.[11] Frank Sanborn developed the first portable ECG machine the same year.[12] This was a significant development in the miniaturization of ECG recording. Further research started focusing on finer points of ECG that can help to glean more useful and corroborative information regarding mechanisms and cardiac activity during AF. The atrial cycle length has been studied as a predictor of paroxysmal AF and of recurrence after cardioversion. This is done using frequency analysis of fibrillatory ECG.[13] Further studies have led to elucidation of initiating mechanisms for AF. In 1998, the PVs assumed an important role as the triggers driving paroxysmal AF. Ablation in the region of the PVs also rewardingly treated AF, leading to an exciting chase to identify the anatomic and electrical characteristics of these veins better. Certain ECG morphologies of the P waves can predict paroxysmal AF and identify the culprit PV.[14,15] Newer technologies, such as the 65-lead ECG mapping system (Resolution Medical, Inc., Pleasanton, CA), can facilitate noninvasive localization of AF trigger sites by matching the P wave integral map morphology of a premature atrial contraction with the reference database of 34 mean paced P wave integral map patterns.[16] AF

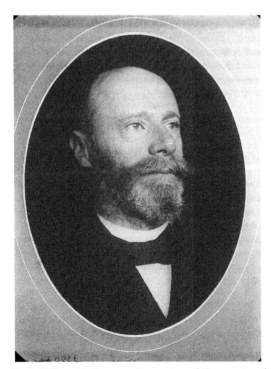

Fig. 1. Willem Einthoven when rector of the senate of the university in 1906. (*Courtesy of* The Einthoven Foundation, Leiden, The Netherlands; with permission.)

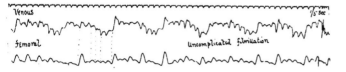

Fig. 3. Venous and femoral artery tracings from a dog during AF show a completely irregular pulse. (*From* Lewis T. The reaction of the heart to digitalis when the auricle is fibrillating. BMJ 1910;2:1670; with permission.)

was also later appreciated on intracardiac ECG.[17,18] Algorithms have been developed that can help to localize PV activity using intracardiac recordings during spontaneous and paced PV activity.[19] Time-frequency analysis of surface ECG has been reported to aid noninvasive monitoring of effects of antiarrhythmic drugs on fibrillatory rate and waveform.[20] We have come a long way since Einthoven but still use the same basic principles of ECG diagnosis of AF. Many more advances are likely to occur in understanding AF, but ECG is always likely to remain a trusted, economic, and noninvasive source of invaluable information that assists in clinical decision making.

PATHOPHYSIOLOGY: WHAT CAUSES ATRIAL FIBRILLATION?

The understanding of mechanisms underlying the initiation and maintenance of AF has evolved over the past decades. The earliest concept of re-entry proposed by Winterberg in 1906[21] and by Lewis and Schleiter[22] in 1912 advocated that rapid focal activity from one or more centers accounted for AF. In 1913, Mines[23] showed that the mechanism of re-entry was an impulse circling a large anatomic obstacle. In 1947, Scherf[24] revived the theory of focal trigger in AF. In the 1960s, Moe and colleagues[25] supported the theory of randomly propagating multiple wavelets as the main mechanism underlying AF. The re-entrant wavelet hypothesis required that the concept of "wavelength" of the arrhythmia circuit be introduced. In the 1970s, Allessie and colleagues[26] introduced the concept of "leading circle re-entry." In a goat model of AF, they demonstrated that the average circuit diameter was 20 to 30 mm and that a minimum of five to eight random wavelets was required to sustain AF. All these theories of random re-entry wavelets explained the sustenance of AF, but how it was initiated was also warranted. Allessie and colleagues[27] offered several possible explanations: a "stable background circuit" capable of initiating new AF when the earlier episode dies out, abnormal focal trigger sites in the atria, and the possibility of an echo beat from the AV node or from an accessory pathway. The present understanding is that AF requires a "critical atrial mass" needed to maintain the arrhythmia and that there is a critical rate greater than which

organized atrial activity cannot continue. Thus, at a certain rate, organized atrial activity can disintegrate into AF provided that the critical tissue mass is available to sustain it. Recent studies in isolated human atrial preparations showed that a single meandering functional re-entrant wavefront produced AF.[28] Recent work by Jalife and colleagues[29] questions the randomness of atrial activity in AF. Their study suggests the presence of a possible "mother circuit" that serves as a periodic background focus; the presence of anatomic obstacles (eg, scar, orifices) serves to break up the wavefront from the mother circuit into multiple wavelets that spread in various directions. Wu and colleagues[30] have proposed the role of pectinate muscles as obstacles that break the activation wave, thus promoting re-entry. They may also serve as an anchoring site for the wave, leading to rotor-like activity. The likelihood that focal activation plays some role in AF is now well accepted. In 1966, in an anatomic study of the left atrium–PV junction in human hearts, Nathan and Eliakim[31] reported that the proximal portion of the PV has a sleeve of myocardium that is a direct extension from the adjacent atrial tissue and is electrically coupled to the atrium. Haissaguerre and colleagues[32] reported arrhythmogenicity of the PVs as possible focal triggers in some cases of AF. The myocardial sleeves that extend from the left atrium onto the PVs seem to be the pathologic correlate of the arrhythmogenic focus. Since then, multiple other foci of AF have been discovered in the thoracic venous structures connected to the atria, including the superior vena cava,[33] coronary sinus,[34] and vein of Marshall.[35] The autonomic basis of AF was also explored by Coumel,[36] who classified AF as adrenergic or vagally mediated. There has also been research implicating genes that predispose to AF.

GENETICS OF ATRIAL FIBRILLATION: BORN WITH IT?

Genetics has excitingly permeated every domain of medicine, and cardiac electrophysiology is no exception. Interest in the genetic basis of AF was driven by the occurrence of AF in families and its association with other arrhythmic conditions with genetic bases, such as Wolff-Parkinson-White (WPW) syndrome[37] and hypertrophic cardiomyopathy.[38] Familial AF was first reported in 1943.[39] Recent studies show that routinely encountered AF may have a genetic basis more commonly than previously considered.[40] In 1997, Brugada and colleagues[41] reported the first monogenic basis for familial AF implicating a gene on chromosome 10. Ellinor and colleagues[42] mapped a gene for familial AF to chromosome 6. Genes coding for potassium channels have been discovered to date that are held responsible for AF.[43] More genes are likely to be discovered, and, although remote at this time, genetic therapy may someday be a means to cure or prevent AF in those predisposed.

MAPPING ATRIAL FIBRILLATION: LOCALIZING THE ORIGIN OF ATRIAL FIBRILLATION

The development of mapping techniques[44] is central to appreciating the success we have today in treating AF with ablation. Mapping AF has helped to clarify its mechanism and localize possible anatomic sites for effective radiofrequency (RF) ablation. Conventionally, this has been done by correlation of 12-lead surface ECG with intracardiac data. Three-dimensional imaging of the triggering foci and correlation with the activation sequence can better localize therapy. Electroanatomic or CARTO mapping is a nonfluoroscopic mapping system that uses magnetic technology to determine the location and orientation of the mapping and ablation catheter accurately while simultaneously recording local electrograms from the catheter tip. Noncontact mapping is performed using the EnSite3000 (Endocardial Solutions, St. Paul, Minnesota) mapping system, consisting of a balloon or multielectrode array that detects endocardial activation recorded by noncontact intracavitary electrodes. The activation points are displayed as computed electrograms or isopotential maps.[45] Other techniques used include the basket (EPT; Boston Scientific, Natick, MA) and amplification technique. The electrodes are coupled to achieve bipolar recordings, and each electrode couple is then amplified and filtered separately for every channel (CardioLab System; Prucka Engineering, Houston, Texas). Intracardiac echocardiography can be a valuable tool in localizing anatomic areas for ablation. It allows for assessment of wall contact of ablation catheters for creation of long linear lesions for catheter ablative treatment of AF.[46] Inverse ECG images the activation time map on the entire surface of the heart from ECG mapping data, enabling reconstruction of unifocal, multifocal, and more distributed activation patterns.[47,48] MRI has also shown promise in demonstrating pulmonary venous anatomy, which is central to the technique of RF ablation of focal AF.[49] Since the focus on PVs as triggers for AF, there is an increasing need to identify their anatomy and electrical functionality correctly. Ablation in the region of the PVs is fraught with risks,[50] mandating that this procedure be made as successful yet safe as possible. Newer technology aims at precisely doing this. One of the most logically developed technologies seems to be superimposition of a three-dimensional anatomic image with the image of the ablating catheter while correlating it with the electrical activation maps. This has been successfully achieved using multislice multidetector CT combined with three-dimensional electroanatomic mapping.[51] The PV anatomy has also been studied using high-frequency intravascular ultrasound.[52] The other recent advances have been the use of remote navigation combined with electroanatomic mapping[53] and the use of robotic surgery.[54] Mapping technology should continue to evolve, making ablation techniques safer and more successful. These should also become more noninvasive, allowing ablations to become technically easier and analytically simpler, thus reducing procedure times.

DRUGS FOR ATRIAL FIBRILLATION: FROM DIGITALIS TO DRONEDARONE

Medical therapy for AF is still the primary modality of treatment, although ablation may become a first-line therapy in well-chosen patients in the future. Digitalis was probably the first drug available to treat AF. Digitalis was discovered in 1785 by William Withering (**Fig. 4**),[55] who described its various qualities and uses. Quinidine was likely the next antiarrhythmic medication; it was used in 1951 to treat AF.[56] Amiodarone and disopyramide were explored in the 1970s to treat AF. Multiple studies regarding the efficacy of amiodarone in AF showed that it is useful and effective.[57,58] Disopyramide was reported to be as effective as quinidine in double-blind trials conducted in 1980.[59] Vaughan Williams[60] first classified antiarrhythmic drugs into four classes based on their pharmacologic actions in 1984. The class IC agent encainide was tried for treatment of AF in 1988 and was noted to have a 27% incidence of proarrhythmia.[61] After data from the Cardiac Arrhythmia Suppression Trial (CAST)[62] were reported, the class IA and IC agents were relegated to treatment of AF in patients exclusively without structural heart disease. Flecainide and propafenone recently made a comeback as effective medications for a "pill-in-the-pocket" approach to treating AF.[63] Sotalol was a class III drug that has received much approval for use in AF. It was known that sotalol

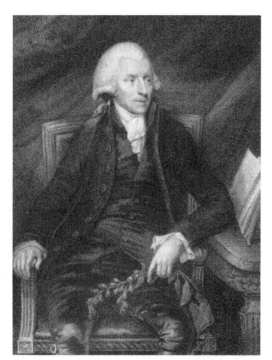

Fig. 4. William Withering, discoverer of the medicinal use of digitalis, in 1775.

had electrophysiologic properties in addition to beta-receptor blockade.[64] Intravenous infusion of sotalol was initially reported as ineffective in restoration of sinus rhythm but as effective in rate control in AF;[65] later, its antiarrhythmic efficacy was also proved. Dofetilide and ibutilide are the newer class III agents that were studied in 1992 to 1993 as options in treating AF.[66,67] The toxicity of long-term amiodarone use has led to the discovery of a congener drug, dronedarone. Dronedarone, azimilide, tedisamal, and trecetilide (class III agents) are still awaiting US Food and Drug Administration approval pending long-term safety data regarding their clinical use. Future drug development and use are likely to be guided by a better molecular understanding of the electrical basis of AF. The long-standing battle of rate versus rhythm control strategy has been subdued, although not put to rest, after the results of the recent Atrial Fibrillation Follow-up Investigation of Rhythm Management (AFFIRM)[68] and Rate Control Versus Electrical Cardioversion (RACE)[69] trials were published. These trials showed the noninferiority of rate control to rhythm control, but this division is not so clear when it involves patients with heart failure or symptomatic AF. AF portends a considerable risk for thromboembolism; this was reported as early as 1958 in a patient with paroxysmal AF and a normal heart.[70] Fisher[71] reported using anticoagulants for cerebral thrombosis in the same year. Today, it is considered standard of care to treat high-risk patients with anticoagulants and low-risk patients with antiplatelet therapy. This is facilitated by the $CHADS_2$ (Congestive Heart Failure, Hypertension, Age > 75 years, Diabetes mellitus and previous Stroke) score.[72] The inflammatory nature of AF (as evinced by elevated C-reactive protein levels) is another pathophysiologic aspect of AF that is being explored because it may have significant clinical and therapeutic implications.

CARDIOVERSION: BEATING ELECTRICITY WITH ELECTRICITY

Cardioversion is the process of restoration of normal sinus rhythm by application of a synchronized external or internal current to the heart. It can be considered as an interim measure in the management of AF because it is more likely to be successful early in the course of AF and may ward off the need for more invasive therapy in some patients if normal sinus rhythm can be maintained on or off pharmacotherapy. In 1962, Lown and colleagues[73] described the first known device for application of electrical energy to the heart for correction of rhythm disturbances. The term *cardioversion* was first used in the next year for electrical correction of AF.[74] In 1963, Lown and colleagues also showed that cardioversion was safer and more effective than quinidine. In 1968, diazepam was the first agent reported as an effective sedative for cardioversion.[75] It was also realized that cardioversion did not obviate the need for anticoagulation if AF was present for more than a week.[76] The next step was to evaluate the long-term success of cardioversion in the management of AF. Within the next few years, longer duration of AF,[77] increased left atrial size,[78,79] and presence of congestive heart failure[80] came to be predictors of lower success rates with cardioversion. Cardioversion was also recognized to be dangerous in the setting of digitalis toxicity.[81] The recognition of atrial stunning for 3 weeks after cardioversion was next recognized by pulsed Doppler studies.[82] These studies underscore the need for optimal anticoagulation that is recommended today in the pericardioversion period. The exact positioning of the external electrodes for successful cardioversion was initially considered as unimportant as long as the current traveled along the long axis of the heart;[83] this has been shown in recent studies as well.[84] If external cardioversion works, so should internal cardioversion. This was the logic behind developing the "atrial cardioverter-atrioverter,"[85] the atrial rhythm control device counterpart of the implantable defibrillator that works so well for ventricular arrhythmias. The atrial cardioverter is still being evaluated as useful therapy for AF because of problems with patient discomfort associated with delivery of the shock. Studies have shown that it is accurate in targeting AF for cardioversion not associated with ventricular proarrhythmias. Today, cardioversion is widely used and works for selected patients, especially when used in combination with or under the cover of antiarrhythmic medications, when attempting conversion to and maintenance of normal sinus rhythm.

ABLATING ATRIAL FIBRILLATION: LEARNING WHILE BURNING

In 1982, Scheinman and colleagues[86] used direct current (DC) energy to treat supraventricular tachycardia. RF energy has since replaced DC energy as a source of energy for catheter ablation of arrhythmias. Once again, the PVs assumed center stage as the target for ablation therapy in AF. Other sites of ablation include the left atrium and the thoracic veins, which have now been identified as sustaining AF after PV ablation. In 1994, Haissaguerre and colleagues[87] reported successful treatment of AF by ablation of the PVs. Since then, multiple techniques have been developed at various leading centers globally, with varying success in curing AF ablation. The use of RF energy has been concerning because it can be thrombogenic and cause complications from damage to underlying structures depending on the site of ablation. Other sources of energy that have been successfully used include cryoenergy (using a freeze-thaw cycle), microwave energy (by generation of frictional heat), ultrasound energy (using oscillation for heat generation), and laser energy (generates heat by harmonic oscillation in water molecules).[88] These energy modalities have been used during surgery utilizing the Maze procedure for successful creation of endocardial lesions, thus interrupting AF. RF energy is still the most commonly used energy source, and the other sources are used only at specific centers that are experienced in their use. Although ablation is not first-line therapy for paroxysmal AF at this time, trials are underway to discuss this further.[89] RF ablation also does not have pristine outcomes at this time; however, improved success rates are being reported. Like any other condition, optimal success rates are only likely to be achieved by correct patient selection; the criteria for selection can only be born out of large randomized controlled trials. Until then, we have to be content with attempting drug therapy first and considering ablation for failed drug therapy. Surgical intervention is only likely to be used in patients undergoing cardiac valve repair or other intracardiac procedures. Catheter

technology also continues to advance, permitting better energy delivery systems that ensure interruption of the AF circuits. When the only available ablation technology was RF energy applied through tip deflectable ablation catheters with a single electrode, long linear atrial lesions could only be made by a "drag" technique.[90] Multielectrode catheters were developed to surmount this problem so that a linear atrial lesion can be produced by placing it against the atrial wall and delivering energy.[91] Lesh and colleagues[92] developed a catheter design integrating a cylindric ultrasound transducer within a water-filled balloon to produce narrow circumferential zones of hyperthermic tissue death at the PV ostia. Newer catheters have been developed that permit the delivery of other energy modalities, leading to better success rates of AF ablation.

THROMBOEMBOLISM IN ATRIAL FIBRILLATION: IS CLOT GOING TO STAY HOME OR NOT?

The thromboembolic risk for AF is now well appreciated, and its prevention is one of the prime goals of therapy, especially in patients in whom achieving sinus rhythm is difficult or not possible. The earliest studies on thromboembolic complications from AF were in patients who had mitral valve disease. The incidence of thrombosis reported was as high as 84% in MS and 9% in mitral insufficiency.[93] In 1958, the National Institute of Neurology and Blindness listed AF as a cause of cerebral infarction of cardiac etiology.[94] At a symposium on thrombosis and anticoagulants in 1960, AF as a risk factor for thrombosis in patients who have rheumatic heart disease and the importance of anticoagulation in this situation were emphasized.[95] In recent years, the presence of a local hypercoagulable state in the left atrium in the setting of AF has been recognized, adding another dimension to the pathogenesis of thromboembolism in AF. This hypercoagulable state has been found to be related to the hematocrit, fibrinogen concentration, left atrial size,[96] various hematologic abnormalities, and endothelial dysfunction.[97,98] Differences in thrombus composition (abundance of fibrin in in situ atrial thrombi versus tissue factor and platelet-leukocyte clusters in embolized clots) have now been revealed using immunohistochemistry. These inherent differences likely decide which thrombus persists in the atrium and which one travels far and wide.[99] Inflammation has been proposed as a possible contributor to thrombogenesis in AF.[100] Paroxysmal AF carries the same risk as persistent or permanent AF.[101] Lone atrial flutter is now known to portend the same thromboembolic risk as that in patients with lone AF (incidence of thrombi as high as 11%–21% and embolic risk ~7%),[102,103] especially in patients with a reduced ejection fraction, thus warranting anticoagulation.[104] Anticoagulation offers the best strategy to combat the stroke risk associated with AF. The management of a patient who had MS and AF with the successful use of quinidine and anticoagulation was reported in the early 1950s.[105] The presence of atrial thrombosis was verified soon thereafter at mitral valve surgery,[106] and multiple reports since then have noted the importance of diagnosing the presence of atrial thrombi and the importance of anticoagulation.[107–111] Historically, warfarin sodium, dicoumarol, and phenindione have been used as anticoagulants in various studies.[112–114] Today, warfarin sodium is the most commonly used anticoagulant in the United States. Its comparison to aspirin in stroke prevention was the subject of many trials; its superiority has been proved beyond doubt in patients at high risk for embolism. Aspirin is still the recommended treatment for low-risk patients with lone AF.[115,116] The issue of when to stop anticoagulation after cardioversion or after AF ablation procedures is currently a matter of debate, with concerns about silent AF recurrences. The details of management of thromboembolism in AF are the subject of a separate article in this issue. The discovery of an ideal alternative to warfarin continues to elude us to date. The hopes raised by such agents as ximelagatran have unfortunately been dashed because of complications of hepatotoxicity.[117] Mechanical devices (eg, Percutaneous Left Atrial Appendage Transcatheter Occlusion [PLAATO system; PLAATO Inc., Plymouth, MN],[118] WATCHMAN, [Atritech Inc., Plymouth, MN],[119] Amplatzer septal occluder)[120] have now been developed that attempt to seal the left atrial appendage, resulting in containment of the thrombus at its most common site of origin (responsible for 90% of left atrial thrombi). These devices are not standard therapy for AF at the current time. The search for an ideal agent with a wide therapeutic window, comparable or greater efficacy than warfarin, a reasonable safety profile, less frequent need for monitoring, yet affordable by the many individuals with AF is a formidable challenge that remains to be overcome.

SURGERY FOR ATRIAL FIBRILLATION: DOWN THE CORRIDOR AND INSIDE THE MAZE

The assumption that the electrophysiologic basis of AF is the multiple random circulating re-entrant wavelets led to the development of the Maze surgical procedure. In 1991, James Cox and colleagues[121] reported their success with the original

Maze procedure. Multiple surgical procedures were devised and tested in dogs, which finally led to a surgical approach that effectively creates an electrical Maze in the atrium. The atrial incisions prevent re-entry and allow sinus impulses to activate the entire atrial myocardium in a channeled manner, thereby preserving atrial transport function after surgery. Thus, there is resolution of the electrical dysfunction and restoration of the atrial mechanical function. The procedure had been tried in 7 patients since 1987 (5 with paroxysmal AF and 2 with chronic AF), with cure from AF and freedom from postoperative antiarrhythmic medications. These researchers went on to present further data on 75 patients in 1992, with a 98% cure rate for AF at an average of 3 months of follow-up.[122] By 1995, it was claimed that the procedure had been standardized to the extent that a good outcome was likely independent of the surgeon and did not depend on mapping guidance.[123] In the same year, the Maze procedure was modified twice, resulting in the Maze III procedure. This was intended to overcome the problems of chronotropic incompetence and left atrial dysfunction seen to result in some patients after the original Maze procedure.[124] The Maze III procedure was then combined with mitral valve surgery, yielding a success rate of 79% for treatment of AF; fine fibrillatory waves and an enlarged left atrium were predictive of failure.[125] Cox and colleagues[125] emphasized that return of atrial mechanical function was key to the success of the Maze procedure. In 1997, Cox[126] reported return of right atrial contractile function in 99% of cases and return of left atrial contractile function in 93% of cases. These success rates were reported to persist 3 years later. In an attempt to restore left atrial function, modifications have been introduced to the Maze III procedure.[127] The Maze III procedure can now be performed through a minimally invasive approach, although there is skepticism about its success.[128] In 1997, Patwardhan and colleagues[129] reported success of the Maze procedure using RF bipolar coagulation in patients who had rheumatic heart disease and AF to produce atrial lesions, with a success rate of 80%. Pulsed wave Doppler evaluation at follow-up showed return of atrial transport function, and presence of "A" wave in all these patients in tricuspid valve flow and in 75% patients in mitral valve flow. Calkins and colleagues[130] performed a Maze-like procedure using the Guidant Heart Rhythm Technologies Linear Ablation System (St. Paul, MN) to create long transmural lesions. Bipolar RF ablation avoids the morbidity of cut-and-sew lesions, reduces procedural time, and increases the likelihood of transmurality and continuity of lesions created compared with unipolar devices.[131] A combination of energy sources has also been used successfully for the Maze procedure.[132] The other surgical technique to treat AF has been the Corridor procedure. The procedure is a surgical open heart procedure designed to isolate a "corridor" from the right and left atrium consisting of the sinus node area, the atrioventricular nodal junction, and the connecting right atrial mass. The principle of this surgery is to channel the electrical impulse from the sinus to the AV node through an atrial area small enough to prevent AF. Between 1987 and 1990, 20 patients with severely disabling symptoms attributable to frequent paroxysmal AF underwent the Corridor operation, with permanent success in 16 patients.[133] The Corridor procedure has been used successfully in patients undergoing surgery for mitral valve disease, with results comparable to the Maze procedure (75% success rate).[134] The surgical options for AF seem to be evolving as well; the focus seems to fluctuate from trying to isolate the trigger to trying to modify the substrate. The other area of focus is to move to a "minimally invasive" mode for achieving successful interventional management of AF.[135,136] Surgical treatment of AF is still extremely rewarding when performed concomitant with surgery for associated surgically amenable cardiac disease.

BACK TO THE FUTURE: WHERE DO WE GO FROM HERE?

We have come a long way in the successful management (treatment for the most part and cure in some cases) of AF. It is only when we look back that we can appreciate how far we have come. Although technology continues to advance, we cannot help but admire the efforts of those who laid the foundation for clinical recognition, physical diagnosis, electrical documentation, drug therapy, and interventional and surgical management of this interesting disorder. The "grandfather arrhythmia" has come a long way; it continues to show us newer mechanisms and presents us with newer challenges in its management. The future holds a lot in store as regards pharmacologic and nonpharmacologic therapies as more advanced molecular biology, imaging, and mapping techniques evolve. Someday, we may finally be ideally equipped to deal with AF, and, eventually, the simple yet complete cure may be in sight.

REFERENCES

1. Lip GYH, Beevers DG. ABC of atrial fibrillation: history, epidemiology and importance of atrial fibrillation. BMJ 1995;311:1361–7.

2. Chauveau A, Marey EJ. Appareils et Expériences Cardiographiques Démonstration Nouvelle du Méchanisme des Mouvements du Coeur par l'Emploi des Instruments Enregistreurs à Indications Continuées. In: Baillière JB, editor. Paris, p. 1863.

3. Flegel KM. From delirium cordis to atrial fibrillation: historical development of a disease concept. Ann Intern Med 1995;122:867–73.

4. Cushny AR, Edmunds CW. Paroxysmal irregularity of the heart and auricular fibrillation. Am J Med Sci 1907;133:66–77.

5. Schweitzer P, Keller S. A history of atrial fibrillation. Vnitr Lek 2002;48(1):24–6.

6. Adams R. Cases of diseases of the heart, accompanied with pathological observations. Dublin Hospital Reports 1827;4:353–453.

7. MacKenzie J. New methods of studying affections of the heart. V. The inception of the rhythm of the heart by the ventricle. Br Med J 1905;1:812–5.

8. Diker E, Aydogdu S, Ozdemir M, et al. Prevalence and predictors of atrial fibrillation in rheumatic valvular heart disease. Am J Cardiol 1996;77:96–8.

9. Einthoven W. Le telecardiogramme. Arch Int Physiol 1906;4:132–64.

10. Lewis T. Auricular fibrillation: a common clinical condition. BMJ 1909;2:1528.

11. Ernestene AC, Levine SA. A comparison of records taken with the Einthoven string galvanometer and the amplifier type electrocardiograph. Am Heart J 1928;4:725–31.

12. Available at: http://www.ecglibrary.com/ecghist.html. Accessed January 3, 2006.

13. Holm M, Pehrson S, Ingemansson M, et al. Non-invasive assessment of the atrial cycle length during atrial fibrillation in man: introducing, validating and illustrating a new ECG method. Cardiovasc Res 1998;38(1):69–81.

14. Dilaveris P, Gialafos E, Sideris S, et al. MD simple electrocardiographic markers for the prediction of paroxysmal idiopathic atrial fibrillation. Am Heart J 1998;135(5):733–8.

15. Rajawat YS, Gerstenfeld EP, Patel VV, et al. ECG criteria for localizing the pulmonary vein origin of spontaneous atrial premature complexes: validation using intracardiac recordings. Pacing Clin Electrophysiol 2004;27(2):182–8.

16. Sippensgroenewegen A, Natale A, Marrouche NF, et al. Potential role of body surface ECG mapping for localization of atrial fibrillation trigger sites. J Electrocardiol 2004;37:47–52.

17. Giraud G, Latour H, Levy A, et al. Endocavitary electrocardiography and the mechanism of auricular fibrillation. Montp Med 1952;41–42(7):625–39.

18. Vitek B, Valenta J. Auricular fibrillation in the intracardiac ECG. Cesk Pediatr 1969;24(5):401–7.

19. O'Donnell D, Bourke JP, Furniss SS. P wave morphology during spontaneous and paced

19. pulmonary vein activity: differences between patients with atrial fibrillation and normal controls. J Electrocardiol 2003;36(1):33–40.
20. Husser D, Stridh M, Cannom DS, et al. Validation and clinical application of time-frequency analysis of atrial fibrillation electrocardiograms. J Cardiovasc Electrophysiol 2007;18(1):41–6.
21. Winterberg H. Ueber Herzflimmern und seine Beeinflussung durch Kampher. Zeitschrift fur Experimentelle Pathologie und Therapie 1906;3:182–208.
22. Lewis T, Schleiter HG. The relation of regular tachycardias of auricular origin to auricular fibrillation. Heart 1912;3:173–93.
23. Mines GR. On dynamic equilibrium in the heart. J Physiol 1913;46:349–82.
24. Scherf D. Studies on auricular tachycardia caused by aconitine administration. Proc Soc Exp Biol Med 1947;64:233–9.
25. Moe GK, Rheinboldt WC, Abildskov JA, et al. A computer model of atrial fibrillation. Am Heart J 1964;67:200–20.
26. Allessie MA, Rensma PL, Brugada J, et al. Pathophysiology of atrial fibrillation. In: Zipes DP, Jalife J, editors. Cardiac electrophysiology: from cell to bedside. Philadelphia: WB Saunders; 1990. p. 548–59.
27. Allessie MA, Boyden PA, Camm AJ, et al. Pathophysiology and prevention of atrial fibrillation. Circulation 2001;10(5):769–77.
28. Ikeda T, Czer L, Trento A, et al. Induction of meandering functional reentrant wavefront in isolated human atrial tissues. Circulation 1997;96: 3013–20.
29. Jalife J, Berenfeld O, Mansour M. Mother rotors and fibrillatory conduction: a mechanism of atrial fibrillation. Cardiovasc Res 2002;54:204–16.
30. Wu TJ, Kim YH, Yashima M, et al. Progressive action potential duration shortening and the conversion from atrial flutter to atrial fibrillation in the isolated canine right atrium. J Am Coll Cardiol 2001;38:1757–65.
31. Nathan H, Eliakim M. The junction between the left atrium and the pulmonary veins. An anatomic study of human hearts. Circulation 1966;34:412–22.
32. Haissaguerre M, Jais P, Shah DC, et al. Spontaneous initiation of atrial fibrillation by ectopic beats originating in the pulmonary veins. N Engl J Med 1998;339:659–66.
33. Li J, Wang L. Catheter ablation of atrial fibrillation originating from superior vena cava. Arch Med Res 2006;37(3):415–8.
34. Haissaguerre M, Hocini M, Sanders P, et al. Localized sources maintaining atrial fibrillation organized by prior ablation. Circulation 2006;113(5): 616–25.
35. Chen PS, Chou CC, Tan AY, et al. The mechanisms of atrial fibrillation. J Cardiovasc Electrophysiol 2006;17(3):S2–7.
36. Coumel P. Paroxysmal atrial fibrillation: a disorder of autonomic tone? Eur Heart J 1994;15(Suppl A): 9–16.
37. Gollob MH, Seger JJ, Gollob TN, et al. Novel PRKAG2 mutation responsible for the genetic syndrome of ventricular preexcitation and conduction system disease with childhood onset and absence of cardiac hypertrophy. Circulation 2001;104(25): 3030–3.
38. Gruver EJ, Fatkin D, Dodds GA, et al. Familial hypertrophic cardiomyopathy and atrial fibrillation caused by Arg663His beta-cardiac myosin heavy chain mutation. Am J Cardiol 1999;83(12A): 13H–8H.
39. Wolff L. Familial auricular fibrillation. N Engl J Med 1943;229:396–7.
40. Darbar D, Herron KJ, Ballew JD, et al. Familial atrial fibrillation is a genetically heterogeneous disorder. J Am Coll Cardiol 2003;41(12):2185–92.
41. Brugada R, Tapscott T, Czernuszewicz GZ, et al. Identification of a genetic locus for familial atrial fibrillation. N Engl J Med 1997;336(13): 905–11.
42. Ellinor PT, Shin JT, Moore RK, et al. Locus for atrial fibrillation maps to chromosome 6q14-16. Circulation 2003;107(23):2880–3.
43. Chen YH, Xu SJ, Bendahhou S, et al. KCNQ1 gain-of function mutation in familial atrial fibrillation. Science 2003;299(5604):251–4.
44. Sra Jasbir, Thomas JM. New techniques for mapping cardiac arrhythmias. Indian Heart J 2001;53: 423–44.
45. Schneider MA, Schmitt C. Non-contact mapping: a simultaneous spatial detection in the diagnosis of arrhythmias. Z Kardiol 2000;89(3):177–85.
46. Epstein LM, Mitchell MA, Smith TW, et al. Comparative study of fluoroscopy and intracardiac echocardiographic guidance for the creation of linear atrial lesions. Circulation 1998;98:1796–801.
47. Tilg B, Fischer G, Modre R, et al. Electrocardiographic imaging of atrial and ventricular electrical activation. Med Image Anal 2003;7:391–8.
48. Modre R, Tilg B, Fischer G, et al. Noninvasive myocardial activation time imaging: a novel inverse algorithm applied to clinical ECG mapping data. IEEE Trans Biomed Eng 2002;49:1153–61.
49. Wittkampf FH, Vonken EJ, Derksen R, et al. Pulmonary vein ostium geometry: analysis by magnetic resonance angiography. Circulation 2003;107: 21–3.
50. Wellens HJ. Pulmonary vein ablation in atrial fibrillation: hype or hope? Circulation 2000;102(21): 2562–4.
51. Martinek M, Nesser HJ, Aichinger J, et al. Impact of integration of multislice computed tomography imaging into three-dimensional electroanatomic mapping on clinical outcomes, safety, and efficacy

using radiofrequency ablation for atrial fibrillation. Pacing Clin Electrophysiol 2007;30(10):1215–23.

52. Cabrera JA, Sanchez-Quintana D, Farre J, et al. Ultrasonic characterization of the pulmonary venous wall: echographic and histological correlation. Circulation 2002;106:968–73.

53. Pappone C, Santinelli V. Remote navigation and ablation of atrial fibrillation. J Cardiovasc Electrophysiol 2007;18(1):S18–20.

54. Pappone C, Vicedomini G, Manguso F, et al. Robotic magnetic navigation for atrial fibrillation ablation. J Am Coll Cardiol 2006;47(7): 1390–400.

55. Withering W. An account of the foxglove and some of its medical uses, with practical remarks on dropsy, and other diseases. In: Willius FA, Keys TE, editors, Classics of cardiology. New York: Dover Publications Inc.; 1941;1:231–52.

56. Fischermann K, Schleisner P. Quinidine sulphate therapy of chronic auricular fibrillation in patients over fifty. Nord Med 1950;43(17):705–6.

57. Zagatti G, Benzoni A, Caturelli G. Cordarone in the maintenance of sinus rhythm: prevention of paroxysmal atrial fibrillation and of supraventricular paroxysmal tachycardia. Arch Maragliano Patol Clin 1974;30(2):245–9.

58. Santos AL, Aleixo AM, Landeiro J, et al. Conversion of atrial fibrillation to sinus rhythm with amiodarone. Acta Med Port 1979;1:15–23.

59. Kimura E, Mashima S, Tanaka T. Clinical evaluation of antiarrhythmic effects of disopyramide by multi-clinical controlled double-blind methods. Int J Clin Pharmacol Ther Toxicol 1980;18(8):338–43.

60. Vaughan Williams EM. A classification of antiarrhythmic actions reassessed after a decade of new drugs. J Clin Pharmacol 1984;24:129–47.

61. Rinkenberger RL, Naccarelli GV, Berns E, et al. Efficacy and safety of class IC antiarrhythmic agents for the treatment of coexisting supraventricular and ventricular tachycardia. Am J Cardiol 1988;62(6):44D–55D.

62. Preliminary report: effect of encainide and flecainide on mortality in a randomized trial of arrhythmia suppression after myocardial infarction. The Cardiac Arrhythmia Suppression Trial (CAST) investigators. N Engl J Med 1989; 321(6):406–12.

63. Alboni P, Botto GL, Baldi N, et al. Outpatient treatment of recent-onset atrial fibrillation with the "pill-in-the-pocket" approach. N Engl J Med 2004; 351(23):2384–91.

64. Simon A, Berman E. Long-term sotalol therapy in patients with arrhythmias. J Clin Pharmacol 1979; 19(8–9 Pt 2):547–56.

65. Teo KK, Harte M, Horgan JH. Sotalol infusion in the treatment of supraventricular tachyarrhythmias. Chest 1985;87(1):113–8.

66. Rasmussen HS, Allen MJ, Blackburn KJ, et al. Dofetilide, a novel class III antiarrhythmic agent. J Cardiovasc Pharmacol 1992;20(2):S96–105.

67. Nabih MA, Prcevski P, Fromm BS, et al. Effect of ibutilide, a new class III agent, on sustained atrial fibrillation in a canine model of acute ischemia and myocardial dysfunction induced by microembolization. Pacing Clin Electrophysiol 1993;16(10): 1975–83.

68. Wyse DG, Waldo AL, DiMarco JP, et al. A comparison of rate control and rhythm control in patients with atrial fibrillation. N Engl J Med 2002;347(23): 1825–33.

69. Hagens VE, Ranchor AV, Van Sonderen E, et al. Effect of rate or rhythm control on quality of life in persistent atrial fibrillation. Results from the Rate Control Versus Electrical Cardioversion (RACE) study. J Am Coll Cardiol 2004;43(2): 241–7.

70. Weintraub G, Sprecace G. Paroxysmal atrial fibrillation and cerebral embolism with apparently normal heart. N Engl J Med 1958;259(18):875–6.

71. Fisher CM. The use of anticoagulants in cerebral thrombosis. Neurology 1958;8(5):311–32.

72. Gage BF, Waterman AD, Shannon W, et al. Validation of clinical classification schemes for predicting stroke: results from the National Registry of Atrial Fibrillation. JAMA 2001;285(22):2864–70.

73. Lown B, Amarasingham R, Neuman J. New method for terminating cardiac arrhythmias: use of synchronized capacitor discharge. JAMA 1962;182: 548–55.

74. Lown B, Perlroth MG, Kaidbey S, et al. "Cardioversion" of atrial fibrillation. A report on the treatment of 65 episodes in 50 patients. N Engl J Med 1963;269:325–31.

75. Winters WL Jr, McDonough MT, Hafer J, et al. A useful hypnotic drug for direct-current cardioversion. JAMA 1968;204:926–8.

76. DeSilva RA, Lown B. Cardioversion for atrial fibrillation—indications and complications. In: Kulbertus HE, Olsson SB, Schlepper M. Atrial fibrillation. Hassle: Mondal 1994; 231–9.

77. Wikland B, Edhag O, Eliasch H. Atrial fibrillation and flutter treated with synchronized DC shock. A study on immediate and long term results. Acta Med Scand 1967;182:665–71.

78. Fisher RD, Mason DT, Morrow AG. Restoration of normal sinus rhythm after mitral valve replacement. Correlations with left atrial pressure and size. Circulation 1968;37(2):173–7.

79. Hoglund C, Rosenhamer G. Echocardiographic left atrial dimension as a predictor of maintaining sinus rhythm after conversion of atrial fibrillation. Acta Med Scand 1985;217:411–5.

80. Futral AA, McGuire LB. Reversion of chronic atrial fibrillation. JAMA 1967;199:885–8.

81. Kleiger R, Lown B. Cardioversion and digitalis. II. Clinical studies. Circulation 1966;33:878–87.

82. Manning WJ, Leeman DE, Gotch PJ, et al. Pulse Doppler evaluation of atrial mechanical function after electrical cardioversion of atrial fibrillation. J Am Coll Cardiol 1989;13:617–23.

83. Kerber RE, Jensen SR, Grayzel J, et al. Elective cardioversion: influence of paddle-electrode location and size on success rates and energy requirements. N Engl J Med 1981;305:658–62.

84. Siaplaouras S, Buob A, Rotter C, et al. Randomized comparison of anterolateral versus anteroposterior electrode position for biphasic external cardioversion of atrial fibrillation. Am Heart J 2005;150(1):150–2.

85. Wellens HJ, Lau CP, Luderitz B, et al. Atrioverter: an implantable device for the treatment of atrial fibrillation. Circulation 1998;98(16):1651–6.

86. Scheinman MM, Morady F, Hess DS, et al. Catheter-induced ablation of the atrioventricular junction to control refractory supraventricular arrhythmias. JAMA 1982;248:851–5.

87. Haissaguerre M, Marcus FI, Fischer B, et al. Radiofrequency catheter ablation in unusual mechanisms of atrial fibrillation: report of three cases. J Cardiovasc Electrophysiol 1994;5(9):743–51.

88. Yiu KH, Lau CP, Lee KL, et al. Emerging energy sources for catheter ablation of atrial fibrillation. J Cardiovasc Electrophysiol 2006;17(3):S56–61.

89. Wazni OM, Marrouche NF, Martin DO, et al. Radiofrequency ablation vs antiarrhythmic drugs as first-line treatment of symptomatic atrial fibrillation: a randomized trial. JAMA 2005;293(21):2634–40.

90. Swartz JF, Pellersells G, Silvers J, et al. A catheter-based curative approach to atrial fibrillation in humans. Circulation 1994;90(Suppl 1):335.

91. Olgin JE, Kalman JM, Chin M, et al. Electrophysiological effects of long, linear atrial lesions placed under intracardiac ultrasound guidance. Circulation 1997;96(8):2715–21.

92. Lesh MD, Guerra P, Roithinger FX, et al. Novel catheter technology for ablative cure of atrial fibrillation. J Interv Card Electrophysiol 2000;4(1):127–39.

93. Storer J, Lisan P, Delmonico JE, et al. Physiopathological concepts of mitral valvular disease. JAMA 1954;155:103.

94. Adams RD. Recent developments in cerebrovascular diseases. Br Med J 1958;1(5074):785–8.

95. Thrombosis and anticoagulants. Br Med J 1960; 2(5206):1153–5.

96. Black IW, Chesterman CN, Hopkins AP, et al. Hematologic correlates of left atrial spontaneous echo contrast and thromboembolism in nonvalvular atrial fibrillation. J Am Coll Cardiol 1993;21(2):451–7.

97. Yamashita T, Sekiguchi A, Iwasaki YK, et al. Thrombomodulin and tissue factor pathway inhibitor in endocardium of rapidly paced rat atria. Circulation 2003;108(20):2450–2.

98. Akar JG, Jeske W, Wilber DJ. Acute onset human atrial fibrillation is associated with local cardiac platelet activation and endothelial dysfunction. J Am Coll Cardiol 2008;51(18):1790–3.

99. Wysokinski WE, Owen WG, Fass DN, et al. Atrial fibrillation and thrombosis: immunohistochemical differences between in situ and embolized thrombi. J Thromb Haemost 2004;2(9):1637–44.

100. Conway DS, Buggins P, Hughes E, et al. Relation of interleukin-6, C-reactive protein, and the prothrombotic state to transesophageal echocardiographic findings in atrial fibrillation. Am J Cardiol 2004;93(11):1368–73.

101. Nieuwlaat R, Dinh T, Olsson SB, et al. Should we abandon the common practice of withholding oral anticoagulation in paroxysmal atrial fibrillation? Eur Heart J 2008;29(7):915–22.

102. Bikkina M, Alpert MA, Mulekar M, et al. Prevalence of intraatrial thrombus in patients with atrial flutter. Am J Cardiol 1995;76(3):186–9.

103. Seidl K, Hauer B, Schwick NG, et al. Risk of thromboembolic events in patients with atrial flutter. Am J Cardiol 1998;82:580–3.

104. Scholten MF, Thornton AS, Mekel JM, et al. Anticoagulation in atrial fibrillation and flutter. Europace 2005;7(5):492–9.

105. Lackay H, Housel EL. The arrest of recurrent embolism due to auricular fibrillation with mitral stenosis by quinidine-anticoagulant therapy. Ann Intern Med 1951;35(5):1143–9.

106. McGoon DC, Henly WS. The significance of auricular fibrillation and auricular thrombosis in mitral valve surgery. Bull Johns Hopkins Hosp 1952;91(6):419–26.

107. Brock R. The technique of mitral valvotomy. lecture delivered at the Royal College of Surgeons of England on 16th April 1956. Ann R Coll Surg Engl 1956;19(1):1–22.

108. Bakoulas G, Mullard K. Mitral valvotomy and embolism. Thorax 1966;21:43–6.

109. Duclos F, Zambrano A. Myocardial infarct caused by probable embolism in a case of mitral stenosis with recent auricular fibrillation. Arch Inst Cardiol Mex 1961;31:770–80.

110. Somerville W, Chambers RJ. Systemic embolism in mitral stenosis: relation to the size of the left atrial appendage. Br Med J 1964;2(5418):1167–9.

111. Embolism in mitral valve disease. Br Med J 1964; 2(5418):1149–50.

112. Glenn F, Holswade GR. Emboli in the surgical treatment of mitral stenosis. Surg Gynecol Obstet 1960; 111:289–96.

113. Dahlgren S, Bjork VO. Thromboembolic complications in connection with mitral commissurotomy after discontinuation of anticoagulant therapy. J Thorac Cardiovasc Surg 1962;43:780–4.

114. Uglov FG, Potashov LV. The prophylaxis of thromboembolic complications in surgery for mitral stenosis. J Thorac Cardiovasc Surg 1962;44:408.

115. Wyse DG. Anticoagulation in atrial fibrillation: a contemporary viewpoint. Heart Rhythm 2007;4(Suppl 3):S34–9.

116. Fuster V, Ryden LE, Cannom DS, et al. ACC/AHA/ESC 2006 guidelines for management of patients with atrial fibrillation: a report of the American College of Cardiology/American Heart Association Task Force on Practice Guidelines and the European Society of Cardiology Committee for Practice Guidelines (Writing Committee to Revise the 2001 Guidelines for Management of Patients with Atrial Fibrillation). Circulation 2006;114:e257–354.

117. Agnelli G, Eriksson BI, Cohen AT, et al. Safety assessment of new antithrombotic agents: lessons from the EXTEND study on ximelagatran. Thromb Res 2008 May 14.

118. Sievert H, Lesh MD, Trepels T, et al. Percutaneous left atrial appendage transcatheter occlusion to prevent stroke in high-risk patients with atrial fibrillation: early clinical experience. Circulation 2002;105:1887–9.

119. Fountain RB, Holmes DR, Chandrasekaran K, et al. The PROTECT AF (WATCHMAN Left Atrial Appendage System for Embolic PROTECTion in patients with atrial fibrillation) trial. Am Heart J 2006; 151(5):956–61.

120. Meier B, Palacios I, Windecker S, et al. Transcatheter left atrial appendage occlusion with Amplatzer devices to obviate anticoagulation in patients with atrial fibrillation. Catheter Cardiovasc Interv 2003; 60(3):417–22.

121. Cox JL, Schuessler RB, D'Agostino HJ Jr, et al. The surgical treatment of atrial fibrillation. III. Development of a definitive surgical procedure. J Thorac Cardiovasc Surg 1991;101(4):569–83.

122. Cox JL, Boineau JP, Schuessler RB, et al. Five-year experience with the maze procedure for atrial fibrillation. Ann Thorac Surg 1993;56(4):814–23.

123. Cox JL, Boineau JP, Schuessler RB, et al. Electrophysiologic basis, surgical development, and clinical results of the maze procedure for atrial flutter and atrial fibrillation. Adv Card Surg 1995;6:1–67.

124. Cox JL, Boineau JP, Schuessler RB, et al. Modification of the maze procedure for atrial flutter and atrial fibrillation. I. Rationale and surgical results. J Thorac Cardiovasc Surg 1995;110(2):473–84.

125. Kamata J, Kawazoe K, Izumoto H, et al. Predictors of sinus rhythm restoration after Cox maze procedure concomitant with other cardiac operations. Ann Thorac Surg 1997;64(2):394–8.

126. Cox JL. Atrial transport function after the maze procedure for atrial fibrillation: a 10-year clinical experience. Am Heart J 1998;136(6):934–6.

127. Kim KB, Huh JH, Kang CH, et al. Modifications of the Cox-maze III procedure. Ann Thorac Surg 2001;71(3):816–22.

128. Damiano RJ, Voeller RK. Surgical and minimally invasive ablation for atrial fibrillation. Curr Treat Options Cardiovasc Med 2006;8(5):371–6.

129. Patwardhan AM, Dave HH, Tamhane AA, et al. Intraoperative radiofrequency microbipolar coagulation to replace incisions of Maze III procedure for correcting atrial fibrillation in patients with rheumatic valvular disease. Eur J Cardiothorac Surg 1997;12:627–33.

130. Calkins H, Hall J, Ellenbogen K, et al. A new system for catheter ablation of atrial fibrillation. Am J Cardiol 1999;83:227D–36D.

131. Yii M, Yap CH, Nixon I, et al. Modification of the Cox-maze III procedure using bipolar radiofrequency ablation. Heart Lung Circ 2007;16(1): 37–49.

132. Sternik L, Ghosh P, Luria D, et al. Mid-term results of the 'hybrid maze': a combination of bipolar radiofrequency and cryoablation for surgical treatment of atrial fibrillation. J Heart Valve Dis 2006; 15(5):664–70.

133. Defauw JJ, Guiraudon GM, van Hemel NM, et al. Surgical therapy of paroxysmal atrial fibrillation with the "corridor" operation. Ann Thorac Surg 1992;53(4):564–70.

134. Velimirovic DB, Petrovic P, Djukic P, et al. Corridor procedure—surgical option for treatment of chronic atrial fibrillation in patients undergoing mitral valve replacement. Cardiovasc Surg 1997; 5(3):320–7.

135. Skanes AC, Klein GJ, Guiraudon G, et al. Hybrid approach for minimally-invasive operative therapy of arrhythmias. J Interv Card Electrophysiol 2003; 9(2):289–94.

136. Guiraudon G, Jones DL, Skanes AC, et al. En bloc exclusion of the pulmonary vein region in the pig using off pump, beating, intra-cardiac surgery: a pilot study of minimally invasive surgery for atrial fibrillation. Ann Thorac Surg 2005;80(4):1417–23.

Current Perceptions of the Epidemiology of Atrial Fibrillation

William B. Kannel, MD, MPH, FACC[a,b],*,
Emelia J. Benjamin, MD, ScM[b,c]

KEYWORDS

- Atrial fibrillation • Epidemiology • Prognosis
- Risk factors • Cohort study

INCIDENCE, PREVALENCE, AND SECULAR TRENDS

Atrial fibrillation (AF) is a common, growing, and serious cardiac rhythm disturbance that is responsible for considerable morbidity and mortality in the population. The currently diagnosed estimate of 2.3 million people in the United States with it is expected to increase to 5.6 million by 2050. Its prevalence doubles with each decade of age, reaching almost 9% at the age of 80 to 89 years. Its population prevalence has reached epidemic proportions. This doubling with each decade of age occurs independent of the known predisposing conditions. Cardiovascular Health Study and Framingham Study data indicate that the incidence of AF per 1000 person-years in those younger than the age 64 years is 3.1 in men and 1.9 in women, increasing sharply to approximately 19.2 per 1000 person-years in those aged 65 to 74 years and to as high as 31.4 to 38 in octogenarians.[1,2] The estimated general population prevalence of AF is 0.4% to 1%, increasing with advancing age.[3,4] AF is uncommon before 60 years of age, but its prevalence increases markedly thereafter, afflicting approximately 10% of the population by 80 years of age.[4] Approximately one third of all patients who have AF are aged 80 years or older, and it is estimated that by 2050, half of patients who have AF are likely to be in this age group.[4]

There is a male preponderance of risk for reasons currently unknown.[5] The increase in incidence with age may involve age-related cardiac abnormalities, including gradual loss of nodal fibers and increased fibrous and adipose tissue in the sinoatrial node, decreased ventricular compliance from myocardial fibrosis resulting in atrial dilatation that predisposes to AF, and extensive senile amyloid infiltration of the sinoatrial node.[6–8] There also seems to be an age-related prothrombotic diathesis. Age is a more potent AF risk factor if it is combined with other risk factors.[9] Also, aging reflects longer exposure to predisposing conditions for AF, and even in advanced age, some individuals are clearly more vulnerable to its development than others.

Most reports on the epidemiology of AF are based on white North Americans or Europeans.[10] Based on limited data, the age-adjusted risk for AF in African Americans appears to be about half that of whites.[1,9,11] AF also is less common in African-American than in white heart failure patients.[12]

Because of the more than half-century surveillance of the Framingham Study cohort, it was possible to determine the lifetime risk for developing AF, which is 1 in 4 for men and women aged 40 years and older.[13] These lifetime risks for AF are 1 in 6 even in the absence of predisposing

A version of this article originally appeared in *Medical Clinics of North America*, volume 92, issue 1.
Funding for this study was provided by grants N01-HC 25195, RO1 HL076784, 1R01 AG028321, and 6R01-NS 17950.
[a] National Heart Lung and Blood Institute's Framingham Heart Study, MA, USA
[b] Boston University School of Medicine's Framingham Heart Study, 73 Mount Wayte Avenue, Suite 2, Framingham, MA 01702–5827, USA
[c] School of Public Health, Boston University School of Medicine, MA, USA
* Corresponding author. The Framingham Study, 73 Mount Wayte Avenue #2, Framingham, MA 01702–5827.
E-mail address: billkannel@yahoo.com (W.B. Kannel).

cardiac conditions (**Table 1**). The prospective Rotterdam Study also found a similarly high lifetime AF risk (22%–24% at the age of 40 years).[14] These alarming lifetime risks highlight the important public health liability posed by AF and the urgent necessity to continue investigation of predisposing conditions, preventive strategies, and more effective therapies.

The most credible explanation for the increasing prevalence of AF is that the current elderly population has more predisposing conditions, such as diabetes, obesity, heart failure, coronary and valvular heart disease, and prior cardiac surgery. This trend, brought about by advances in treatment of cardiovascular disease, has produced a population of elderly survivors containing more candidates for AF than formerly. The Rochester study, however, observed only modest increases in the prevalence of these predisposing conditions over 3 decades, which only partially explained the observed magnitude of the increased AF prevalence.[15]

CARDIOVASCULAR RISK FACTORS

Based on Framingham Study data, men have a 1.5-fold age- and risk factor–adjusted greater risk for AF than women. Of the standard cardiovascular risk factors, hypertension, diabetes, and obesity are the significant independent AF predictors. Because of its greater prevalence, hypertension is responsible for more AF in the population (14%) than any other risk factor

(**Table 2**).[2] Cigarette smoking was a significant risk factor in women adjusting only for age (odds ratio [OR] = 1.4) but was just short of significance on adjustment for other risk factors. Neither obesity nor alcohol intake seemed to be independently associated with the short-term risk for AF incidence in either gender. In other studies with sufficient power and numbers of individuals who consume alcohol in large amounts, however, it seems that alcohol abuse is a risk for AF occurrence.[16,17]

Obesity is associated with long-term AF risk, which seems to be partially mediated by left atrial enlargement. The prevalence of obesity, diabetes, and the metabolic syndrome has reached major proportions worldwide. A retrospective analysis of AF incidence in relation to body mass index (BMI) in consecutive patients undergoing cardiac surgery found obesity to be an important determinant of new-onset AF after cardiac surgery.[18] It is uncertain to what extent cardiovascular risk factors mediate the association between obesity and AF. A population-based Veterans Administration case-control study found that the association of AF with BMI seemed mediated partially by diabetes but only minimally through other cardiovascular risk factors.[19] Obesity is associated with atrial enlargement and ventricular diastolic dysfunction, which are established predictors of AF.

Interrelations among AF risk factors, such as obesity, diabetes, and the "metabolic syndrome," suggest that an insulin-resistant state is operative. A prospective analysis of consecutive hospitalized

Table 1
Lifetime risk for atrial fibrillation in the absence of antecedent or concurrent diagnosis of congestive heart failure or myocardial infarction

Index Age, Years	Men	Women
Lifetime risk for AF without antecedent or concurrent congestive heart failure		
40	20.5	17.0
50	20.5	17.3
60	20.3	17.4
70	19.1	17.0
80	17.6	15.9
Lifetime risk for AF without antecedent or concurrent congestive heart failure or myocardial infarction		
40	16.3	15.6
50	16.6	15.9
60	16.8	16.1
70	16.5	15.9
80	16.0	14.8

All values are percentages.
Data from Lloyd-Jones DM, Wang TJ, Leip E, et al. Lifetime risk for development of atrial fibrillation: the Framingham Heart Study. Circulation 2004;110:1042–6.

Table 2
Cardiovascular risk factors for atrial fibrillation in a 38-year follow-up: Framingham Study

	Odds Ratios			
	Age-Adjusted		Risk Factor–Adjusted	
Risk Factors	Men	Women	Men	Women
Diabetes	1.7**	2.1***	1.4*	1.6**
ECG LV hypertrophy	3.0**	3.8**	1.4	1.3
Hypertension	1.8**	1.7**	1.0**	1.4*
Cigarettes	1.0	1.4*	1.1	1.4
BMI	1.03	1.02	—	—
Alcohol	1.01	0.95	—	—

Abbreviations: BMI, body mass index; ECG, electrocardiography; LV, left ventricular; —, not retained in the model.
*P<.05; **P<.01; ***P<.001.
Data from Benjamin EJ, Levy D, Vaziri SM, et al. Independent risk factors for atrial fibrillation in a population-based cohort: the Framingham Heart Study. JAMA 1994;271:840–4.

patients without obvious heart disease comparing subjects with and without the metabolic syndrome found that paroxysmal AF or atrial flutter occurred in 9% of patients with the syndrome and in only 4% of patients without it (P = .02). Multivariable analysis indicated that the metabolic syndrome remained a significant risk factor independent of left atrial diameter or age (OR = 2.8; P<.01). Among the five components of the metabolic syndrome, BMI was the most strongly associated with AF or atrial flutter (OR = 3.0; P = .02). It was concluded that the metabolic syndrome is strongly associated with AF or atrial flutter in patients without heart disease and that obesity may be an important underlying mechanism.[20]

The Framingham Study prospectively investigated BMI as a long-term risk for new onset of AF.[21] During a mean follow-up of 13.7 years, age-adjusted incidence rates for AF increased across BMI categories (normal, overweight, and obese) in men (9.7, 10.7, and 14.3 per 1000 person-years) and women (5.1, 8.6, and 9.9 per 1000 person-years). On adjustment for cardiovascular risk factors and interim myocardial infarction or heart failure, a 4% increase in AF risk per unit increase in BMI was observed in men and women. The adjusted hazard ratios (HRs) for AF associated with obesity were 1.5 for men and women compared with normal BMI. After adjustment for echocardiographic left atrial diameter in addition to clinical risk factors, BMI no longer was associated with AF risk. It was concluded that obesity is an important and potentially modifiable risk factor for AF, the excess risk for which seems to be mediated chiefly by left atrial dilatation. These data suggest that weight control may reduce the population burden of AF.

For men and women, respectively, diabetes conferred a 1.4- and 1.6-fold AF risk and hypertension conferred a 1.5- and 1.4-fold risk after adjusting for other associated conditions. Diabetes was also found to be a significant independent predictor of AF in four other studies, associated with an average relative risk (RR) of 1.8; however, in two other studies, it was not.[9] Because the strength of diabetes as a predictor seems to be greater in lower risk patients who have AF, it is speculated that it also may be associated with noncardioembolic strokes. Diabetes is a less powerful independent predictor than prior stroke or transient ischemic attack (TIA), hypertension, or age, but further analysis is needed to refine its predictive value for thromboembolism in patients who have AF. The reduction in stroke in warfarin-treated patients who had diabetes was lower than average in two studies.[9]

Because of its high prevalence, hypertension seems to be responsible for more AF in the population (14%) than any other risk factor.[2,5] Increased pulse pressure, a reflection of aortic stiffness, increases the cardiac load and, in the Framingham Study, increased AF risk.[22] Cumulative 20-year AF incidence rates were 5.6% for subjects who had a pulse pressure of 40 mm Hg or less (twenty-fifth percentile) and 23.3% for those who had a pulse pressure greater than 61 mm Hg (seventy-fifth percentile). Even adjusting for age; gender; baseline and time-dependent change in mean arterial pressure; and clinical risk factors for AF, including BMI, smoking, valvular heart disease, diabetes, electrocardiography (ECG) left ventricular (LV) hypertrophy, hypertension treatment, and prevalent myocardial infarction or heart failure, pulse pressure was associated with an increased risk for AF (adjusted HR = 1.26 per 20–mm Hg increment; P = .001). Systolic pressure was also significantly related to AF (HR = 1.14 per 20–mm Hg increment; P = .006). When diastolic pressure was added, the model fit improved and the diastolic relation was inverse (adjusted HR = 0.87 per 10–mm Hg increment), consistent with a pulse pressure effect. Furthermore, the association between pulse pressure and AF persisted in models that adjusted for baseline left atrial dimension, LV mass, and LV fractional shortening (adjusted HR = 1.23, 95% confidence interval [CI]: 1.09–1.39; P = .001). It seems that pulse pressure is an important risk factor for incident AF. Further research is needed to determine whether or not interventions that reduce pulse pressure can help to retard the growing incidence of AF.

CARDIOVASCULAR CONDITIONS

Persons who develop AF usually are elderly and more likely than persons of the same age to have predisposing cardiac abnormalities.[2,5] Adjusting for cardiovascular risk factors, valvular heart disease, myocardial infarction, and heart failure substantially increases AF occurrence. Echocardiographic predictors of AF include left atrial enlargement, LV fractional shortening, LV wall thickness, and mitral annular calcification, offering prognostic information for AF beyond traditional clinical risk factors.

Approximately 20% of men and 30% of women with AF have valvular heart disease, approximately a quarter of both genders have heart failure, and 26% of men and 13% of women have myocardial infarctions. Prospectively, these overt cardiac conditions impose a substantial risk for AF. Adjusting for other relevant conditions, heart failure is associated with a 4.5- and 5.9-fold risk and valvular heart disease with a 1.8- and 3.4-fold risk for AF in men and women, respectively. Myocardial

infarction significantly increased the risk factor–adjusted likelihood of AF by 40% in men only (**Table 3**).

Mitral annular calcification is associated with adverse cardiovascular disease outcomes and stroke. Prospective data are limited on the association of mitral annular calcification with AF in particular. The Framingham Study investigated the association between mitral annular calcification and long-term (>16 years of follow-up) risk for AF in the original cohort attending routine examinations between 1979 and 1981.[23] In multivariable-adjusted analyses, mitral annular calcification was associated with a 1.6-fold increased risk for AF. This association was attenuated somewhat on further adjustment for left atrial size (HR = 1.4, 95% CI, 0.9–2.0), suggesting that the association between mitral annular calcification and AF is mediated partially through left atrial enlargement.[23]

ECG LV hypertrophy seems to predispose to AF. In a double-blind, randomized, parallel-group study of subjects who had hypertension and ECG LV hypertrophy enrolled in the Losartan Intervention for Endpoint Reduction in Hypertension Study, occurrence of new-onset AF was investigated in relation to in-treatment regression or continued absence of ECG LV hypertrophy.[24] Quantified regression of ECG LV hypertrophy was associated with a reduced likelihood of acquiring AF, independent of blood pressure lowering and treatment.

ECHOCARDIOGRAPHIC ABNORMALITIES

Echocardiographic enlargement of the left atrial dimension and abnormal mitral or aortic valve function were each associated independently with increased prevalence and incidence of AF in the Cardiovascular Health Study.[1,11] In the Framingham Study, echocardiographic predictors of AF include left atrial enlargement (39% increase in risk

Table 3
Risk for atrial fibrillation by specified cardiac conditions in subjects aged 55 to 94 years: Framingham Study

| | Odds Ratios | | | |
| | Age-Adjusted | | Risk Factor–Adjusted | |
Cardiac Conditions	Men	Women	Men	Women
Myocardial infarction	2.2**	2.4**	1.4*	1.2
Heart failure	6.1***	8.1***	4.5***	5.9***
Valve disease	2.2***	3.6***	1.8**	3.4***

*P<.05; **P<.01; ***P<.001.
Data from Benjamin EJ, et al. Independent risk factors for atrial fibrillation in a population-based cohort: the Framingham Heart Study. JAMA 1994;271:840–4.

per 5-mm increment), LV fractional shortening (34% per 5% decrement), and LV wall thickness (28% per 4-mm increment) (**Table 4**). These echocardiographic features offer prognostic information for AF beyond the traditional clinical risk factors.[5,25]

CLINICAL MANIFESTATIONS

AF can cause palpitations, fatigue, lightheadedness, and exertional dyspnea by precipitating myocardial decompensation. When there is underlying coronary disease, it can bring on or aggravate angina because of an often associated rapid heart rate. AF is often undetected, however, because of lack of symptoms it often is first detected by routine ECG examination in the course of a myocardial infarction or stroke, on implanted pacemakers, or on ambulatory ECG monitoring.

AF was diagnosed incidentally in 12% of patients in the Cardiovascular Health Study[1] and in 45% of patients in the Stroke Prevention in Atrial Fibrillation Trials[26] having ECG for unrelated reasons. In a study of patients with paroxysmal AF, there were 12 times more asymptomatic than symptomatic episodes of AF and 38% of the patients with implanted pacemakers who experienced AF for more than 48 hours were unaware of it.[27] The 1.6% prevalence of AF in the absence of clinical and subclinical cardiovascular disease in the Cardiovascular Health Study indicates that "lone AF" is fairly uncommon in the elderly.[11]

PROGNOSIS

AF is associated with an increased long-term risk for stroke, heart failure, and all-cause mortality, particularly in women.[28] The doubled mortality rate of patients who have AF is linked to the severity of the underlying heart disease.[29–31] Approximately two thirds of the 3.7% mortality over 8.6 months in the Activité Liberale la Fibrillation Auriculaire study was attributed to cardiovascular causes.[32] AF also independently predicts excess mortality and an increased incidence of embolic stroke, however, accounting for between 75,000 and 100,000 strokes per year in the United States.[3] AF is, per se, a powerful risk factor for stroke among older patients. The epidemic of AF in the twenty-first century seems to be occurring in conjunction with an increasing prevalence of heart failure, obesity, type 2 diabetes mellitus, and the prediabetic metabolic syndrome.[33]

Framingham Study data indicate that AF and heart failure often coexist and that each may have an adverse impact on the other.[34] The decreased survival rate associated with AF occurs across a wide age range and is partially attributable to the vulnerability of patients who have AF to heart failure. Reported differences in mortality attributable to AF among studies may be influenced by the proportion of deaths from heart failure and thromboembolism. In large trials of heart failure, AF is a strong independent risk factor for mortality and major morbidity. In the Carvedilol or Metoprolol European Trial (COMET), there was no difference in all-cause mortality in subjects with AF at entry, but mortality increased in those who developed AF during follow-up.[35] In the Valsartan Heart Failure Trial of patients with chronic heart failure, development of AF was associated with significantly worse outcomes.[36] Managing AF in conjunction with heart failure is a major challenge requiring more trial data to guide and optimize its management.

The chief and most feared consequence of AF is a stroke, the risk for which is increased four- to fivefold.[37] AF assumes greater importance as a stroke hazard with advancing age, and by the ninth decade of life, it becomes the dominant factor. The attributable risk for stroke associated with AF increases steeply from 1.5% at the age of 50 to 59 years to 23.5% at the age of 80 to 89 years. The decreased survival rate associated with AF occurs across a wide age range.

AF is an established major independent risk factor for embolic stroke or TIA, but there is also evidence that a stroke may precipitate the onset of AF because of its hemodynamic and autonomic

Table 4	
Echocardiographic predictors of atrial fibrillation in subjects aged 50 to 59 years: Framingham Study	
Echocardiographic Feature	**Atrial Fibrillation Risk**
Left atrial diameter, mm	39% increase per 5 mm
Fractional shortening, %	34% increase per 5% decrease
LV wall thickness	28% increase per 4 mm
Two or more of previous features versus none	17% versus 3.7%

Data from Vaziri SM, Larson MG, Benjamin EJ, et al. Echocardiographic predictors of nonrheumatic atrial fibrillation. The Framingham Heart Study. Circulation 1994;89:724–30.

consequences. Approximately half of elderly patients with AF have hypertension as a concomitant major risk factor for stroke. Hypertension is a powerful independent predictor of stroke in AF and an important risk factor for developing AF. The strong association between AF, hypertension, and stroke could depend on reduced aortic compliance, LV hypertrophy, diastolic dysfunction, and left atrial dilatation, giving rise to stasis and thrombus formation.[26,38,39]

AF accounts for approximately 45% of all embolic strokes. The reported risk for stroke in placebo-treated patients in randomized warfarin trials is 4.5% per year.[38,40] Collaborative analysis of five randomized trials by the Atrial Fibrillation Investigators identified five major risk factors for stroke in patients who have AF: advanced age, prior stroke or TIA, a history of hypertension, heart failure, and diabetes.[39] Stroke risk increases at least fivefold in patients who have clinical risk factors, Other factors, such as female gender, systolic blood pressure (>160 mm Hg), and LV dysfunction, are also linked variably to stroke in patients who have AF. In patients aged 80 to 89 years, 36% of strokes occur in those who have AF. The annual risk for stroke in octogenarians who have AF ranges from 3% to 8% per year, depending on the burden of associated stroke risk factors.[37]

Ischemic stroke and systemic arterial occlusion in AF are generally attributed to embolism of a thrombus from the fibrillating left atrium; however, up to 25% of strokes in patients who have AF may result from intrinsic cerebrovascular disease, other cardiac sources of embolism, or atherosclerotic pathologic findings in the proximal aorta.[9,38] Although 12% harbor carotid artery stenosis, carotid atherosclerosis is not substantially more common in patients with AF who have a stroke, and therefore seems to be a minor contributing factor.[41,42]

In the distant past, paroxysmal AF was considered more dangerous than persistent AF, with the former postulated to be more likely to embolize. The Framingham Study found chronic sustained AF to be at least as dangerous.[43] Analyses of pooled data from five randomized controlled trials suggest that paroxysmal and chronic AF have similar risks for stroke.[39]

Before the Framingham Study report in 1982, there were many misconceptions about AF.[43] Its prognosis was believed to depend entirely on the underlying cardiac condition rather than on AF per se. AF unassociated with overt cardiovascular disease was considered to be a benign condition. Risk for embolism was not considered excessive unless AF was intermittent or associated with mitral stenosis. The Framingham Study report established that AF further increased stroke risk associated with coronary heart disease and heart failure.[43]

AF is responsible for substantial morbidity and mortality in the general population, chiefly from stroke, and leads to more hospital admissions than any other dysrhythmia.[37,44,45] In addition to often disabling symptoms and impaired quality of life, AF can precipitate heart failure and trigger potentially fatal ventricular dysrhythmias. Reflecting this widespread epidemic of AF, data from US, Scottish, and Danish studies reported a 2- to 2.5-fold increase in hospitalization rates for AF between the 1980s and 1990s.[46–48]

PUBLIC HEALTH BURDEN AND COST

AF, first described in 1909, has acquired increasing clinical and public health importance because of the expanding elderly population containing vulnerable candidates.[47] Data from a National Hospital Discharge Survey indicate that hospital admissions resulting from AF increased two- to threefold from 1985 to 1999. During this period, hospitalizations listing AF increased from fewer than 800,000 to more than 2 million, predominantly in the elderly and men. Coyne and colleagues,[49] assessing direct costs of treating AF in the United States, list AF as one of the principal discharge diagnoses for 350,000 hospitalizations and 5 million office visits in 2001. The total costs in 2005 dollars were estimated at $6.65 billion, including $2.93 billion for hospitalizations.

Thus, AF is a costly public health problem.[50] Many factors contribute to the high cost of AF, with hospitalizations constituting the major contributor (52%), followed by drugs (23%), consultations (9%), further investigations (8%), loss of work (6%), and paramedical procedures (2%). The annual cost per patient is close to $3600. Considering the prevalence of AF, the total economic burden is huge.[9]

THYROID DISEASE

For decades, hyperthyroidism has been an undisputed condition predisposing to AF. The prevalence of AF reported in patients at the time of diagnosis of overt hyperthyroidism varies from 2% to 30%.[51–53] Approximately 10% to 15% of persons who have overt hyperthyroid disease with AF are reported to have an arterial embolic event.[54–56] Studies also suggest that subclinical abnormalities of thyroid-stimulating hormone have detrimental effects on the cardiovascular system.[57] Although AF is an acknowledged manifestation of hyperthyroidism, older people in whom AF is common do not often have overt hyperthyroidism.

It was not firmly established that subclinical hyperthyroidism imposed a risk for AF until the Framingham Study investigated this hypothesis prospectively in relation to serum thyrotropin concentrations over 10 years in participants older than the age of 60 years. A low-serum thyrotropin level (<0.1 mU/L) was found to be associated with a threefold higher risk for developing AF over a decade, even after adjusting for other known risk factors.[58]

The increased AF risk for hyperthyroidism was confirmed in the Cardiovascular Health Study of subjects aged 65 years or older.[59] Eighty-two percent of participants had normal thyroid function, 15% had subclinical hypothyroidism, 1.6% had overt hypothyroidism, and 1.5% had subclinical hyperthyroidism. Individuals with subclinical hyperthyroidism had a twofold adjusted greater incidence of AF compared with those with normal thyroid function. No differences were seen in the subclinical hyperthyroidism and euthyroidism groups for incident coronary heart disease, stroke, cardiovascular death, or all-cause mortality. Likewise, there were no differences in the subclinical hypothyroidism or overt hypothyroidism group versus the euthyroidism group for cardiovascular outcomes or mortality. These data show an association between subclinical hyperthyroidism and development of AF but do not support the hypothesis that unrecognized subclinical hyperthyroidism or subclinical hypothyroidism is associated with other cardiovascular disorders that might predispose to AF.

NOVEL RISK FACTORS

Many novel modifiable and nonmodifiable risk factors for AF have been identified. These include reduced vascular compliance, atherosclerosis, insulin resistance, environmental factors, inflammatory markers, the obesity-induced metabolic syndrome, thrombogenic tendencies, sleep apnea, decreased arterial compliance, left atrial volume, diastolic dysfunction, and natriuretic peptides. There is emerging evidence that genetic variation also contributes to the risk for AF.

An inflammatory contribution for AF is supported by its frequent occurrence after cardiac surgery (25%–40%) and its association with pericarditis and myocarditis. The time course of AF after cardiac surgery parallels activation of the complement system and release of proinflammatory cytokines.[60,61] C-reactive protein, a marker of inflammation, predicts adverse cardiac events linked to AF.[60,61] In the Cardiovascular Health Study, C-reactive protein was associated independently with AF at baseline and predicted an increased risk for developing future AF.[62] It seems likely that indices of inflammation are markers for the underlying inflammatory atherosclerotic vascular disease.[62–64]

There is other evidence suggesting a role of inflammation. A cross-sectional, community-based, Swedish observational study in a primary health care facility investigated AF prevalence in patients who had hypertension and type 2 diabetes, seeking possible mechanisms for its occurrence in these conditions. AF was found to be significantly associated with combined hypertension and type 2 diabetes even after adjusting for other cardiovascular risk factors. The BMI AF risk was attenuated on adjustment for ischemic ECG findings and lost significance with adjustment for insulin resistance (OR = 1.3, 95% CI: 0.5–3.1), suggesting that AF may be associated with the diabetes-hypertension combination because of insulin resistance.[65] The insulin-resistant "metabolic syndrome" is considered to be proinflammatory, and AF is linked to inflammation. The finding that new-onset AF is related significantly to BMI in multivariate analysis, adjusting for age and gender, also has some credibility because obesity is an independent predictor of diastolic dysfunction, which is also a major determinant of AF.[66]

Obesity-promoted natriuretic peptides secreted from cardiomyocytes have a fundamental role in cardiovascular remodeling, volume homeostasis, and response to ischemia. Framingham Study investigation of the relation of B-type natriuretic peptide and N-terminal proatrial natriuretic peptide indicates that these natriuretic peptides are linked with an increased risk for AF and its predisposing cardiovascular conditions, such as heart failure and stroke (**Table 5**).[67]

There is a well-documented relation between obesity and sleep apnea. A high recurrence rate of AF after cardioversion and AF recurrences in general is more common in untreated than treated obstructive sleep apnea. Patients undergoing cardioversion are reported to have a 49% prevalence of sleep apnea compared with a 39% frequency among other cardiac patients without AF. This is not attributable to other predisposing conditions.[68,69] Postulated mechanisms include hypoxia, hypercarbia, autonomic imbalance, atrial stretching, and LV wall stress. Increased right-sided cardiac pressure stimulates the atrial natriuretic peptide release that is encountered in AF. Prospective studies of the relation of sleep-disordered breathing to AF are needed, however, taking into account its relation to obesity, metabolic syndrome, coronary artery disease, heart failure, and stroke.[70,71]

Table 5
Plasma B-type natriuretic peptides and risk for cardiovascular disease and atrial fibrillation: Framingham Study

Outcome	Adjusted Hazard Ratio per 1-SD Increment in log B-type Natriuretic Peptide Values (%)	Adjusted Hazard Ratio for B-type Natriuretic Peptide Values Greater than Eightieth Percentile
Heart failure[b,c]	1.8***	3.1**
AF[c]	1.7***	1.9*
Stroke or TIA[a,b]	1.5**	2.0*
First cardiovascular event[b]	1.3*	1.8*
Death[a]	1.3**	1.6*

Adjusted for age, gender, hypertension, total/high-density lipoprotein cholesterol, smoking, diabetes, BMI, and serum creatinine. Eightieth percentile: women 23.3 pg/mL, men 20 pg/mL. Peptide levels not significantly related to coronary heart disease.

*$P<.05$; **$P<.01$; ***$P<.001$.

[a] Analysis was also adjusted for prevalent cardiovascular disease.
[b] Analysis was also adjusted for prevalent AF.
[c] Analysis was also adjusted for valvular disease and prevalent myocardial infarction.

Data from Wang TJ, Larson MG, Levy D, et al. Plasma natriuretic peptide levels and the risk of cardiovascular events and death. N Engl J Med 2004;350:655–63.

Diastolic dysfunction commonly accompanies aging, hypertension, obesity, diabetes, heart failure, and coronary artery disease in the elderly. There is a graded relation of diastolic dysfunction to AF occurrence. On echocardiographic examination, elderly patients developed new-onset AF at a 1% rate with mild diastolic dysfunction compared with 12% with moderate diastolic dysfunction and 20% with severe diastolic dysfunction. Diastolic dysfunction provides incremental predictive information for the development of AF over that obtained from clinical risk factors. As left atrial volumes increase, diastolic function deteriorates, providing predictive information for the development of AF and stroke. Furthermore, left atrial volume is a predictor of other cardiovascular events, including myocardial infarction, stroke, and coronary revascularization, all of which predispose to AF.[72,73]

GENETIC INFLUENCES

Alleged genetically determined risk factors, such as blood pressure, obesity, and greater stature, predispose to AF. It is uncertain how these constitutional factors promote AF, but metabolic disorders and genetic factors may be implicated. A familial occurrence of AF has been recognized but is considered uncommon. The Framingham Study confirmed that observed parental AF increases its risk for offspring two- to threefold after excluding persons with predisposing conditions. This observation supports a genetic susceptibility for this dysrhythmia.[74] In such AF families, familial linkage studies are beginning to explore the genetics of AF, particularly in younger persons.[75–77] Identification of a gene defect linked to chromosome 10q in a Spanish family, nearly half the members of which had AF, supports the hypothesis of familial AF.[76,78] Most patients with AF in these families are younger than the age of 65 years, however, suggesting that the postulated genes causing AF may not be involved directly in the elderly.

The National Heart Lung and Blood Institute is sponsoring projects to examine the genetic contribution to AF and other cardiovascular phenotypes in the community. Two studies in particular plan to genotype thousands of candidate genes (Candidate Gene Association Resource project) and a 550,000 genome-wide scan of genetic polymorphisms (SNP Health Association Resource [SHARe]), with thousands of participants across many of the institute's cohort studies. Data from these studies should be available for analysis by investigators who have approved projects and ethical oversight. The aggregate results of these studies is to be posted on the Web.[79] Over the next decade, the advent of large-scale genotyping efforts should lead to advances in understanding the contribution of common complex genetic variation to AF in the community.

MULTIVARIABLE RISK ASSESSMENT

Multivariable risk assessment for stroke in patients who have AF is desirable for selecting those who most and least need aggressive anticoagulant therapy. The number needed to treat to prevent one event is inversely related to the level of risk;

thus, estimating the risk for stroke for individual patients with AF is crucial for the decision to prescribe anticoagulation therapy. The threshold risk warranting anticoagulation remains controversial, however. Patients who have a stroke risk of 2% or less per year do not benefit to a large extent from oral anticoagulation, and it would require treating 100 or more patients for 1 year to prevent a single stroke.[9] For high-risk patients with AF, who have stroke rates of 6% per year or greater, the comparable needed-to-treat number is 25 or less, strongly favoring anticoagulation. For patients at intermediate stroke risk (annual rate from 3% to 5%), opinion about routine anticoagulation remains divided.

AF is a major component of the Framingham Study stroke risk prediction algorithm.[80] Framingham Study investigators sought to stratify risk further and elucidate which individuals who had AF were at particularly increased risk for stroke or stroke and death.[80] Their multivariable analysis examined risk factors for stroke among 705 patients who had recently detected AF, excluding those who had sustained an ischemic stroke, TIA, or death within 30 days of diagnosis The significant predictors of ischemic stroke in subjects with AF were age (RR = 1.3 per decade), female gender (RR = 1.9), prior stroke or TIA (RR = 1.9), and diabetes (RR = 1.8). Systolic blood pressure became a significant predictor of stroke if warfarin was included in a time-dependent Cox proportional hazards model. With a scoring system based on age, gender, systolic hypertension, diabetes, and prior stroke or TIA, the proportion of patients classified as low risk varied from 14.3% to 30.6% depending on whether or not selected stroke rate thresholds were less than 1.5% per year or less than 2% per year.

SUMMARY

We are faced with a burgeoning epidemic of AF, which urgently demands improved prevention and treatment of this condition and its cardiovascular substrate. AF and the left atrial enlargement associated with it are likely direct causes of embolic stroke, requiring early detection and treatment. Targeted multivariable profile screening to detect persons who are likely candidates for AF is needed.

Disappointing results of therapy to suppress or eliminate the rhythm disturbance have justifiably focused greater attention on preventive treatment. Many AF risk factors also predispose to cardiovascular diseases that beget its development. Treatment of modifiable risk factors specific for AF in high-risk candidates enables early intervention,

when preventative or corrective measures are most effective. In the future, identification of genetic and biologic markers for AF and its complications may provide pathophysiologic insights and improve risk stratification for more personalized and targeted therapy.

Use of multivariable risk profiles to prevent a stroke, coronary disease, or cardiovascular disease in general should carry a bonus of prevention of AF. Therapies for predisposing factors using angiotensin-converting enzyme inhibitors and angiotensin receptor blockers recommended for hypertensive cardiovascular disease seem to reduce the rate of recurrence of AF after cardioversion and to protect against development of AF in patients with LV dysfunction.[81–83] They also may inhibit the proinflammatory and sympathetic effects of angiotensin and interfere with the triggers and substrate of AF.[9]

Warfarin anticoagulant therapy is highly effective for prevention of stroke in patients who have AF.[26,38] Meta-analysis, according to the principle of intention to treat, shows that adjusted-dose oral anticoagulation is highly efficacious for primary and secondary and disabling stroke prevention, with a risk reduction of 62% versus placebo.[39] Using "on-treatment analysis," the preventive efficacy of oral anticoagulation exceeds 80%. Despite this, a survey of treatment for patients having cerebrovascular disease indicates that only 50% are being treated to recommended standards of care. The deficits found in adherence to recommended processes for basic care for cardiovascular disease in general and for AF in particular pose serious threats to the health of the population. Strategies to reduce these deficits in care are urgently needed.

REFERENCES

1. Psaty BM, Manolio TA, Kuller LH, et al. Incidence of and risk factors for atrial fibrillation in older adults. Circulation 1997;96:2455–61.
2. Benjamin EJ, Levy D, Vaziri SM, et al. Independent risk factors for atrial fibrillation in a population-based cohort: the Framingham Heart Study. J Am Med Assoc 1994;271:840–4.
3. Feinberg WM, Blackshear JL, Laupacis A, et al. Prevalence, age distribution and gender of patients with atrial fibrillation: analysis and implications. Arch Intern Med 1995;155:469–73.
4. Go AS, Hylek EM, Phillips KA, et al. Prevalence of diagnosed atrial fibrillation in adults: national implications for rhythm management and stroke prevention: the Anticoagulation and Risk Factors in Atrial Fibrillation (ATRIA) study. J Am Med Assoc 2001;285:2370–5.

5. Kannel WB, Wolf PA, Benjamin EJ, et al. Prevalence, incidence, prognosis, and predisposing conditions for atrial fibrillation: population-based estimates. Am J Cardiol 1998;82:2N–9N.

6. Falk RH. Etiology and complications of atrial fibrillation: insights from pathology studies. Am J Cardiol 1998;82:10N–7N.

7. Manyari DE, Patterson C, Johnson D, et al. Atrial and ventricular arrhythmias in asymptomatic elderly subjects. Correlation with left atrial size and left ventricular mass. Am Heart J 1990;119:1069–76.

8. Lie JT, Hammond PI. Pathology of the senescent heart: anatomic observations on 237 autopsy studies of patients 90 to 105 years old. Mayo Clin Proc 1988;63:552–64.

9. Fuster V, Ryden LE, Cannom DS, et al. ACC/AHA/ESC 2006 guidelines for the management of patients with atrial fibrillation: a report of the American College of Cardiology/American Heart Association Task Force on Practice Guidelines and the European Society of Cardiology Committee for Practice Guidelines (Writing Committee to Revise the 2001 Guidelines for the Management of Patients with Atrial Fibrillation): developed in collaboration with the European Heart Rhythm Association and the Heart Rhythm Society. Circulation 2006;114:e257–354.

10. Ryder KM, Benjamin EJ. Epidemiology and significance of atrial fibrillation. Am J Cardiol 1999;84:131R–8R.

11. Furberg CD, Psaty BM, Manolio TA, et al. Prevalence of atrial fibrillation in elderly subjects (the Cardiovascular Health Study). Am J Cardiol 1994;74:236–41.

12. Ruo B, Capra AM, Jensvold NG, et al. Racial variation in the prevalence of atrial fibrillation among patients with heart failure: the epidemiology, practice, outcomes, and costs of heart failure (EPOCH) study. J Am Coll Cardiol 2004;43:429–35.

13. Lloyd-Jones DM, Wang TJ, Leip E, et al. Lifetime risk for development of atrial fibrillation: the Framingham Heart Study. Circulation 2004;110:1042–6.

14. Heeringa J, van der Kuip DA, Hofman A, et al. Prevalence, incidence and lifetime risk of atrial fibrillation: the Rotterdam study. Eur Heart J 2006;27:949–53.

15. Tsang TS, Petty GW, Barnes ME, et al. The prevalence of atrial fibrillation in incident stroke cases and matched population controls in Rochester, Minnesota: changes over three decades. J Am Coll Cardiol 2003;42:93–100.

16. Mukamal KJ, Tolstrup JS, Friberg J, et al. Alcohol consumption and risk of atrial fibrillation in men and women: the Copenhagen City Heart study. Circulation 2005;112:1736–42.

17. Djousse L, Levy D, Benjamin EJ, et al. Long-term alcohol consumption and the risk of atrial fibrillation in the Framingham Study. Am J Cardiol 2004;93:710–3.

18. Zacharias A, Schwann TA, Riordan CJ, et al. Obesity and risk of new-onset atrial fibrillation after cardiac surgery. Circulation 2005;112:3247–55.

19. Dublin S, French B, Glazer NL, et al. Risk of new-onset atrial fibrillation in relation to body mass index. Arch Intern Med 2006;166:2322–8.

20. Umetani K, Kodama Y, Nakamura T, et al. High prevalence of paroxysmal atrial fibrillation and/or atrial flutter in metabolic syndrome. Circ J 2007;71:252–5.

21. Wang TJ, Parise H, Levy D, et al. Obesity and the risk of new onset atrial fibrillation. JAMA 2004;292:2471–7.

22. Mitchell GF, Vasan RS, Keyes MJ, et al. Pulse pressure and risk of new onset atrial fibrillation. J Am Med Assoc 2007;297:709–15.

23. Fox CS, Parise H, Vasan R, et al. Mitral annular calcification is a predictor for incident atrial fibrillation. Atherosclerosis 2004;173:291–4.

24. Okin PM, Wachtell K, Devereux RB, et al. Regression of electrocardiographic left ventricular hypertrophy and decreased incidence of new-onset atrial fibrillation in patients with hypertension. J Am Med Assoc 2006;296:1242–8.

25. Vaziri SM, Larson MG, Benjamin EJ, et al. Echocardiographic predictors of nonrheumatic atrial fibrillation. The Framingham Heart Study. Circulation 1994;89:724–30.

26. The SPAF III. Writing Committee for the Stroke Prevention in Atrial Fibrillation Investigators. The SPAF III Writing Committee for the Stroke Prevention in Atrial Fibrillation Investigators. Patients with nonvalvular atrial fibrillation at low risk of stroke during treatment with aspirin: Stroke Prevention in Atrial Fibrillation III Study. J Am Med Assoc 1998;279:1273–7.

27. Israel CW, Gronefeld G, Ehrlich JR, et al. Long-term risk of recurrent atrial fibrillation as documented by an implantable monitoring device: implications for optimal patient care. J Am Coll Cardiol 2004;43:47–52.

28. Stewart S, Hart CL, Hole DJ, et al. A population-based study of the long-term risks associated with atrial fibrillation: 20-year follow-up of the Renfrew/Paisley study. Am J Med 2002;113:359–64.

29. Kannel WB, Abbott RD, Savage DD, et al. Coronary heart disease and atrial fibrillation: the Framingham Study. Am Heart J 1983;106:389–96.

30. Krahn AD, Manfreda J, Tate RB, et al. The natural history of atrial fibrillation: incidence, risk factors, and prognosis in the Manitoba Follow-Up study. Am J Med 1995;98:476–84.

31. Flegel KM, Shipley MJ, Rose G. Risk of stroke in nonrheumatic atrial fibrillation. [published erratum appears in Lancet 1987;1:878]. Lancet 1987;l:526–9.

32. Levy S, Maarek M, Coumel P, et al. Characterization of different subsets of atrial fibrillation in general practice in France: the ALFA study. The College of French Cardiologists. Circulation 1999;99:3028–35.

33. Braunwald E. Shattuck lecture—cardiovascular medicine at the turn of the millennium: triumphs, concerns, and opportunities. N Engl J Med 1997; 337:1360–9.

34. Wang TJ, Larson MG, Levy D, et al. Temporal relations of atrial fibrillation and congestive heart failure and their joint influence on mortality: the Framingham Heart Study. Circulation 2003;107:2920–5.

35. Swedberg K, Olsson LG, Charlesworth A, et al. Prognostic relevance of atrial fibrillation in patients with chronic heart failure on long-term treatment with beta-blockers. Eur Heart J 2005;26:1303–8.

36. Maggioni AP, Latini R, Carson PE, et al. Valsartan reduces the incidence of atrial fibrillation in patients with heart failure: results from the Valsartan Heart Failure Trial (Val-HeFT). Am Heart J 2005;149:1–10.

37. Wolf PA, Abbot RD, Kannel WB. Atrial fibrillation as independent risk factor for stroke: the Framingham Study. Stroke 1991;22:983–8.

38. Gersh BJ, Tsang TSM, Barnes ME, et al. The changing epidemiology of non-valvular atrial fibrillation: the role of novel risk factors. Eur Heart J Suppl 2005;7:C5–C11.

39. Risk factors for stroke and efficacy of antithrombotic therapy in atrial fibrillation. Analysis of pooled data from five randomized, controlled trials. Arch Intern Med 1994;154:1449–57.

40. Krahn AD, Manfreda J, Tate RB, et al. The natural history of atrial fibrillation: incidence, risk factors, and prognosis in the Manitoba follow-up study. J Am Med Assoc 1994;98:476–84.

41. Kanter MC, Tegeler CH, Pearce LA, et al. Carotid stenosis in patients with atrial fibrillation. Prevalence, risk factors, and relationship to stroke in the Stroke Prevention in Atrial Fibrillation study. Arch Intern Med 1994;154:1372–7.

42. Hart RG, Halperin JL. Atrial fibrillation and stroke: concepts and controversies. Stroke 2001;32:803–8.

43. Kannel WB, Abbott RD, Savage DD, et al. Epidemiologic features of chronic atrial fibrillation: the Framingham Study. N Engl J Med 1982;306:1018–22.

44. Benjamin EJ, Wolf PA, D'Agostino RB, et al. Impact of atrial fibrillation on risk of death: the Framingham Study. Circulation 1999;98:946–52.

45. Bailey D, Lehnmann MH, Schumacher DN, et al. Hospitalization for arrhythmias in the United States. Importance of atrial fibrillation. J Am Coll Cardiol 1992;19:41A [abstract].

46. Wolf PA, Benjamin EJ, Belanger AJ, et al. Secular trends in the prevalence of atrial fibrillation: the Framingham study. Am Heart J 1996;131:790–5.

47. Stewart S, MacIntyre K, MacLeod MM, et al. Trends in hospital activity, morbidity and case fatality related to atrial fibrillation in Scotland, 1986–1996. Eur Heart J 2001;22:693–701.

48. Frost L, Engholm G, Møller H, et al. Decrease in mortality in patients with a hospital diagnosis of atrial fibrillation in Denmark during the period 1980–1993. Eur Heart J 1999;20:1592–9.

49. Coyne KS, Paramore C, Grandy S, et al. Assessing the direct costs of treating nonvalvular atrial fibrillation in the United States. Value Health 2006;9: 348–56.

50. Stewart S, Murphy N, Walker A, et al. Cost of an emerging epidemic: an economic analysis of atrial fibrillation in the UK. Heart 2004;90:286–92.

51. White PD, Aub JC. The electrocardiogram in thyroid disease. Arch Intern Med 1918;22:766–9.

52. Sandler G, Wilson GM. The nature and prognosis of heart disease in thyrotoxicosis: a review of 150 patients with 131I. QJM 1959;52:347–69.

53. Peterson P, Hansen JM. Stroke in thyrotoxicosis with atrial fibrillation. Stroke 1988;19:15–8.

54. Nordyke RA, Gilbert FI, Harada AS, et al. Disease: influence of age on clinical findings. Arch Intern Med 1988;148:626–31.

55. Presti CF, Hart RG. Thyrotoxicosis, atrial fibrillation and embolism revisited. Am Heart J 1989;117: 976–7.

56. Singer DE. Randomized trials of warfarin for atrial fibrillation. N Engl J Med 1992;327: 1451–3.

57. Tenerz A, Forberg R, Jansson R. Is a more active attitude warranted in patients with subclinical thyrotoxicosis? J Intern Med 1990;228:229–33.

58. Sawin CT, Geller A, Wolf PA, et al. Low serum thyrotropin concentrations as a risk factor for atrial fibrillation in older persons. N Engl J Med 1994;331: 1249–52.

59. Cappola AR, Fried LP, Arnold AM, et al. Thyroid status, cardiovascular risk and mortality in older adults. J Am Med Assoc 2006;295:1033–41.

60. Falk RH. Atrial fibrillation. N Engl J Med 2001;344: 1067–78.

61. Bruins P, Velthuis H, Yazdanbakhsh AP, et al. Activation of the complement system during and after cardiopulmonary bypass surgery: postsurgery activation involves C-reactive protein and is associated with postoperative arrhythmia. Circulation 1997;96:3542–8.

62. Aviles RJ, Martin DO, Apperson-Hansen C, et al. Inflammation as a risk factor for atrial fibrillation. Circulation 2003;108:3006–10.

63. Boss CJ, Lip GY. The role of inflammation in atrial fibrillation. Int J Clin Pract 2005;59(8):870–2.

64. Chung MK, Martin DO, Sprecher D, et al. C-reactive protein elevation in patients with atrial arrhythmias: inflammatory mechanisms and persistence of atrial fibrillation. Circulation 2001;104:2886–91.

65. Powell BD, Redfield MM, Bybee KA, et al. Association of obesity with left ventricular remodeling and diastolic dysfunction in patients without coronary artery disease. Am J Cardiol 2006;98:116–20.

Available at: http://www.ajconline.org/medline/record/ivp_00029149_98_116.

66. Hanna IR, Heeke B, Bush H. The relationship between stature and the prevalence of atrial fibrillation in patients with left ventricular dysfunction. J Am Coll Cardiol 2006;47:1683–8.

67. Wang TJ, Larson MG, Levy D, et al. Plasma natriuretic peptide levels and the risk of cardiovascular events and death. N Engl J Med 2004;350:655–63.

68. Kanagala R, Murali NS, Friedman PA, et al. Obstructive sleep apnea and the recurrence of atrial fibrillation. Circulation 2003;107:2589–94.

69. Gami AS, Pressman G, Caples SM, et al. Association of atrial fibrillation and obstructive sleep apnea. Circulation 2004;110:364–7.

70. Shamsuzzaman AS, Gersh BJ, Somers VK. Obstructive sleep apnea: implications for cardiac and vascular disease. J Am Med Assoc 2003;290:1906–14.

71. Krieger J, Laks L, Wilcox I, et al. Atrial natriuretic peptide release during sleep in patients with obstructive sleep apnea before and after treatment with nasal continuous positive airway pressure. Clin Sci 1989;77:407–11.

72. Tsang TS, Gersh BJ, Appleton CP. Left ventricular diastolic dysfunction as a predictor of the first diagnosed nonvalvular atrial fibrillation in 840 elderly men and women. J Am Coll Cardiol 2002;40:1636–44.

73. Benjamin EJ, D'Agostino RB, Belanger AJ, et al. Left atrial size and the risk of stroke and death. The Framingham Heart Study. Circulation 1995;92:835–41.

74. Fox CS, Parise H, D'Agostino RB, et al. Parental atrial fibrillation as a risk factor for atrial fibrillation in offspring. J Am Med Assoc 2004;291:2851–5.

75. Darbar D, Herron KJ, Ballew JD, et al. Familial atrial fibrillation is a genetically heterogeneous disorder. J Am Coll Cardiol 2003;41:2185–92.

76. Brugada R, Tapscott T, Czernuszewicz GZ, et al. Identification of a genetic locus for familial atrial fibrillation. N Engl J Med 1997;366:905–11.

77. Crenshaw BS, Ward SR, Granger CB, et al. Atrial fibrillation in the setting of acute myocardial infarction: the GUSTO-I experience. J Am Coll Cardiol 1997;30:406–13.

78. Chen YH, Xu SJ, Bendahhou S. KCNQ1 gain-of-function mutation in familial atrial fibrillation. Science 2003;299:251–4.

79. Available at: http://www.ncbi.nlm.nih.gov/projects/gap/cgi-bin/study.cgi?study_id=phs000007.v3.p2. Accessed November 17, 2008..

80. Wang TJ, Massaro JM, Levy D, et al. A risk score for predicting stroke or death in individuals with new onset atrial fibrillation in the community: the Framingham Heart Study. J Am Med Assoc 2003;290:1049–56.

81. Vermes E, Tardif JC, Bourassa MG. Enalapril decreases the incidence of atrial fibrillation in patients with left ventricular dysfunction: insight from the Studies of Left Ventricular Dysfunction (SOLVD) trials. Circulation 2003;107:2926–31.

82. Klein HU, Goette A. Blockade of atrial angiotensin II type 1 receptors: a novel antiarrhythmic strategy to prevent atrial fibrillation? J Am Coll Cardiol 2003;41:2205–6.

83. Rowan SB, Bailey DN, Bublitz CE, et al. Trends in anticoagulation for atrial fibrillation in the U.S.: an analysis of the national ambulatory medical care survey database. J Am Coll Cardiol 2007;49:1561–5.

Genetics of Atrial Fibrillation

Steven A. Lubitz, MD[a,b], B. Alexander Yi, MD, PhD[c],
Patrick T. Ellinor, MD, PhD[d,e],*

KEYWORDS

- Atrial fibrillation • Arrhythmia
- Mutation • Gene • Genetics

Atrial fibrillation (AF) is the most common arrhythmia encountered in clinical practice, and is increasing in both incidence and prevalence.[1,2] More than 2 million Americans currently have AF, and estimates project that between 5 and 12 million will be affected by 2050.[1,2] AF is associated with substantial morbidity, including one third of all strokes in patients older than 65[3] and a twofold increased risk of mortality.[4,5] The costs attributable to the care of individuals with AF are in excess of $6.4 billion per year.[3]

AF is often associated with hypertension and structural heart disease, and traditionally has not been considered a genetic condition. However, a number of recent studies have demonstrated that AF and in particular, lone AF, have a substantial genetic basis.[6–9] Mutations in several ion channels have been identified in individuals with familial AF,[10–17] although they appear to be rare causes of the arrhythmia.[18,19] Recently, a genome-wide association study has led to the identification of genetic variants associated with common forms of AF. In the course of this review we will discuss the heritability of AF, the methods used to identify causal variants underlying AF, and our current understanding of genetic variation implicated in AF.

ATRIAL FIBRILLATION IS A HERITABLE CONDITION

While familial forms of AF have long been reported,[20] a genetic predisposition for more common forms of AF has only recently been recognized. In 2003, Fox and coworkers[8] studied more than 5000 individuals whose parents were enrolled in the original Framingham Heart Study. Over a 19-year follow-up period, they found that the development of AF in the offspring was independently associated with parental AF, particularly if the offspring cohort was restricted to those younger than 75 and without antecedent heart disease. Having a parent with AF approximately doubled the 4-year risk of developing AF, even after adjustment for risk factors such as hypertension, diabetes mellitus, and myocardial infarction.

Arnar and colleagues[6] similarly described a genetic predisposition to AF in a study of more than 5000 Icelanders in 2006. After assessing relatedness from a nationwide genealogical database, 80% of those with AF were related to another individual with AF. The relative risk of AF for first-degree relatives of a family member with AF was 1.77, when compared with individuals in the general population. The relative risk for AF increased to 4.67 when the sample was restricted to individuals less than 60 years old.

A version of this article originally appeared in *Medical Clinics of North America*, volume 92, issue 1.
[a] Cardiovascular Institute, Mount Sinai School of Medicine, New York, NY 10029, USA
[b] Division of Preventive Medicine, Brigham and Women's Hospital, Boston, MA 02446, USA
[c] Cardiology Division, Massachusetts General Hospital and Harvard Medical School, Boston, MA 02114, USA
[d] Cardiac Arrhythmia Service, Massachusetts General Hospital and Harvard Medical School, Boston, MA 02114, USA
[e] Cardiovascular Research Center, Massachusetts General Hospital and Harvard Medical School, Boston, MA 02114, USA
* Corresponding author. Cardiac Arrhythmia Service, Massachusetts General Hospital and Harvard Medical School, Boston, MA 02114.
E-mail address: pellinor@partners.org (P. Ellinor).

Further evidence of the heritability of AF was demonstrated in a chart review of more than 2000 patients with AF referred for evaluation at the Mayo Clinic.[9] Five percent of subjects had a family history of AF, and the number was as high as 15% among those with lone AF. In 2005, we found that nearly 40% of individuals with lone AF referred to the Arrhythmia Service at Massachusetts General Hospital had at least one relative with the arrhythmia, and a substantial number reported having multiple affected relatives.[7] In over 90% of cases, AF in the relatives could be verified. To obtain a crude index of heritability, we determined the prevalence of AF among each class of relative compared with that among age- and sex-matched subjects. The relative risk of AF was increased among family members, and ranged from twofold in fathers to nearly 70 fold in male siblings.

GENETIC STUDIES IN ATRIAL FIBRILLATION

Once a condition is found to be heritable, there are several techniques that are commonly used to identify the genetic basis of a disease. These include linkage analysis, candidate gene resequencing, and association studies. We will discuss each of these methods in the context of their application to AF.

Linkage Analysis

The genes that underlie simple monogenic disorders with a Mendelian pattern of inheritance can be identified using linkage analysis. When passed from generation to generation, genetic markers that lie close together on the same chromosome are likely to be transmitted en bloc in proportion to their proximity to each other. A genome-wide search for groups of markers that co-segregate with the disease as it travels through a family tree is performed to identify the approximate location of a genetic disease locus. Linkage studies report a logarithm of the odds, or LOD score, that reflects the likelihood of two markers or a marker and disease co-segregating when compared to chance alone. A LOD score of 3 or more (or odds of greater than 1000:1) is considered statistically significant. Traditionally, restriction enzyme sites and microsatellite repeats have been used as genetic markers, but more recently, it has become possible to use single nucleotide polymorphisms, or SNPs.[21] The ease of use in genotyping has made SNPs the most widely used genetic markers today.

Linkage analysis can be used to narrow the search for a causative gene to a chromosomal locus, or relatively small region of the human genome associated with disease. However, this limited region may still contain hundreds of genes spread over millions of base pairs. Once a genetic locus is identified, online data from human genome databases developed as a result of the Human Genome Project are used to identify candidate genes within the locus. These genes are then sequenced in affected individuals in an attempt to identify the sequence variants that correlate with the disease.

Once a base pair change is identified, it is important to differentiate between a mutation and a genetic polymorphism, or common variant in the genome. For a sequence alteration to be considered a mutation it must segregate with the disease, have a plausible mechanism, and not be found in healthy controls. Ultimately, the mutation should be sufficient to cause the phenotype, either in a human kindred or in a genetic model organism.

Although several genetic loci have been reported in kindreds with Mendelian AF in which specific genetic mutations have yet to be identified (**Table 1**),[22–25] linkage analysis has facilitated the identification of individual mutations in several cases of familial AF.[10,26]

In one such family of Chinese descent, Chen and coworkers[10] identified a mutation in *KCNQ1*, which encodes a potassium channel that underlies the slowly repolarizing current in cardiomyocytes known as I_{Ks} (**Fig. 1**). The investigators were able to map the disease locus to a 12-megabase region on the short arm of chromosome 11, in a four-generation family with AF. The *KCNQ1* gene was located within this region, and sequencing revealed a serine to glycine missense mutation at position 140 (S140G) in affected family members. The S140G mutation is located in the first transmembrane-spanning segment[27] at the outer edges of the voltage-sensing domain and far from the pore-forming region of the potassium channel structure. The S140G mutation results in a gain of channel function, in contrast to mutations in *KCNQ1* associated with the long QT syndrome that typically result in a loss of channel function. In cultured cells, expression of the S140G mutant channel resulted in dramatically enhanced potassium channel currents and markedly altered potassium channel gating kinetics, which would be predicted to increase I_{Ks}. Such an increase would be expected to lead to a shortening of the action potential duration and thus predispose atrial myocytes to reentry and subsequent AF (see **Fig. 1**).

While the identification of this mutation provided an initial inroad into the pathogenesis of AF, this family also illustrates our limited understanding of the role of the KCNQ1 channel in atrial versus ventricular repolarization. Specifically, it remains unclear why a mutation that results in an in vitro gain of function in KCNQ1 is associated with delayed ventricular repolarization, as manifested by

Table 1
Genes and loci implicated in familial atrial fibrillation

		Genes		
11p15.5	KCNQ1/KvLQT1	Increases I_{Ks}, Expected to shorten APD	AD	10,14
21q22.1	KCNE2/MiRP1	Increases I_{Ks}	AD	11
17q23.1-24.2	KCNJ2	Increases I_{K1}; Expected to shorten APD	AD	12
12p13	KCNA5	Loss of I_{Kur}; prolongs APD	AD	13
3p21	SCN5A	Hyperpolarizing shift of resting membrane potential; Expected to prolong APD	AD	15–17
1p36-p35	NPPA	Results in mutant atrial natriuretic peptide; associated with shortened APD	AD	26
Genetic Loci				
Chr	Gene	Comments	Inheritance	Reference
5p13	Unknown	Associated with sudden death	AR	24
6q14-q16	Unknown	Overlaps with locus for DCM	AD	23
10q22-q24	Unknown	Overlaps with locus for DCM	AD	22
10p11-q21	Unknown		AD	25

Abbreviations: Chr, Chromosome; AD, autosomal dominant; AR, autosomal recessive; DCM, dilated cardiomyopathy.

a prolonged QT interval, in more than half of the individuals with the S140G mutation.

Other gain of function mutations in *KCNQ1* have been associated with the short QT syndrome.[28] Hong and colleagues[29] reported an unusual case of AF detected in utero and confirmed on electrocardiogram upon delivery of the newborn. The infant's electrocardiogram also displayed a short QT interval. Based on this association, they sequenced the *KCNQ1* gene and found a valine to methionine mutation in position 141 (adjacent to the mutated position found by Chen and colleagues). Like the S140G mutation, in vitro expression of V141M mutant channels displayed markedly enhanced current density and altered gating kinetics.

More recently, Hodgson-Zingman and colleagues[26] identified a frameshift mutation in *NPPA* in a family with AF. The mutation in *NPPA*, which encodes atrial natriuretic peptide, resulted in increased levels of a circulating mutant peptide. Electrophysiological assessment in a rat heart model revealed decreased action potential

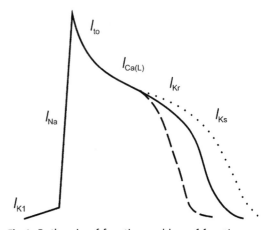

Fig. 1. Both gain of function and loss of function mutations in I_{Ks} have been associated with AF. Mutations in *KCNQ1* and *KCNE2* increase the current I_{Ks}, which is predicted to shorten the action potential (*dashed line*) in cardiac myocytes and render atrial myocytes susceptible to reentrant arrhythmias. Mutations in *KCNA5* (encodes Kv1.5) that are predicted to prolong the action potential duration (*dotted line*) have also been associated with AF.

duration, consistent with known mechanisms of reentrant mediated AF.[30]

Candidate Gene Studies

A candidate gene can be any gene that is hypothesized to cause a disease. Based on the work relating KCNQ1 to AF, investigators have considered other potassium channels as potential candidate genes for AF and screened for mutations in these genes in cohorts of subjects with AF.

Otway and colleagues[14] examined 50 kindreds with AF and amplified the genes for KCNQ1 and KCNE1-3, which encode accessory subunits of KCNQ1. They found a single mutation in KCNQ1 in only one family—an arginine to cysteine change at amino acid position 14 (R14C) in KCNQ1. Unlike the S140G mutation discovered by Chen and colleagues,[10] R14C had no significant effect on KCNQ1/KCNE1 current amplitudes in cultured cells at baseline. However, upon exposure to hypotonic solution, mutant channels exhibited a marked increase in currents compared with wild type channels. Interestingly, of those who carried the R14C mutation, only those with left atrial dilatation had AF, leading the authors to propose a "two-hit" hypothesis for AF. They also identified a mutation in KCNE2 in two of the kindreds. Like the S140G mutation in KCNQ1 the mutation in KCNE2 (R27C) dramatically increased the amplitude of I_{Ks}.[11]

Finally, other work has suggested that the relationship between potassium channels and AF extends beyond I_{Ks}. The work of Xia and colleagues[12] may also implicate KCNJ2 which encodes, an inward rectifier potassium channel that underlies the I_{K1} current, in AF. In their work, a V93I mutation was found in all affected members in one kindred with familial AF. The V93I also leads to gain of function KCNJ2 channels, which increase potassium current amplitudes. However, there is still an incomplete understanding of how an increase in the background current I_{K1} might lead to atrial arrhythmias.

We have screened our cohort with lone AF for mutations in KCNQ1, KCNJ2 and KCNE1-5 and were unable to find any mutations in these genes.[18] These findings suggest that potassium channels are an uncommon cause of AF and there is much more to be learned about the diversity of molecular pathways that lead to this arrhythmia.

The genes encoding connexins, gap-junction proteins that mediate the spread of action potentials between cardiac myocytes, have also been examined as potential candidates for AF. Prior work has shown that mice with null alleles of GJA5, the gene for connexin40, exhibit atrial reentrant arrhythmias.[31] From this work, Gollob and coworkers[32] considered this gene as a potential candidate in individuals with idiopathic AF who underwent pulmonary vein isolation surgery. An analysis of DNA isolated from their cardiac tissue showed that 4 of the 15 subjects had mutations in GJA5 that markedly interfered with the electrical coupling between cells. In three of the patients, DNA isolated from their lymphocytes lacked the same mutation in GJA5 indicating that the connexin40 mutations had been acquired after fertilization or was a somatic mutation. One of the four individuals carried the mutation in both cardiac tissue and lymphocytes consistent with a germline rather than somatic mutation. However, more information about the transmission of AF in relatives of these individuals was not available.

Association Studies

Although traditional methods such as linkage analysis can be applied to families where the phenotype and pattern of inheritance are consistent with a monogenic disorder, the mode of transmission for AF is less clear. Association studies have been used in an attempt to identify the genetic basis of AF and other apparently complex traits. In an association study the frequency of a genetic marker, such as a SNP, is compared between individuals with an outcome (cases) and those without an outcome (controls). Over the past 10 years, many case-control and cohort studies have been performed in subjects with AF, leading to the identification of variants associated with disease. These studies have typically tested a small number of variants and have been directed at candidate genes previously believed to be involved in AF. Examples include genes encoding products involved in regulation of the renin-angiotensin-aldosterone axis[33–40] and calcium handling,[41] as well as neurohormonal[39] and lipoprotein[42] pathways. Additionally, genes encoding gap junction proteins,[43,44] ion channels,[15,45–49] interleukins,[50,51] signaling molecules,[34,45,52] and mediators of other molecular pathways[53] have been examined (summarized in **Table 2**). Unfortunately, these studies have been limited by a low prior probability of any polymorphism truly being associated with AF. Further complicating these analyses are the small sample sizes and a lack of replication in distinct populations, as well as phenotypic and genetic heterogeneity.

In recent years, genome-wide association studies (GWAS) have been made possible by advancements in genotyping technology that allow investigators to assay hundreds of thousands of SNPs spread over the entire human genome. The studies are typically executed using a case-control

Table 2
Polymorphisms associated with atrial fibrillation

Gene	Variant	Cases	Controls	OR	P Value	Replicated?	Comments	Reference
—	rs2200733	3913	22,092	1.72	3.3×10^{-41}	Yes	Identified in GWAS	62
—	rs10033464	3913	22,092	1.39	6.9×10^{-11}	Yes	Identified in GWAS	62
ACE	D/D	51	289	1.5	.016	Yes	In patients with CHF	34
ACE	D/D	404	520	1.89	<.001	Yes		36
CYP11B2	T-344C	63	133	2.65	.03	No	In patients with CHF	40
AGT	M235T	250	250	2.5	<.001	No		33
AGT	G-6A	250	250	3.3	.005	No		33
AGT	G-217A	250	250	2.0	.002	No		33
AGT	T174M	968	8267	1.2	.05	No		37
AGT	20 C/C	968	8267	1.5	.01	No		37
CETP	Taq1B	97	97	0.35	.05	No		42
GJA5	-44A	14	16	5.3	.0019	Yes		44
GJA5	-44A, +71G	173	232	1.514	<.006	Yes (for -44A only)		43
EDN2	A985G	26	84	5.89	.018	No	In patients with HCM	39
NOS3	894T/T	51	289	3.2	.001	No	In patients with CHF	34
NOS3	T-786C	331	441	1.4	.05	No		45
GNB3	C825T	291	292	0.46	.02	No		52
hsp70	Met439Thr	48	194	2.43	.016	No	In postoperative CABG patients	53
IL6	G-174C	26	84	3.25	.006	No	In postoperative CABG patients	50
IL10	A-592C	196	873	0.32	3.70×10^{-03}	No	Lone AF	51
KCNE4	E145D	142	238	1.66	.044	No		49
KCNE5	97T	158	96	0.52	.007	No		48
KCNH2	K897T	1207	2475	1.25	.00033	No		46
MinK/KCNE1	38G	108	108	1.8	.024	Yes		47
MinK/KCNE1	38G	331	441	1.73	<.005	Yes		45
MMP2	C1306T	196	873	8.1	1.26×10^{-02}	No	Lone AF	51
SLN	G-65C	147	92	1.98	.011	No		41

Abbreviations: ACE, Angiotensin I converting enzyme; AF, atrial fibrillation; AGT, Angiotensinogen; CABG, coronary artery bypass graft; CETP, cholesteryl ester transfer protein; CHF, congestive heart failure; CYP11B2, Aldosterone synthase; EDN2, endothelin 2; GJA5, connexin 40; GNB3, guanine nucleotide binding protein; GWAS, genome-wide association study; HCM, hypertrophic cardiomyopathy; hsp70, heat shock protein 70; IL6, interleukin 6; IL10, interleukin 10; NOS3, nitric oxide synthase 3; SLN, sarcolipin gene.

study design.[54] GWAS attempt to identify novel genetic polymorphisms that are significantly more or less common in a group with a disease as compared with a control group. Since the markers are spread over the entire genome, these experiments give no weight to existing candidate genes. Such studies have been used successfully in the past several years to identify potential novel pathways for diabetes,[55] obesity,[56] coronary heart disease,[57,58] macular degeneration,[59] and repolarization.[60]

Although GWAS have the potential to identify new pathways for disease, they also have a number of limitations. In particular, with hundreds of thousands of individual associations being tested, these studies have a high likelihood of producing false-positive associations. There is still discussion within the field of what the threshold level should be for genome-wide significance.[61] False-positive results can also emerge from population stratification or the failure to properly control for ethnicity, thus resulting in over- or underrepresentation of spurious ethnic-specific markers. Although variations in study design have been proposed in an effort to eliminate false associations, ultimately replication of the associations in other populations is the best method of validation.[54]

The biological significance of the identified variants is another concern. Most variants found in genetic association studies have been associated with relatively weak effects, with typical odds ratios ranging from approximately 1.3 to 1.5. Although such variants may generate new ideas about disease pathogenesis, understanding the biological mechanisms by which the majority of variants confer disease susceptibility remains challenging.

Recently, a team led by the researchers at de-CODE genetics have reported the results of a GWAS for AF. Gudbjartsson and colleagues[62] examined over 300,000 SNPs and identified two polymorphisms on the long arm of chromosome 4 (4q25) that were highly associated (rs2200733 and rs10033464, $P = 3.3 \times 10^{-41}$ and 6.9×10^{-11}, respectively) with AF or atrial flutter in a group of Icelanders. To improve both the validity and generalizability of the findings, the study was replicated in other populations in Iceland, Sweden, the United States, and Hong Kong. Neither variant was correlated with obesity, hypertension, or myocardial infarction suggesting that the genetic variants are not associated with AF by affecting those risk factors.

How do the variants on chromosome 4 lead to AF? At present, the mechanism of action of these variants is unclear. Interestingly, these SNPs lie upstream from a gene that could plausibly play a role in the pathogenesis of AF, the paired-like homeodomain transcription factor 2, PITX2. This gene is known to be critical in the development of the left atrium,[63–66] pulmonary myocardium,[67] and in the suppression of left atrial pacemakers cells in early development.[68] One can speculate that these variants may alter the function of PITX2 either in early development or in adulthood and thus predispose to AF. However, currently there is no direct link between the PITX2 gene and these noncoding variants more than 50,000 base pairs away. Future work examining the correlation between these variants and PITX2 RNA levels, protein levels, or tissue specificity will hopefully clarify the mechanism underlying the association of these SNPs with AF.

REFINING GENETIC STUDIES OF ATRIAL FIBRILLATION

To continue to improve upon the utility of genetic studies for AF we will need to overcome a number of obstacles. A critical step in any genetic study is the ability to correctly assign the diagnosis. AF represents a particular challenge because many individuals are asymptomatic, some have paroxysmal disease, and yet others develop AF late in life. Genotypic and phenotypic heterogeneity further complicate the classification of AF. Rather than a single entity, AF may represent the final common pathway for a number of distinct pathogenic insults such as heart failure, hypertension, or thyroid abnormalities.

To address these challenges, we will have to continue to improve upon the characterization and classification of AF. The identification of endophenotypes, or subtle, heritable traits that co-segregate with AF, may help to refine ongoing genetic studies. For AF, endophenotypes such as specific P-wave morphologies, pulmonary venous anatomy as assessed by CT or MRI, or biomarkers that are heritable and easily detectable may be helpful.

SUMMARY

Recent studies of AF have identified mutations in a series of ion channels; however, these mutations appear to be relatively rare causes of AF. A genome-wide association study has identified novel variants on chromosome 4 associated with AF, although the mechanisms of action for these variants remain unknown. Ultimately, a greater understanding of the genetics of AF should yield insights into novel pathways, therapeutic targets, and diagnostic testing for this common arrhythmia.

ACKNOWLEDGMENTS

This work was supported by a grant from the Disque Deane Foundation to Dr. Ellinor and a National Institutes of Health training grant (5T32HL007575) to Dr. Lubitz.

REFERENCES

1. Miyasaka Y, Barnes ME, Gersh BJ, et al. Secular trends in incidence of atrial fibrillation in Olmsted County, Minnesota, 1980 to 2000, and implications on the projections for future prevalence. Circulation 2006;114(2):119–25.
2. Go AS, Hylek EM, Phillips KA, et al. Prevalence of diagnosed atrial fibrillation in adults: national implications for rhythm management and stroke prevention: the AnTicoagulation and Risk Factors in Atrial Fibrillation (ATRIA) study. JAMA 2001;285(18):2370–5.
3. Coyne KS, Paramore C, Grandy S, et al. Assessing the direct costs of treating nonvalvular atrial fibrillation in the United States. Value Health 2006;9(5):348–56.
4. Benjamin EJ, Wolf PA, D'Agostino RB, et al. Impact of atrial fibrillation on the risk of death: the Framingham heart study. Circulation 1998;98(10):946–52.
5. Gajewski J, Singer RB. Mortality in an insured population with atrial fibrillation. JAMA 1981;245(15):1540–4.
6. Arnar DO, Thorvaldsson S, Manolio TA, et al. Familial aggregation of atrial fibrillation in Iceland. Eur Heart J 2006;27(6):708–12.
7. Ellinor PT, Yoerger DM, Ruskin JN, et al. Familial aggregation in lone atrial fibrillation. Hum Genet 2005;118(2):179–84.
8. Fox CS, Parise H, D'Agostino RB Sr, et al. Parental atrial fibrillation as a risk factor for atrial fibrillation in offspring. JAMA 2004;291(23):2851–5.
9. Darbar D, Herron KJ, Ballew JD, et al. Familial atrial fibrillation is a genetically heterogeneous disorder. [comment]. J Am Coll Cardiol 2003;41(12):2185–92.
10. Chen YH, Xu SJ, Bendahhou S, et al. KCNQ1 gain-of-function mutation in familial atrial fibrillation. Science 2003;299(5604):251–4.
11. Yang Y, Xia M, Jin Q, et al. Identification of a KCNE2 gain-of-function mutation in patients with familial atrial fibrillation. Am J Hum Genet 2004;75(5):899–905.
12. Xia M, Jin Q, Bendahhou S, et al. A Kir2.1 gain-of-function mutation underlies familial atrial fibrillation. Biochem Biophys Res Commun 2005;332(4):1012–9.
13. Olson TM, Alekseev AE, Liu XK, et al. Kv1.5 channelopathy due to KCNA5 loss-of-function mutation causes human atrial fibrillation. Hum Mol Genet 2006;15(14):2185–91.
14. Otway R, Vandenberg JI, Guo G, et al. Stretch-sensitive KCNQ1 mutation A link between genetic and environmental factors in the pathogenesis of atrial fibrillation? J Am Coll Cardiol 2007;49(5):578–86.
15. Chen LY, Ballew JD, Herron KJ, et al. A common polymorphism in SCN5A is associated with lone atrial fibrillation. Clin Pharmacol Ther 2007;81(1):35–41.
16. Darbar D, Kannankeril PJ, Donahue BS, et al. Cardiac sodium channel (SCN5A) variants associated with atrial fibrillation. Circulation 2008;117(15):1927–35.
17. Ellinor PT, Nam EG, Shea MA, et al. Cardiac sodium channel mutation in atrial fibrillation. J Neurosci 2008;5(1):99–105.
18. Ellinor PT, Moore RK, Patton KK, et al. Mutations in the long QT gene, KCNQ1, are an uncommon cause of atrial fibrillation. Heart 2004;90(12):1487–8.
19. Ellinor PT, Petrov-Kondratov VI, Zakharova E, et al. Potassium channel gene mutations rarely cause atrial fibrillation. BMC Med Genet 2006;7:70.
20. Wolff L. Familial auricular fibrillation. N Engl J Med 1943;229:396–8.
21. Consortium TIH. A haplotype map of the human genome. Nature 2005;437(7063):1299–320.
22. Brugada R, Tapscott T, Czernuszewicz GZ, et al. Identification of a genetic locus for familial atrial fibrillation. N Engl J Med 1997;336(13):905–11.
23. Ellinor PT, Shin JT, Moore RK, et al. Locus for atrial fibrillation maps to chromosome 6q14-16. Circulation 2003;107(23):2880–3.
24. Oberti C, Wang L, Li L, et al. Genome-wide linkage scan identifies a novel genetic locus on chromosome 5p13 for neonatal atrial fibrillation associated with sudden death and variable cardiomyopathy. Circulation 2004;110(25):3753–9.
25. Volders PG, Zhu Q, Timmermans C, et al. Mapping a novel locus for familial atrial fibrillation on chromosome 10p11-q21. Heart Rhythm 2007;4(4):469–75.
26. Hodgson-Zingman DM, Karst ML, Zingman LV, et al. Atrial natriuretic peptide frameshift mutation in familial atrial fibrillation. N Engl J Med 2008;359(2):158–65.
27. Schenzer A, Friedrich T, Pusch M, et al. Molecular determinants of KCNQ (Kv7) K+ channel sensitivity to the anticonvulsant retigabine. J Neurosci 2005;25(20):5051–60.
28. Bellocq C, van Ginneken ACG, Bezzina CR, et al. Mutation in the KCNQ1 gene leading to the short QT-interval syndrome. Circulation 2004;109:2394–7.
29. Hong K, Piper DR, Diaz-Valdecantos A, et al. De novo KCNQ1 mutation responsible for atrial fibrillation and short QT syndrome in utero. Cardiovasc Res 2005;68(3):433–40.
30. Nattel S. New ideas about atrial fibrillation 50 years on. Nature 2002;415(6868):219–26.
31. Hagendorff A, Schumacher B, Kirchhoff S, et al. Conduction disturbances and increased atrial vulnerability in connexin40-deficient mice analyzed by transesophageal stimulation. Circulation 1999;99:1508–15.
32. Gollob MH, Jones DL, Krahn AD, et al. Somatic mutations in the connexin 40 gene (GJA5) in atrial fibrillation. N Engl J Med 2006;354(25):2677–88.

33. Tsai CT, Lai LP, Lin JL, et al. Renin-angiotensin system gene polymorphisms and atrial fibrillation. Circulation 2004;109(13):1640–6.

34. Bedi M, McNamara D, London B, et al. Genetic susceptibility to atrial fibrillation in patients with congestive heart failure. Heart Rhythm 2006;3(7):808–12.

35. Yamashita T, Hayami N, Ajiki K, et al. Is ACE gene polymorphism associated with lone atrial fibrillation? Jpn Heart J 1997;38(5):637–41.

36. Fatini C, Sticchi E, Gensini F, et al. Lone and secondary nonvalvular atrial fibrillation: role of a genetic susceptibility. Int J Cardiol 2007;120(1):59–65.

37. Ravn LS, Benn M, Nordestgaard BG, et al. Angiotensinogen and ACE gene polymorphisms and risk of atrial fibrillation in the general population. Pharmacogenet Genomics 2008;18(6):525–33.

38. Tsai CT, Hwang JJ, Chiang FT, et al. Renin-angiotensin system gene polymorphisms and atrial fibrillation: a regression approach for the detection of gene-gene interactions in a large hospitalized population. Cardiology 2008;111(1):1–7.

39. Nagai T, Ogimoto A, Okayama H, et al. A985G polymorphism of the endothelin-2 gene and atrial fibrillation in patients with hypertrophic cardiomyopathy. Circ J 2007;71(12):1932–6.

40. Amir O, Amir RE, Paz H, et al. Aldosterone synthase gene polymorphism as a determinant of atrial fibrillation in patients with heart failure. Am J Cardiol 2008;102(3):326–9.

41. Nyberg MT, Stoevring B, Behr ER, et al. The variation of the sarcolipin gene (SLN) in atrial fibrillation, long QT syndrome and sudden arrhythmic death syndrome. Clin Chim Acta 2007;375(1-2):87–91.

42. Asselbergs FW, Moore JH, van den Berg MP, et al. A role for CETP TaqIB polymorphism in determining susceptibility to atrial fibrillation: a nested case control study. BMC Med Genet 2006;7:39.

43. Juang JM, Chern YR, Tsai CT, et al. The association of human connexin 40 genetic polymorphisms with atrial fibrillation. Int J Cardiol 2007;116(1):107–12.

44. Firouzi M, Ramanna H, Kok B, et al. Association of human connexin40 gene polymorphisms with atrial vulnerability as a risk factor for idiopathic atrial fibrillation. Circ Res 2004;95(4):e29–33.

45. Fatini C, Sticchi E, Genuardi M, et al. Analysis of minK and eNOS genes as candidate loci for predisposition to non-valvular atrial fibrillation. Eur Heart J 2006;27(14):1712–8.

46. Sinner MF, Pfeufer A, Akyol M, et al. The non-synonymous coding IKr-channel variant KCNH2-K897T is associated with atrial fibrillation: results from a systematic candidate gene-based analysis of KCNH2 (HERG). Eur Heart J 2008;7:907–14.

47. Lai LP, Su MJ, Yeh HM, et al. Association of the human minK gene 38G allele with atrial fibrillation: evidence of possible genetic control on the pathogenesis of atrial fibrillation. Am Heart J 2002; 144(3):485–90.

48. Ravn LS, Hofman-Bang J, Dixen U, et al. Relation of 97T polymorphism in KCNE5 to risk of atrial fibrillation. Am J Cardiol 2005;96(3):405–7.

49. Zeng Z, Tan C, Teng S, et al. The single nucleotide polymorphisms of I(Ks) potassium channel genes and their association with atrial fibrillation in a Chinese population. Cardiology 2007;108(2):97–103.

50. Gaudino M, Andreotti F, Zamparelli R, et al. The -174G/C interleukin-6 polymorphism influences postoperative interleukin-6 levels and postoperative atrial fibrillation. Is atrial fibrillation an inflammatory complication? Circulation 2003;108(Suppl 1): II195–9.

51. Kato K, Oguri M, Hibino T, et al. Genetic factors for lone atrial fibrillation. Int J Mol Med 2007;19(6): 933–9.

52. Schreieck J, Dostal S, von Beckerath N, et al. C825T polymorphism of the G-protein beta3 subunit gene and atrial fibrillation: association of the TT genotype with a reduced risk for atrial fibrillation. Am Heart J 2004;148(3):545–50.

53. Afzal AR, Mandal K, Nyamweya S, et al. Association of Met439Thr substitution in heat shock protein 70 gene with postoperative atrial fibrillation and serum HSP70 protein levels. Cardiology 2008;110(1): 45–52.

54. Risch NJ. Searching for genetic determinants in the new millennium. Nature 2000;405(6788):847–56.

55. Saxena R, Voight BF, Lyssenko V, et al. Genome-wide association analysis identifies loci for type 2 diabetes and triglyceride levels. Science 2007; 316(5829):1331–6.

56. Frayling TM, Timpson NJ, Weedon MN, et al. A common variant in the FTO gene is associated with body mass index and predisposes to childhood and adult obesity. Science 2007;316(5826):889–94.

57. McPherson R, Pertsemlidis A, Kavaslar N, et al. A common allele on chromosome 9 associated with coronary heart disease. Science 2007;316(5830): 1488–91.

58. Helgadottir A, Thorleifsson G, Manolescu A, et al. A common variant on chromosome 9p21 affects the risk of myocardial infarction. Science 2007; 316(5830):1491–3.

59. Dewan A, Liu M, Hartman S, et al. HTRA1 promoter polymorphism in wet age-related macular degeneration. Science 2006;314(5801):989–92.

60. Arking DE, Pfeufer A, Post W, et al. A common genetic variant in the NOS1 regulator NOS1AP modulates cardiac repolarization. Nat Genet 2006;38(6): 644–51.

61. Hunter DJ, Kraft P. Drinking from the fire hose—statistical issues in genomewide association studies. N Engl J Med 2007;357(5):436–9.

62. Gudbjartsson DF, Arnar DO, Helgadottir A, et al. Variants conferring risk of atrial fibrillation on chromosome 4q25. Nature 2007;448(7151):353–7.

63. Gage PJ, Suh H, Camper SA. Dosage requirement of Pitx2 for development of multiple organs. Development 1999;126(20):4643–51.

64. Campione M, Ros MA, Icardo JM, et al. Pitx2 expression defines a left cardiac lineage of cells: evidence for atrial and ventricular molecular isomerism in the iv/iv mice. Dev Biol 2001;231(1):252–64.

65. Franco D, Campione M. The role of Pitx2 during cardiac development. Linking left-right signaing and congenital heart diseases. Trends Cardiovasc Med 2003;13:157–63.

66. Logan M, Pagan-Westphal SM, Smith DM, et al. The transcription factor Pitx2 mediates situs-specific morphogenesis in response to left-right asymmetric signals. Cell 1998;94(3):307–17.

67. Mommersteeg MT, Brown NA, Prall OW, et al. Pitx2c and Nkx2-5 are required for the formation and identity of the pulmonary myocardium. Circ Res 2007;101(9):902–9.

68. Mommersteeg MT, Hoogaars WM, Prall OW, et al. Molecular pathway for the localized formation of the sinoatrial node. Circ Res 2007;100(3):354–62.

New Concepts in Atrial Fibrillation: Neural Mechanisms and Calcium Dynamics

Chung-Chuan Chou, MD[a],*, Peng-Sheng Chen, MD[b]

KEYWORDS

- Atrium • Calcium • Fibrillation • Nervous system
- Autonomic

Atrial fibrillation (AF) is a complex disease with multiple possible mechanisms.[1] Many studies indicate that the arrhythmogenic foci within the thoracic veins are AF initiators. Once initiated, AF alters atrial electrical and structural properties (atrial remodeling) in a way that promotes its own maintenance and recurrences and may alter the response to antiarrhythmic drugs. The exact mechanisms through which the arrhythmogenic foci are triggered remain elusive, however. One possible immediate trigger is the paroxysmal autonomic nervous system (ANS) discharge. In normal dogs, sympathetic nerve stimulation rarely triggers AF. In dogs that undergo chronic rapid atrial pacing, however, sympathetic stimulation can lead to rapid repetitive activations in the isolated canine pulmonary vein (PV) and vein of Marshall preparations.[2,3]

Sharifov and colleagues[4] reported that a combined isoproterenol and acetylcholine infusion is more effective than acetylcholine alone in inducing AF. Clinically, alterations of autonomic tone, involving the sympathetic and parasympathetic nervous systems, are implicated in initiating paroxysmal AF.[5] These results suggest that simultaneous sympathetic and parasympathetic (sympathovagal) discharge is particularly profibrillatory. Also, evidence shows heightened atrial sympathetic innervation in patients who have persistent AF,[6] suggesting that potential autonomic

substrate modification may be part of a remodeled atrial substrate for AF maintenance.

PATTERNS OF ACTIVATION AT THE PULMONARY VEIN AND PULMONARY VEIN–LEFT ATRIAL JUNCTION DURING SUSTAINED ATRIAL FIBRILLATION

AF is characterized by the coexistence of multiple activation wavelets within the atria. The mechanisms through which multiple wavefronts occur have been debated for many years. The focal source hypothesis states that a single rapidly focal driver underlies the mechanisms of AF. Alternatively, the multiple wavelet hypothesis posits that heterogeneous dispersion of repolarization is responsible for wavebreaks and the generation of multiple wavelets that sustain AF.[7]

Zipes and Knope,[8] Spach and colleagues,[9] and Scherlag and colleagues[10] provided the first pieces of evidence supporting the importance of thoracic veins in the generation of electrical activity. The importance of these original works were proven by Haissaguerre and colleagues,[11] who showed the critical role of PV in the generation and maintenance of AF in humans.

Hamabe and colleagues[12] reported that the PV–left atrial (LA) junction has segmental muscle disconnection and differential muscle narrowing in dogs.

A version of this article originally appeared in *Medical Clinics of North America*, volume 92, issue 1.
[a] The Second Section of Cardiology, Chang Gung Memorial Hospital, 199 Tung Hwa North Road, Taipei 10591, Taiwan
[b] Department of Medicine, Indiana University School of Medicine, 1801 North Capitol Avenue, E475, Indianapolis, IN 46202, USA
* Corresponding author.
E-mail address: 2867@adm.cgmh.org.tw (C-C. Chou).

doi:10.1016/j.ccl.2008.09.003
0733-8651/08/$ – see front matter © 2009 Elsevier Inc. All rights reserved.

Combined with the complex fiber orientations within the PV, these changes provide robust anatomic bases for generating conduction disturbances at the PV–LA junction and complex intra-PV conduction patterns, to facilitate reentry formation.

High-density (1-mm resolution) computerized mapping techniques have shown that rapid PV focal discharges[13–15] and PV–LA junction microreentry[15] are present during sustained AF induced by rapid LA pacing (**Fig. 1**). **Fig. 1**A shows the activation snapshots of right superior PV during sustained AF, showing three consecutive focal discharges (6081, 6203, and 6316 ms). The focal discharge wavefronts meet lines of functional conduction block (dotted lines) followed by the formation of complete reentry loops (6409–6595 ms). The wavefronts from LA also encountered a functional line of block, followed by the formation of reentry. After infusion of ibutilide (**Fig. 1**B), a typical class III antiarrhythmic drug that can prolong the effective refractory period of atria, focal discharges (6344 and 6582 ms) and reentrant wavefronts (6035–6296 ms) activated at slower rates. The conducted wavefronts between the PV and

LA were reduced significantly by ibutilide. The overall incidence of focal discharge in the PVs was not suppressed, however. A high dose of ibutilide may terminate all reentrant activity completely, thereby converting AF to PV tachycardia before conversion to sinus rhythm. These findings suggest that sustained AF is the result of a combination of PV focal discharge and PV–LA reentrant activity.

A recent computational simulation study[16] showed that up-regulation of the L-type Ca^{2+} current steepened restitution curves of the action potential duration (APD) and the conduction velocity. Spontaneous firing of ectopic foci, coupled with sinus activity, produced dynamic spatial dispersion of repolarization, including discordant alternans, which facilitated unidirectional conduction block and initiated reentrant atrial flutter or AF. The size of vulnerable window was larger for PV ectopic foci than for right atrial foci. These findings imply that the ectopic beats originated from the PV are more likely to trigger AF than ectopic beats from elsewhere in the atria.

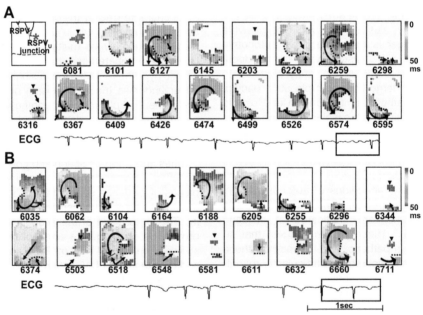

Fig. 1. Patterns of activation during sustained AF induced by chronic rapid atrial pacing. (A) Snapshots of focal discharge and reentrant activation patterns within right super PV at baseline AF. Asterisk in the left upper corner indicates the anatomic location of focal discharge at the proximal right superior PV. Black horizontal dotted line indicates the PV–LA junction. The number below each snapshot represents the time in milliseconds, with the beginning of data acquisition as time zero. In snapshots, red color represents the wavefront; black arrows, the direction of wave propagation; black dotted line, line of block; arrowhead, site of focal discharge. The color bar on the right shows the time scale (0–50 ms). (B) Snapshots of focal discharge and reentrant activation patterns within right superior PV after ibutilide infusion (0.02 mg/kg). A rectangle toward the end of the ECG tracings shows the period corresponding to the snapshots in (A) and (B). (*From* Chou CC, Zhou S, Tan AY, et al. High-density mapping of pulmonary veins and left atrium during ibutilide administration in a canine model of sustained atrial fibrillation. Am J Physiol Heart Circ Physiol 2005;289:H2704; with permission).

ANATOMIC AND NEURAL SUBSTRATES IN THE PULMONARY VEINS

Zipes and Knope[8] conclude that not only did atrial muscle extend for some distance into these the thoracic veins but also these muscle sleeves received vagal innervation. Both the autonomic nerves and atrial muscles in the PVs may have been important in triggering AF. Subsequent works showed significant heterogeneity of the cell types within the PV muscle sleeves. Masani and colleagues[17] showed that node-like cells were present in the myocardial layer of the PV of rats. Among the ordinary myocardial cells resembling those of the atrial myocardium, clear cells with structural features similar to those of sinus node cells were identified. They appeared singly or in small groups among ordinary myocardial cells.

Cheung[18] reported that isolated PVs were capable of independent pacemaking activity. Light and electron microscope studies suggest that cells morphologically akin to specialized conduction cells were present in human PVs.[19] Chou and colleagues[20] reported that canine PVs had a layer of large, pale, periodic acid-Schiff (PAS)–positive cells at the site of focal discharge, supporting the notion that Purkinje-like cells were present in the PVs.

A distinguishing feature of the sinus node, compared with other parts of the atria, is the presence of rich autonomic innervation.[21–23] In comparison, Tan and colleagues[24] identified abundant sympathetic nerve fibers within the PV using immunohistochemical staining techniques. These findings are consistent with those reported by Masani,[17] who observed that in PVs, nerve fibers containing small and large vesicles with and without dense cores were juxtaposed with the node-like cells. The close interaction between the nerve structures and the specialized muscle cells might play a role in the generation of ectopic activities.

CARDIAC AUTONOMIC INNERVATION

Kawashima[25] performed detailed anatomic studies of human cardiac autonomic innervation. The cardiac sympathetic ganglia include a superior cervical ganglion that communicates with C1 through C3, and the cervicothoracic (stellate) ganglion, which communicates with C7 through T2. In addition, the thoracic ganglia (as low as the seventh thoracic ganglion) also contribute to the sympathetic innervation to the heart. The superior, middle, and inferior cardiac nerves from these ganglia innervate the heart by following a simple course along the brachiocephalic trunk, common carotid, and subclavian arteries. Alternatively, the thoracic cardiac nerves in the posterior mediastinum follow a complex course to reach the heart in the middle mediastinum. Parasympathetic innervation is supplied by the vagus nerve and is divided into superior, middle, and inferior branches. Although both sides of the autonomic branches run through the ventral and dorsal aspects of the aortic arch, the right autonomic cardiac nerves tend to follow a ventral course.

Many investigators have studied the macroscopic and microscopic anatomy of cardiac autonomic nerves within the atria. Among those that focused on PV autonomic nerves, Armour and colleagues[26] provided a detailed map of autonomic nerve distributions in human hearts. They found that autonomic nerves were concentrated in ganglionic plexi around great vessels, such as the PVs. Chiou and colleagues[27] determined that these nerves converged functionally onto fat pads located around the superior vena cava–aortic junction, and that catheter ablation of this fat pad effectively denervated many regions of the atria but preserved innervation of the ventricle.

On a more microscopic scale, Chevalier and colleagues[28] discovered several gradients of PV autonomic innervation, with nerves more abundant in the proximal PV than distal PV and more abundant in the epicardium than endocardium. The PV–LA junction is rich in autonomic innervation.[24] Stimulation of the ganglionic plexi at this junction can convert PV focal discharges into AF,[29] and radiofrequency ablation at these sites can potentially result in successful denervation and prevent AF inducibility.[30,31]

A recent experimental vagal AF study in canines[31] reported that ablation of the autonomic ganglia at the base of the PVs suppresses the effective refractory period–abbreviating and AF-promoting effects of cervical vagal stimulation, suggesting that ganglionic plexi ablation may contribute to the effectiveness of PV-directed ablation.

VAGAL INFLUENCES ON CARDIAC ELECTROPHYSIOLOGY

It is well-known that vagal nerve stimulation and acetylcholine infusion can result in significant changes of cardiac electrophysiology, including heterogeneous effects on atrial refractory period,[32] pacemaker activity and atrioventricular conduction,[33] and induction of AF.[34] Cervical vagal stimulation shortens the atrial effective refractory period primarily in the high right atrium and facilitates induction of AF through single premature extrastimulus.[35] Coumel and colleagues[36] reported that vagal activity might predispose patients to paroxysmal atrial arrhythmias. In 18 human cases (mostly middle-aged men, 30 ~ 50 years old), the investigators discovered sinus slowing often preceded the onset of atrial arrhythmias. The investigators proposed that vagal activation might induce shortening of the APD, facilitating reentrant atrial arrhythmias.

SYMPATHETIC ACTIVATION AND THE "CALCIUM-TRANSIENT TRIGGERING" HYPOTHESIS

Two recent works have enhanced understanding of the mechanisms through which sympathovagal activation facilitates the onset of paroxysmal AF. Burashnikov and Antzelevitch[37] infused acetylcholine to abbreviate atrial APD and permit rapid pacing in an isolated coronary-perfused canine right atrium, which led to intracellular calcium (Ca_i) accumulation. If this practice is coupled with a long pause (such as that occurred after AF), then a large Ca^{2+} release from the sarcoplasmic reticulum could induce the late phase 3 early afterdepolarizations (EADs) and extrasystoles that initiated AF. This novel late phase 3 EAD mechanism is observed only in association with marked APD abbreviation.

Patterson and colleagues[38] showed that simultaneous infusion of norepinephrine and acetylcholine during rapid pacing facilitated the development of EADs and triggered atrial tachycardias. They also measured tension development and discovered that the persistent diastolic elevation of tension was associated with EADs. Assuming that tension is a good measure of Ca_i, then diastolic Ca_i elevation underlies the mechanisms of EADs. The investigators termed this phenomenon *Ca_i transient triggering* and suggested that increased forward Na^+-Ca^{2+} exchanger current might contribute to the generation of EADs.

The muscle sleeves of thoracic veins are capable of developing automaticity and triggered activity during sympathetic stimulation.[39] Ryanodine at low concentrations (0.5–2 µmol/L) causes a calcium-independent Ca_i release and facilitates the development of pacemaker activity in rabbit PVs.[40] The importance of Ca_i transient in atrial arrhythmogenesis is supported by a study that used isolated Langendorff-perfused canine PV–LA preparations and two cameras to map membrane potential and Ca_i simultaneously.[20] Rapid PV firing was induced by rapid atrial pacing and low-dose ryanodine and isoproterenol infusion, and the rise of Ca_i preceded the action potential upstroke during focal discharge. A clustering of PAS-positive large cells was seen around the PV focal discharge sites.

To determine the interaction between sympathetic nerves and PAS-positive cells, Tan and colleagues[41] performed a study in normal dogs. After sinus node crushing, left stellate ganglion stimulation caused PV tachycardias. The focus of tachycardia was determined by multichannel computerized mapping. PAS staining at the site of PV ectopy showed abundant pale-looking, glycogen-rich specialized conducting (Purkinje) cells. In addition, immunostaining showed abundant sympathetic (tyrosine hydroxylase–positive) nerves at those sites. These results support the notion that sympathetic simulation induced PV focal discharge from sites, with juxtapositioning of specialized conducting cells and autonomic nerves.

STRUCTURAL ANATOMY OF THE ATRIAL AND PULMONARY VEIN AUTONOMIC NERVES

Pappone and colleagues[42] hypothesized that bradycardia induction was caused by vagal nerve stimulation, whereas its abolition with continued radiofrequency application suggests vagal denervation. The distribution of adrenergic and cholinergic nerves in this region were not delineated, however, and therefore whether sympathetic nerves were also eliminated during radiofrequency application is unclear.

Tan and colleagues[24] performed immunostaining of 192 PV–LA segments harvested from 32 veins of eight human autopsied hearts using antityrosine hydroxylase antibodies to label adrenergic nerves and anticholine acetyltransferase antibodies to label cholinergic nerves. Nerve densities were analyzed along the longitudinal and circumferential axes of the PV–LA junction. Longitudinally, adrenergic and cholinergic nerve densities were highest in the LA within 5 mm from the PV–LA junction versus further distally in the PV or more proximally in the LA proper. Circumferentially, both nerve densities were higher in the superior aspect of the left superior PV, anterosuperior aspect of the right superior PV, and inferior aspects of both inferior PVs than diametrically opposite, and higher in the epicardium than endocardium.

Significantly, the investigators noted no area of discrete adrenergic or cholinergic predominance.[24] Instead, both nerve types have similar macroscopic distributions in and around PVs. Additionally, confocal microscopy of dual-stained sections showed that at cellular levels, up to 25% of all nerve fiber bundles contained adrenergic and cholinergic nerves, more than 90% of ganglia contain adrenergic and cholinergic elements within the same ganglion, and up to 30% of ganglion cell bodies may express adrenergic and cholinergic enzymes simultaneously within the neuroplasm. These data indicate that adrenergic and cholinergic nerves are highly colocated not only at tissue but also at cellular levels.

IMPLICATIONS OF NEURAL ANATOMY OF THE PULMONARY VEIN

If sympathetic and parasympathetic nerves are costimulated or ablated, why is bradycardia the dominant response elicited during ganglionic stimulation or ablation rather than tachycardia? Several explanations are proposed. First, complex extracardiac neural pathways[27,43] involved in the generation of bradycardic reflexes during stimulation or ablation around the PVs, project to vagal nuclei centrally but do not involve sympathetic tracts.[43] Second, a paracrine mechanism might be in operation, because ganglion cells predominantly are cholinergic[24] and release mostly acetylcholine when stimulated or ablated. Third, adrenergic nerves are distributed more widely than cholinergic nerves.[24,44] Hence, radiofrequency ablation is more likely to eliminate adrenergic nerves than cholinergic nerves, resulting in a heightened vagal tone and bradycardia. Clinical reports[30,42] show that autonomic reflexes are elicited most commonly within approximately 1 cm of the PV–LA junction. The anatomic colocalization of adrenergic and cholinergic innervations implies that it would be almost impossible to eliminate only sympathetic or parasympathetic nerves during catheter ablation of AF. The coexistence of adrenergic and cholinergic phenotypes within ganglionic cell neuroplasm also suggests that when ganglion cells are stimulated, adrenergic and cholinergic mediators may be released simultaneously, affecting cellular electrophysiology in ways that may predispose to triggered activity.[38]

AUTONOMIC NERVOUS SYSTEM AND ATRIAL FIBRILLATION IN HUMANS

Several observations suggest that the ANS plays an important role in the initiation and maintenance of AF in humans. Most patients who have idiopathic paroxysmal AF seem vagally dependent, with a heightened susceptibility to vasovagal cardiovascular response. In contrast, in most patients who have organic heart diseases, the paroxysmal AF episodes seem more sympathetically dependent.[45] A shift toward an increase in sympathetic tone or a loss of vagal tone has been observed before postoperative paroxysmal AF,[46] the onset of atrial flutter,[47] and paroxysmal AF occurring during sleep,[48] whereas a shift toward vagal predominance had been observed in young patients who

have lone AF and nocturnal episodes of paroxysmal AF.[49] More recently, three studies reported a primary increase in adrenergic drive followed by marked modulation toward vagal predominance immediately before the onset of paroxysmal AF.[5,50,51] The ANS activity in all of these studies was evaluated indirectly, however, through analysis of heart rate variability parameters on continuous ECG recordings. Heart rate variability measures changes in the relative degree of ANS, not the absolute level of sympathetic or parasympathetic discharges. Therefore, sympathetic and vagal nerve activity must be recorded directly to prove or disprove these observations in ambulatory animals.

SYMPATHETIC NERVE RECORDINGS IN ANIMAL MODELS OF PAROXYSMAL ATRIAL FIBRILLATION

Barrett and colleagues[52] first reported successful continuous recording of renal sympathetic nerve activity in conscious rabbits for more than 7 days. The renal sympathetic nerve activity may not predict the cardiac sympathetic nerve activity, however.

To record cardiac sympathetic nerve activity, Jung and colleagues[53] used Data Sciences International transmitters to record stellate ganglion nerve activity, 24 h/d, 7 d/wk, for an average of 41.5 ± 16.6 days in normal ambulatory dogs. The results showed a circadian variation of sympathetic outflow. Normal dogs rarely develop paroxysmal AF, however. To test the hypothesis that spontaneous ANS discharges can serve as triggers of paroxysmal AF, an animal model of paroxysmal AF must be developed.

Wijffels and colleagues[54] showed that intermittent rapid pacing could induce progressively increased electrophysiological remodeling, leading to persistent AF. Rapid atrial pacing also causes significant neural remodeling characterized by heterogeneous increase of sympathetic innervation[55] and extensive nerve sprouting.[56]

Tan and colleagues[57] implanted Data Sciences International transmitters to directly record left stellate ganglion nerve activity, left vagal nerve activity, and LA local bipolar electrograms or surface ECG simultaneously in ambulatory dogs over several weeks. Intermittent rapid atrial pacing was performed and ANS activity was monitored when the pacemaker was turned off. Paroxysmal atrial tachycardia and paroxysmal AF were documented and the investigators found that simultaneous sympathovagal discharges were the most common triggers of paroxysmal atrial tachycardia and paroxysmal AF. Cryoablation of the stellate ganglia and the superior cardiac branches of vagal nerve eliminated all episodes of paroxysmal AF and atrial tachycardias.

These results further support the hypothesis that ANS activity is important in the generation of paroxysmal AF. Histologic examinations of cryoablated dogs showed cardiac nerve sprouting and sympathetic hyperinnervation in the atria. These findings suggest decentralization rather than denervation of the sympathovagal nerves underlies the antiarrhythmic mechanism of stellate ganglion and vagal nerve ablation.

CA$_i$ DYNAMICS AND VAGAL ATRIAL FIBRILLATION IN HEART FAILURE

The Framingham Heart Study[58] concluded that in subjects experiencing heart failure, late development of AF was associated with increased mortality. Heart failure–related atrial arrhythmias seem to arise from macroreentrant sources, primarily by increasing atrial size and promoting interstitial fibrosis.[59] In addition to macroreentry, Stambler and colleagues[60] reported that triggered activity induced by delayed afterdepolarizations may also be a mechanism of focal atrial tachycardias in pacing-induced dogs with heart failure.

Okuyama and colleagues[61] showed that some AF episodes were characterized by focal activations in the PVs and vein of Marshall, and by complex fractionated wavefronts within the PVs in a canine heart failure model, suggesting the occurrence of significant proarrhythmic remodeling in the PVs during heart failure. A major arrhythmogenic mechanism in heart failure results from altered ryanodine receptor function.[62] A combination of abnormal ryanodine receptor and increased sympathetic tone during exercise can cause triggered activity.[63]

Alternatively, direct autonomic nerve recordings in a canine heart failure model showed that not only sympathetic but also vagal nerve discharges were increased in dogs with heart failure, and simultaneous sympathovagal discharges were common triggers of atrial arrhythmias.[64] A computer simulation study[65] suggested that vagal AF may arise from acetylcholine-induced stabilization of the primary spiralwave generator and disorganization of propagation by repolarization gradient that causes fibrillatory dynamics.

Because acetylcholine-dependent potassium channel (I$_{KACh}$) activation shortens APD and hyperpolarizes the cell membrane, Atienza and colleagues[66] reported that adenosine activates I$_{KACh}$ and accelerates AF through promoting reentry rather than triggered activity in human. However, Chou and colleagues[67] reported that acetylcholine facilitates both PV focal discharges and PV–LA microreentry during vagal AF in a canine heart failure model.

Using isolated, Langendorff-perfused canine PV–LA preparations and two cameras to map membrane potential and Ca$_i$ simultaneously, investigators showed that pause-related large Ca$_i$ elevation is associated with focal discharges in the PVs.[37] A long preceding pause increases the Ca$_i$ accumulation, causing a greater release of Ca^{2+} from the sarcoplasmic reticulum at the first beat after the pause. Because the APD was reduced by acetylcholine, this large rise of Ca$_i$ resulted in persistent Ca$_i$ elevation into late phase 3, to induce late phase 3 EADs and PV focal discharges.[37,38,68] These triggered beats, followed by sustained PV–LA microreentry, can induce atrial tachycardia and AF, suggesting that both triggered and reentrant activities are important during vagal AF.

Failing hearts have increased sodium-calcium exchanger channel current (I$_{NCX}$),[69] which renders them more susceptible to the late phase 3 EADs. Acetylcholine may increase Na$^+$ conductance and intracellular Na$^+$ activity, leading to altered I$_{NCX}$, reduced Ca$_i$ efflux[70,71] and further enhanced Ca$_i$ accumulation. The hypothesis is also supported by the suppression of late phase 3 EADs by ryanodine and thapsigargin infusion.

Parasympathetic activation and acetylcholine release could be important mechanisms in the pathophysiology and atrial arrhythmogenesis of heart failure. Livanis and colleagues[72] reported that neurally mediated mechanisms may be implicated in the pathophysiology of syncope in patients who have dilated cardiomyopathy. In that study, sympathetic and parasympathetic heart rate parameters were markedly stimulated.

NEURAL MODULATION AS A POTENTIAL THERAPEUTIC STRATEGY

The effectiveness of autonomic modulation as an adjunctive therapeutic strategy to catheter ablation of AF has been inconsistent. Although favorable results have been reported by Nakagawa and colleagues[30] and Pappone and colleagues,[42] others found no beneficial[73] or deleterious[74] outcomes in patients who had denervation compared with those who did not, a finding also underlined by animal studies by Hirose and colleagues,[35] in which partial vagal denervation of the high right atrium was found to increase inducibility of AF. These conflicting studies suggest that the interactions between the ANS and AF are more complex than currently understood. Perhaps a degree of individual variability accounts for these discrepancies, with some patients having more pronounced autonomic triggers than others. As an illustration, Scanavacca and colleagues[75] recently found that in a small number of patients who had "autonomic" paroxysmal AF, denervation alone without substrate modification in the atria effectively prevented AF recurrence in 2 of 11 patients, with these patients having the most pronounced and persistent changes in heart rate variability. In summary, current evidence suggests that autonomic modulation has an adjunctive role to play in catheter AF ablation, especially when applied selectively. Further mechanistic and clinical studies are warranted before a wider application can be recommended.

REFERENCES

1. Allessie MA, Boyden PA, Camm AJ, et al. Pathophysiology and prevention of atrial fibrillation. Circulation 2001;103(5):769–77.
2. Chen YJ, Chen SA, Chang MS, et al. Arrhythmogenic activity of cardiac muscle in pulmonary veins of the dog: implication for the genesis of atrial fibrillation. Cardiovasc Res 2000;48(2):265–73.
3. Doshi RN, Wu T-J, Yashima M, et al. Relation between ligament of Marshall and adrenergic atrial tachyarrhythmia. Circulation 1999;100:876–83.
4. Sharifov OF, Fedorov VV, Beloshapko GG, et al. Roles of adrenergic and cholinergic stimulation in spontaneous atrial fibrillation in dogs. J Am Coll Cardiol 2004;43(3):483–90.
5. Bettoni M, Zimmermann M. Autonomic tone variations before the onset of paroxysmal atrial fibrillation. Circulation 2002;105(23):2753–9.
6. Gould PA, Yii M, McLean C, et al. Evidence for increased atrial sympathetic innervation in persistent human atrial fibrillation. Pacing Clin Electrophysiol 2006;29(8):821–9.
7. Moe GK, Abildskov JA. Atrial fibrillation as a self-sustaining arrhythmia independent of focal discharge. Am Heart J 1959;58(1):59–70.
8. Zipes DP, Knope RF. Electrical properties of the thoracic veins. Am J Cardiol 1972;29:372–6.
9. Spach MS, Barr RC, Jewett PH. Spread of excitation from the atrium into thoracic veins in human beings and dogs. Am J Cardiol 1972;30:844–54.
10. Scherlag BJ, Yeh BK, Robinson MJ. Inferior interatrial pathway in the dog. Circ Res 1972;31:18–35.
11. Haissaguerre M, Jais P, Shah DC, et al. Spontaneous initiation of atrial fibrillation by ectopic beats originating in the pulmonary veins. N Engl J Med 1998;339:659–66.
12. Hamabe A, Okuyama Y, Miyauchi Y, et al. Correlation between anatomy and electrical activation in canine pulmonary veins. Circulation 2003;107:1550–5.
13. Zhou S, Chang C-M, Wu T-J, et al. Nonreentrant focal activations in pulmonary veins in canine model

14. Chou CC, Zhou S, Miyauchi Y, et al. Effects of procainamide on electrical activity in thoracic veins and atria in canine model of sustained atrial fibrillation. Am J Physiol Heart Circ Physiol 2004;286(5): H1936–45.
15. Chou CC, Zhou S, Tan AY, et al. High density mapping of pulmonary veins and left atrium during ibutilide administration in a canine model of sustained atrial fibrillation. Am J Physiol Heart Circ Physiol 2005;289:H2704–13.
16. Gong Y, Xie F, Stein KM, et al. Mechanism underlying initiation of paroxysmal atrial flutter/atrial fibrillation by ectopic foci: a simulation study. Circulation 2007;115(16):2094–102.
17. Masani F. Node-like cells in the myocardial layer of the pulmonary vein of rats: an ultrastructural study. J Anat 1986;145:133–42.
18. Cheung DW. Electrical activity of the pulmonary vein and its interaction with the right atrium in the guinea-pig. J Physiol 1981;314:445–56.
19. Perez-Lugones A, McMahon JT, Ratliff NB, et al. Evidence of specialized conduction cells in human pulmonary veins of patients with atrial fibrillation. J Cardiovasc Electrophysiol 2003;14(8):803–9.
20. Chou C-C, Nihei M, Zhou S, et al. Intracellular calcium dynamics and anisotropic reentry in isolated canine pulmonary veins and left atrium. Circulation 2005;111:2889–97.
21. Crick SJ, Sheppard MN, Anderson RH, et al. A quantitative study of nerve distribution in the conduction system of the guinea pig heart. J Anat 1996;188:403–16.
22. Crick SJ, Wharton J, Sheppard MN, et al. Innervation of the human cardiac conduction system. A quantitative immunohistochemical and histochemical study. Circulation 1994;89(4):1697–708.
23. Miyauchi Y, Zhou S, Okuyama Y, et al. Altered atrial electrical restitution and heterogeneous sympathetic hyperinnervation in hearts with chronic left ventricular myocardial infarction: implications for atrial fibrillation. Circulation 2003;108(3):360–6.
24. Tan AY, Li H, Wachsmann-Hogiu S, et al. Autonomic innervation and segmental muscular disconnections at the human pulmonary vein-atrial junction: implications for catheter ablation of atrial-pulmonary vein junction. J Am Coll Cardiol 2006;48:132–43.
25. Kawashima T. The autonomic nervous system of the human heart with special reference to its origin, course, and peripheral distribution. Anat Embryol (Berl) 2005;209(6):425–38.
26. Armour JA, Murphy DA, Yuan BX, et al. Gross and microscopic anatomy of the human intrinsic cardiac nervous system. Anat Rec 1997;247(2):289–98.
27. Chiou C-W, Eble JN, Zipes DP. Efferent vagal innervation of the canine atria and sinus and

atrioventricular nodes—the third fat pad. Circulation 1997;95:2573–84.

28. Chevalier P, Tabib A, Meyronnet D, et al. Quantitative study of nerves of the human left atrium. Heart Rhythm 2005;2(5):518–22.

29. Scherlag BJ, Yamanashi W, Patel U, et al. Autonomically induced conversion of pulmonary vein focal firing into atrial fibrillation. J Am Coll Cardiol 2005; 45(11):1878–86.

30. Nakagawa H, Scherlag BJ, Wu R, et al. Addition of selective ablation of autonomic ganglia to pulmonary vein antrum isolation for treatment of paroxysmal and persistent atrial fibrillation. Circulation 2006;110(III–459) [abstract].

31. Lemola K, Chartier D, Yeh YH, et al. Pulmonary vein region ablation in experimental vagal atrial fibrillation: role of pulmonary veins versus autonomic ganglia. Circulation 2008;117(4):470–7.

32. Zipes DP, Mihalick MJ, Robbins GT. Effects of selective vagal and stellate ganglion stimulation of atrial refractoriness. Cardiovasc Res 1974;8:647–55.

33. Spear JF, Moore EN. Influence of brief vagal and stellate nerve stimulation on pacemaker activity and conduction within the atrioventricular conduction system of the dog. Circ Res 1973;32:27–41.

34. Goldberger AL, Pavelec RS. Vagally-mediated atrial fibrillation in dogs: conversion with bretylium tosylate. Int J Cardiol 1986;13:47–55.

35. Hirose M, Leatmanoratn Z, Laurita KR, et al. Partial vagal denervation increases vulnerability to vagally induced atrial fibrillation. J Cardiovasc Electrophysiol 2002;13(12):1272–9.

36. Coumel P, Attuel P, Lavallee J, et al. The atrial arrhythmia syndrome of vagal origin. Arch Mal Coeur Vaiss 1978;71(6):645–56.

37. Burashnikov A, Antzelevitch C. Reinduction of atrial fibrillation immediately after termination of the arrhythmia is mediated by late phase 3 early afterdepolarization-induced triggered activity. Circulation 2003;107(18):2355–60.

38. Patterson E, Lazzara R, Szabo B, et al. Sodium-calcium exchange initiated by the Ca2+ transient: an arrhythmia trigger within pulmonary veins. J Am Coll Cardiol 2006;47(6):1196–206.

39. Wit AL, Cranefield PF. Triggered and automatic activity in the canine coronary sinus. Circ Res 1977; 41:434–45.

40. Honjo H, Boyett MR, Niwa R, et al. Pacing-induced spontaneous activity in myocardial sleeves of pulmonary veins after treatment with ryanodine. Circulation 2003;107(14):1937–43.

41. Tan AY, Zhou S, Jung B-C, et al. Ectopic atrial arrhythmias arising from canine thoracic veins during in-vivo stellate ganglion stimulation. Am J Physiol Heart Circ Physiol 2008;295:H691–8.

42. Pappone C, Santinelli V, Manguso F, et al. Pulmonary vein denervation enhances long-term benefit after circumferential ablation for paroxysmal atrial fibrillation. Circulation 2004;109(3):327–34.

43. Aviado DM, Guevara AD. The Bezold-Jarisch reflex. A historical perspective of cardiopulmonary reflexes. Ann N Y Acad Sci 2001;940:48–58.

44. Marron K, Wharton J, Sheppard MN, et al. Distribution, morphology, and neurochemistry of endocardial and epicardial nerve terminal arborizations in the human heart. Circulation 1995;92(8):2343–51.

45. Huang JL, Wen ZC, Lee WL, et al. Changes of autonomic tone before the onset of paroxysmal atrial fibrillation. Int J Cardiol 1998;66:275–83.

46. Dimmer C, Tavernier R, Gjorgov N, et al. Variations of autonomic tone preceding onset of atrial fibrillation after coronary artery bypass grafting. Am J Cardiol 1998;82(1):22–5.

47. Wen ZC, Chen SA, Tai CT, et al. Role of autonomic tone in facilitating spontaneous onset of typical atrial flutter. J Am Coll Cardiol 1998;31(3):602–7.

48. Coccagna G, Capucci A, Bauleo S, et al. Paroxysmal atrial fibrillation in sleep. Sleep 1997;20(6): 396–8.

49. Herweg B, Dalal P, Nagy B, et al. Power spectral analysis of heart period variability of preceding sinus rhythm before initiation of paroxysmal atrial fibrillation. Am J Cardiol 1998;82(7):869–74.

50. Zimmermann M, Kalusche D. Fluctuation in autonomic tone is a major determinant of sustained atrial arrhythmias in patients with focal ectopy originating from the pulmonary veins. J Cardiovasc Electrophysiol 2001;12(3):285–91.

51. Amar D, Zhang H, Miodownik S, et al. Competing autonomic mechanisms precede the onset of postoperative atrial fibrillation. J Am Coll Cardiol 2003; 42(7):1262–8.

52. Barrett CJ, Ramchandra R, Guild SJ, et al. What sets the long-term level of renal sympathetic nerve activity: a role for angiotensin II and baroreflexes? Circ Res 2003;92(12):1330–6.

53. Jung B-C, Dave AS, Tan AY, et al. Circadian variations of stellate ganglion nerve activity in ambulatory dogs. Heart Rhythm 2005;3:78–85.

54. Wijffels MC, Kirchhof CJ, Dorland R, et al. Atrial fibrillation begets atrial fibrillation. A study in awake chronically instrumented goats. Circulation 1995; 92:1954–68.

55. Jayachandran JV, Sih HJ, Winkle W, et al. Atrial fibrillation produced by prolonged rapid atrial pacing is associated with heterogeneous changes in atrial sympathetic innervation. Circulation 2000;101: 1185–91.

56. Chang C-M, Wu T-J, Zhou S-M, et al. Nerve sprouting and sympathetic hyperinnervation in a canine model of atrial fibrillation produced by prolonged right atrial pacing. Circulation 2001;103:22–5.

57. Tan AY, Zhou S, Ogawa B-M, et al. Neural mechanisms of paroxysmal atrial fibrillation and

paroxysmal atrial tachycardia in ambulatory canines. Circulation 2008;118:916–25.

58. Wang TJ, Larson MG, Levy D, et al. Temporal relations of atrial fibrillation and congestive heart failure and their joint influence on mortality: the Framingham Heart Study. Circulation 2003;107(23):2920–5.

59. Li D, Fareh S, Leung TK, et al. Promotion of atrial fibrillation by heart failure in dogs: atrial remodeling of a different sort. Circulation 1999;100:87–95.

60. Stambler BS, Fenelon G, Shepard RK, et al. Characterization of sustained atrial tachycardia in dogs with rapid ventricular pacing-induced heart failure. J Cardiovasc Electrophysiol 2003;14(5):499–507.

61. Okuyama Y, Miyauchi Y, Park AM, et al. High resolution mapping of the pulmonary vein and the vein of Marshall during induced atrial fibrillation and atrial tachycardia in a canine model of pacing-induced congestive heart failure. J Am Coll Cardiol 2003;42:348–60.

62. Marx SO, Reiken S, Hisamatsu Y, et al. PKA phosphorylation dissociates FKBP12.6 from the calcium release channel (ryanodine receptor): defective regulation in failing hearts. Cell 2000;101(4):365–76.

63. Wehrens XH, Lehnart SE, Reiken SR, et al. Protection from cardiac arrhythmia through ryanodine receptor-stabilizing protein calstabin2. Science 2004; 304(5668):292–6.

64. Ogawa M, Zhou S, Tan AY, et al. Left stellate ganglion and vagal nerve activity and cardiac arrhythmias in ambulatory dogs with pacing-induced congestive heart failure. J Am Coll Cardiol 2007;50:335–43.

65. Kneller J, Zou R, Vigmond EJ, et al. Cholinergic atrial fibrillation in a computer model of a two-dimensional sheet of canine atrial cells with realistic ionic properties. Circ Res 2002;90(9):E73–87.

66. Atienza F, Almendral J, Moreno J, et al. Activation of inward rectifier potassium channels accelerates atrial fibrillation in humans: evidence for a reentrant mechanism. Circulation 2006;114(23):2434–42.

67. Chou C-C, Nguyen BL, Tan AY, et al. Intracellular calcium dynamics and acetylcholine-induced triggered activity in the pulmonary veins of dogs with pacing-induced heart failure. Heart Rhythm 2008; 5(8):1170–7.

68. Patterson E, Po SS, Scherlag BJ, et al. Triggered firing in pulmonary veins initiated by in vitro autonomic nerve stimulation. Heart Rhythm 2005;2(6):624–31.

69. Li D, Melnyk P, Feng J, et al. Effects of experimental heart failure on atrial cellular and ionic electrophysiology. Circulation 2000;101(22):2631–8.

70. Tajima T, Tsuji Y, Sorota S, et al. Positive vs. negative inotropic effects of carbachol in avian atrial muscle: role of Ni-like protein. Circ Res 1987;61(4 Pt 2):I105–111.

71. Matsumoto K, Pappano AJ. Sodium-dependent membrane current induced by carbachol in single guinea-pig ventricular myocytes. J Physiol 1989; 415:487–502.

72. Livanis EG, Kostopoulou A, Theodorakis GN, et al. Neurocardiogenic mechanisms of unexplained syncope in idiopathic dilated cardiomyopathy. Am J Cardiol 2007;99(4):558–62.

73. Lemery R, Birnie D, Tang AS, et al. Feasibility study of endocardial mapping of ganglionated plexuses during catheter ablation of atrial fibrillation. Heart Rhythm 2006;3(4):387–96.

74. Cummings JE, Gill I, Akhrass R, et al. Preservation of the anterior fat pad paradoxically decreases the incidence of postoperative atrial fibrillation in humans. J Am Coll Cardiol 2004;43(6):994–1000.

75. Scanavacca M, Pisani CF, Hachul D, et al. Selective atrial vagal denervation guided by evoked vagal reflex to treat patients with paroxysmal atrial fibrillation. Circulation 2006;114(9):876–85.

Information Learned from Animal Models of Atrial Fibrillation

J. Emanuel Finet, MD, David S. Rosenbaum, MD,
J. Kevin Donahue, MD*

KEYWORDS

- Cardiac arrhythmia • Atrial fibrillation
- Animal model • Remodeling

Atrial fibrillation (AF) continues to be the most common arrhythmia encountered clinically and is responsible for significant morbidity and health care cost. Therapy for AF has advanced significantly in recent years, mainly because of a better understanding of arrhythmia mechanisms. Several experimental animal models have been designed to study the underlying triggers and substrates that promote and maintain AF (**Table 1**). The present work summarizes notable findings from these various models.

PATHOPHYSIOLOGY OF ATRIAL FIBRILLATION

Chronic AF can be classified into three subtypes: paroxysmal, persistent, and permanent. Paroxysmal AF refers to episodes that start and stop spontaneously, persistent AF is one that requires cardioversion for its termination, and permanent AF denotes one that resists cardioversion or reverts quickly in spite of cardioversion. AF requires a trigger for its initiation and a suitable electrophysiologic or structural substrate for its maintenance. Triggers include atrial premature beats, vagal stimulation, bradycardia, acute atrial stretch, and ischemia, among others.[1–3] Recently, AF initiation from premature beats originating in the pulmonary veins (PVs) has received attention because ablation techniques have been able to cure this AF.[4] The mechanism underlying the PV ectopy is still debated. Enhanced automaticity,

triggered activity, and microreentry have all been proposed as potential mechanisms for these beats.

After triggers propagate into atrial myocardium, fibrillation is maintained by continuation of these trigger beats with breakdown of conduction (so-called "fibrillatory conduction") or by intra-atrial reentrant processes. Fibrillatory conduction occurs when a stimulus site is activating at a rate that cannot be sustained through the mass of tissue; thus, conduction breaks down distal to the initiating site (**Fig. 1**A). Therefore, even though the arrhythmia comes from an organized focal site, the macroscopic appearance is of fractionated inhomogeneous conduction.

Currently, the dominant mechanistic theory for reentry sustaining fibrillation is the spiral wave model. Unlike the traditional concept of reentry that requires two pathways with differing conduction and refractory properties and anatomic separation between the two pathways, spiral wave reentry depends on functional properties of the tissue. Excitation occurs in a vortex spinning around an excitable but unexcited core. Conduction velocity (CV) is determined by the curvature of the spiral; thus, CV is fastest at the periphery of the wave, where curvature is widest. CV slows as the curvature increases closer to the core, and conduction is nonexistent at the core of the spiral, where curvature is essentially infinite (see **Fig. 1**B). This is in contrast to the so-called "leading circle"

Funding for this work was provided by National Institutes of Health (NIH) grants HL67148 and HL93286 (JKD) and NIH grant HL54807 (DSR).
The Heart and Vascular Research Center, Case Western Reserve University, MetroHealth Campus, 2500 MetroHealth Drive, Cleveland, OH 44109–1998, USA
* Corresponding author.
E-mail address: kdonahue@metrohealth.org (J.K. Donahue).

Cardiol Clin 27 (2009) 45–54
doi:10.1016/j.ccl.2008.09.005
0733-8651/08/$ – see front matter © 2009 Elsevier Inc. All rights reserved.

Table 1
Clinical paradigms in animal models of atrial fibrillation

Model	Autonomic Stimulation	Atrial Tachycardia		Heart Failure	Atrial Tachycardia and Heart Failure		Sterile Pericarditis	Aging
Species	Dogs	Goats	Dogs	Dogs	Dogs	Pigs	Dogs	Dogs
AF	Sustained	Sustained	↑ Inducibility	↑ Inducibility	↑ Inducibility	Sustained	↑ Inducibility	↑ Inducibility
Electrophysiologic remodeling								
Functional	↓ AP, ERP ↑ ERP dispersion	↓ ERP Ø ERP rate adapt ± ↔ CV	↓ ERP Ø ERP rate adapt ± ↔ CV	↑ APD, ERP ↔ CV	± ↓ ERP ↓ CV	NYR	ERP CV	↓ AP, ERP ↑ ERP, dispersion ↓ CV of APDs
Ion current densities	↑ IK, ACh (cholinergic) ↑ IKs, ICa(L) (adrenergic)	NYR	↓ Ito, ICa(L), INa Ø IKs, IKr, NCX ↑ IK1, IKACh	↓ Ito, ICa(L), IKs Ø ICa(T), IKr, IKur, IK1 ↑ NCX	↓ ICa(L), ± ↓ Ito, IKs Ø NCX ↑ IK1	NYR	NYR	NYR
mRNA expression	NYR	NYR	↓ KCND3, CACNA1C, SCN5A ↔ KCNO1; KCNH2; KCNJ2, 3, 5; SLCSA1	NYR	NYR	NYR	NYR	NYR
Protein expression	NYR	NYR	↓ Kv4.3, Nav1.5 ↔ Kir3.1, Kir3.4, NCX	NYR	NYR	NYR	NYR	NYR

Structural remodeling

	Normal							
Anatomic	NYR	↑ Atrial size + Hypertrophy, myolysis, glycogen accumulation Fibrosis or apoptosis	↑ Atrial size Ø Fibrosis or hypertrophy	↑ A and V size + Fibrosis, hypertrophy	↑ A and V size	↑ A and V size + Fibrosis or apoptosis, inflammation, hypertrophy, myolysis	Epicardial: Apoptosis, inflammation, necrosis	+ Fibrosis
mRNA expression	NYR	NYR	↔ ECM	↑ Collagen, fibrillin-1, MMP2, TGFβ1, α-SM actin	NYR	↑ Fibronectin-1, fibrillin-1, fibromodulin, MLC-2v, collagen	NYR	NYR
Protein expression	NYR	↑ α-SM actin ↓ Cx40, titin cardiotin, desmin	↔ ECM	↑ Collagen, fibrillin-1, MMP2	NYR	↑ Fibronectin-1, fibrillin-1, MLC-2v fibromodulin, collagen	Epicardial: ↑ Vimentin ↑ α-actinin, ↓ Cx40, Cx43	NYR

Abbreviations: A, atrium; ACh, acetylcholine; AP, action potentia; APD, action potential duration; CV, conduction velocity; Cx, connexin; ECM, extracellular matrix; ERP, effective refractory period; ICa(T)T-type calcium current; IK, delayed rectifier current; MLC-2v, ventricular isoform of myosin regulatory light chain 2; MMP2, matrix metalloproteinase 2; NCX, sodium-calcium exchanger; NYR, not yet reported; SM, smooth muscle; TGFβ1, transforming growth factor-β1; V, ventricle; ±, inconsistent between reports; ↑, increased; ↓, decreased; ↔, unchanged; Ø, presence or gain of.

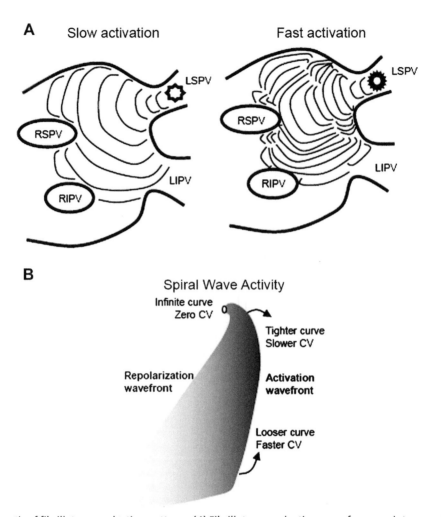

Fig. 1. Schematic of fibrillatory conduction patterns. (*A*) Fibrillatory conduction away from a point source in the left superior pulmonary vein. The schematic depicts normal uniform conduction at slower activation rates, and conduction breakdown as heterogeneities within tissue and curvature around obstacles affects CV at extremely fast activation rates. The breakdown of uniform conduction gives a surface electrocardiographic appearance of disorganization and fibrillation. LIPV, left inferior pulmonary vein; LSPV, left superior pulmonary vein; RIPV, right inferior pulmonary vein; RSPV, right superior pulmonary vein. (*B*) Spiral wave conduction. The angle of curvature is a determinant of CV, in which slow conduction occurs at the tighter portion of the curve and more rapid conduction occurs at the looser portion of the curve. At the core of the spiral, curvature is infinite; thus, conduction is zero.

theory of reentry, in which the central zone of block is unexcitable during reentry,[5] accounting for the ability of spiral waves to meander throughout the atria or remain spatially fixed. Fibrillation can occur with a single spiral (the so-called "mother rotor") if activation is fast enough to cause fibrillatory conduction to occur away from the spiral. More commonly, fibrillation occurs in the presence of multiple spirals that tend to be transient in space and time. Fibrillation is sustained as each spiral progressively spawns other spirals that meander through the tissue.

An important element in sustaining AF is the electrical and structural remodeling caused by AF that promotes AF maintenance and recurrence (AF begets AF).[6,7] This parallels the clinical perception that with time, it becomes more and more difficult to keep patients with AF in sinus rhythm, as expressed by the phrase "domestication of atrial fibrillation," attributed to Mauricio Rosenbaum.[7] Electrophysiologic remodeling includes alteration of ionic current densities, heterogeneous shortening of the effective refractory period (ERP), and decrease of the CV, among others, whereas structural remodeling denotes atrial dilation, interstitial fibrosis, atrial myocyte ultrastructural changes, and altered expression of structural and gap junctional proteins.[8–14] These findings have not been observed in all animal models. Each one is characterized by a unique set of adaptive changes.

Animal Models of Atrial Fibrillation

Autonomic stimulation

Some of the earliest models of AF manipulated autonomic tone in the cardiac atria of dogs. The simplest model involved applying a drop of carbachol to the atrial appendage, which caused sustained AF lasting for the duration of the carbachol exposure.[15] Clamping the appendage separated the fibrillatory source from the substrate, causing cardioversion of the main atrial body but allowing the affected appendage to continue fibrillating. This maneuver supported the idea that fibrillation comes from a rapidly firing point source with fibrillatory conduction away from the stimulus. Atrial muscarinic receptor activation has also been achieved by continuous bilateral electrical stimulation of the cervical vagosympathetic trunks, acetylcholine infusion, or sympathetic denervation, among others.[16–18] The principal electrophysiologic manifestations of parasympathetic stimulation are dramatic shortening of the atrial action potential duration (APD) and ERP caused by activation of the acetylcholine-activated potassium current (IKACh) channel. Point source activation with carbachol causes localized changes, and central stimulation of the vagus causes global, albeit heterogeneous, changes. The novel antiarrhythmic agent NIP-151 potently blocks IKACh with an atrial-specific ERP-prolonging profile, displaying a low proarrhythmic risk, and may be useful for the treatment of AF.[19]

Adrenergic stimulation with isoproterenol or adrenaline also causes AF.[17] Similar to parasympathetic stimulation, the dominant electrophysiologic alteration is shortening of the APD and ERP. The effect of adrenergic stimulation on the ERP is much more spatially homogeneous, and AF induction is much less common when compared with the prominent and reliable effects of parasympathetic stimulation.[20] Increased slow compound of the delayed rectifier potassium current (IKs) channel activity is the likely source for APD alterations with adrenergic stimulation.

Atrial Burst Pacing

Goats

The first reported method for achieving sustained AF in an animal model was developed in the laboratory of Maurits Allessie.[7] He and his colleagues implanted atrial pacing leads in goats and connected the leads to a computer that initiated AF by burst pacing the atria at a frequency of 64 Hz. In later iterations of the model, the computer was replaced by an implanted pacemaker. The computer or pacemaker monitored atrial rate between bursts, and return of sinus rhythm (defined as slowing of atrial rate lower than a programmed set point) initiated further burst pacing. With this treatment, the episodes of nonsustained AF progressively lengthened over time until sustained AF was achieved several weeks after onset of the burst pacing. The concept that "AF begets AF" was first experimentally substantiated in this model. Within 24 hours of burst pacing, the atrial ERP had decreased by 35% without significant change in CV, thus favoring continued fibrillation by shortening the wavelength necessary to sustain reentry. Other electrical changes included a reversion of the physiologic rate adaptation in the ERP and an increase in the rate, inducibility, and stability of AF. Electrical remodeling in this model reversed within 1 week after restoration of sinus rhythm.[21]

Gap junctional remodeling was also observed in the goat AF model.[14] Over a 16-week time course after initiation of burst atrial pacing, connexin 40 (Cx40) expression levels decreased in a heterogeneous fashion (present in some areas of tissue and virtually absent in other areas of the same atrium). Even when Cx40 expression was unaltered, lateralization of connexin expression away from intercalated disks was observed. Expression level and distribution of Cx43 were unaffected. This reduction of Cx40 was found to be completely reversed 4 weeks after return to sinus rhythm.

In addition to the electrical remodeling, structural remodeling was present in the goat. Ausma and colleagues[22] demonstrated that after 9 to 23 weeks, sustained AF led to structural changes in the atrial myocytes similar to those seen in ventricular myocytes from chronic hibernating myocardium. They described myocyte hypertrophy, loss of myofibrils, accumulation of glycogen, changes in mitochondrial shape and size, fragmentation of sarcoplasmic reticulum, and dispersion of nuclear chromatin. No signs of cellular degeneration or changes in the interstitial space were found. The time course of structural remodeling was somewhat variable.[13] Progressive morphologic changes in mitochondria and sarcoplasmic reticulum and homogeneous chromatin distribution peaked 1 week after AF induction, and myolysis and glycogen accumulation were maximal after 8 weeks of AF. Myocyte dedifferentiation has been implicated as an important element in the structural remodeling process. This concept is supported by observation of altered expression patterns of myocyte structural proteins, reexpression of fetal proteins like α-smooth muscle actin, and down-regulation of cardiotin (the A-I junctional part of titin and desmin) at progressive time points that correlate with the ultrastructural observations of structural remodeling. Unlike other animal models (and perhaps the human condition), there is no significant atrial fibrosis in the burst pacing goat model.[13]

The electrical, structural, and gap junctional remodeling in the goat model affect the response to antiarrhythmic drugs.[6] Duytschaever and colleagues[23] compared class I and class III drugs in the AF-induced electrophysiologically remodeled atria of the goat, finding that the effects of flecainide on atrial conduction were not altered after 48 hours of sustained AF, whereas the effects of the rapid component of the delayed rectifier potassium current (IKr) blockers d-sotalol and ibutilide on ERP were lost over the same time course. These data suggest that the kinetics of sodium current (INa) (or at least the interaction with flecainide) are probably not significantly affected by electrical remodeling, although this remains to be determined. In a later work, Blaauw and colleagues[24] demonstrated that AVE0118 administration (blockade of the ultra rapid component of delayed rectifier potassium current [IKur], the transient outward current [ITo], and IKACh) restored the ERP prolonging effects of dofetilide and ibutilide. These data suggest a possible synergy in function of potassium channels that could be exploited therapeutically.

Dogs

Rapid atrial pacing at a rate of 400 or 600 beats per minute (bpm) in dogs increases AF inducibility.[8,9,25] An important element of this model is that it is not a sustained AF model. The pacing emulates sustained atrial tachycardia (AT), although several investigators have shown that episodes of acutely induced AF are progressively longer as a function of time since the start of rapid atrial pacing. Ventricular rate is generally controlled in the model by AV node ablation and ventricular pacemaker implantation.

Like the goat-sustained AF model, electrophysiologic remodeling is prominent in the dog AT model. Gaspo and colleagues[26] demonstrated that rapid atrial pacing decreased CV and the ERP. The ERP changes were maximal within 7 days of pacing onset, but the CV changes did not peak until 42 days after the start of atrial tachypacing. Fareh and colleagues[9] found an increase in the heterogeneity of ERP across the atria in the same model.

In a later work, Yue and colleagues[8] provided a potential molecular basis for these functional effects. They described changes in atrial gene expression at the RNA level that correlated with altered levels of ionic currents. Rapid atrial pacing decreased expression of KV4.3 (a subunit of Ito1), CaV1.2 [a subunit of ICa(L)], and NaV1.5 (a subunit of INa). They observed no changes in KV7.1 (a subunit of IKs), KV11.1 (a subunit of IKr), Kir2.1 (the inward rectifier current [IK1]), or NCX (the sodium-calcium exchanger). Voigt and colleagues[27] recently showed that AT also increases agonist-independent constitutive IKACh single-channel activity by enhancing spontaneous channel opening.

Shiroshita-Takeshita and colleagues[28] evaluated the role of anti-inflammatory drugs in the dog AT model, showing that prednisone, but not ibuprofen or cyclosporine-A, significantly reduced electrophysiologic remodeling. Prednisone was also associated with a decrease of C-reactive protein (CRP) and endothelial nitric oxide synthase levels, suggesting an anti-inflammatory mechanism of action. Evidence also suggests that heat shock proteins (HSPs) may have some protecting role against AF in the dog model. Brundel and colleagues[29] evaluated the effect of HSP induction in this model, demonstrating that HSP induction protects against AT-induced remodeling and that the orally administered HSP inducer geranylgeranylacetone suppressed AF promotion in remodeled atria.

Investigation of structural remodeling has been limited in the dog atrial tachypacing model. The only investigation specifically looking at atrial histology showed no significant increase in fibrosis after 1 week of atrial tachypacing.[11]

Heart Failure

Dogs

Although electrical remodeling seems to be the main determinant for AF promotion in the AT dog model, structural remodeling seems to play the major role in heart failure (HF) models of AF inducibility.[10] HF is generally induced in dogs by right ventricular pacing at 240 bpm for 2 to 3 weeks, followed by pacing at 220 bpm for 3 weeks, generating a tachycardiomyopathy.[30] Reports of cellular electrophysiologic remodeling caused by HF have been inconsistent. Li and colleagues[11] reported no change in average atrial CV or ERP, although they did see heterogeneity in atrial conduction with discrete areas of slow conduction. Cha and colleagues[31] described a 50% increase in the ERP with ventricular tachypacing, and these researchers did not report CV. These functional changes correlated with ionic current changes, including reduced ICa(L), Ito, and IKs, and increased NCX and IK1. These alterations of ionic current densities completely reverse after 4 weeks of recovery.[31]

Structural remodeling, conversely, is currently believed to be the main determinant of induction and maintenance of AF in this model.[10,11,31]

Experimental HF causes hypertrophy of atrial myocytes and extensive interstitial fibrosis. Molecular analyses of atrial tissues reveal upregulation of several extracellular matrix mRNAs after 2 weeks of ventricular tachypacing, including eight collagen genes, fibrillin-1, and matrix metalloproteinase 2 (MMP2).[32] Five weeks after ventricular tachypacing is discontinued, echocardiographic measures of atrial and ventricular structure and function normalize and the duration of induced episodes of AF is decreased. In spite of reversing the HF phenotype, atrial interstitial fibrosis, conduction abnormalities, and AF inducibility are not reversible, at least in the short term.[33]

The effects of combined atrial and ventricular burst pacing in dogs seem to be the average of individual atrial or ventricular burst pacing effects on electrical and structural remodeling. A comparison of dogs exposed to the combined effects of 1 week of atrial tachypacing and 2 weeks of ventricular tachypacing showed increased AF inducibility and increased duration of nonsustained AF episodes after induction.[34] The atrial ERP did not change in this group (in contrast to a 50% increase in the ERP with ventricular tachypacing alone or a 30% decrease in the ERP with atrial tachypacing alone). Ionic current changes in the combined atrial and ventricular tachypacing group also seemed to be the average of effects seen with atrial or ventricular tachypacing alone: Ito decreased 50% with all three models; IKs decreased to same level with ventricular tachypacing and combined tachypacing but did not change with atrial tachypacing; IK1 increased 70% with atrial tachypacing and 37% with combined tachypacing but did not change with ventricular tachypacing; and ICa(L) decreased 31% with ventricular tachypacing, 50% with combined tachypacing, and 60% with atrial tachypacing. The structural effects in the dog model of combined tachypacing have not yet been reported.

Pigs

We reported phenotyping data in the pig model of burst atrial pacing using the Allessie protocol of 64-Hz atrial bursting until sustained AF develops.[7] Unlike the goat model, in which the ventricular rate is not overly fast, the ventricular response rate averages 270 bpm in the pig model. This sustained high rate gives a combined atrial tachyarrhythmia and ventricular HF model. In this model, we found atrial structural remodeling that seemed to be the combined effects reported in the goat AF and dog HF models: the pigs had four-chamber cardiac dilation and dysfunction, cellular hypertrophy, myolysis, inflammation, and fibrosis.[35]

In a similar model, in which the right atrial appendages of pigs were pacing at 600 bpm for 3 to 6 weeks, Lin and colleagues[36] described an increase in the atrial extracellular matrix, correlating with fibronectin-1, fibrillin-1, and fibromodulin gene upregulation. Lai and colleagues[37] demonstrated increases in the ventricular isoform of myosin regulatory light chain 2 (MLC-2v) in atrial tissue in the same pig atrial tachypacing model. The electrophysiologic alterations of the pig model have not yet been evaluated.

Sterile Pericarditis

The dog model of sterile pericarditis was developed in the lab of Al Waldo. These researchers created pericarditis by irritating the pericardium with talcum after sterile mediastinotomy and pericardiotomy. The predominant arrhythmia in the model is atrial flutter, but AF is also induced.[38] Kumagai and colleagues[39] showed that unstable and migratory reentrant circuits of extremely short cycle length, principally involving the atrial septum, seem to be responsible for arrhythmia maintenance. Bachmann's bundle seemed critical to maintenance of the arrhythmia because its ablation terminated or prevented inducibility.[40] Heterogeneous reductions in CV have also been described in the model. The conduction changes correlated with a measurable transmural gradient in Cx40 and Cx43 expression.[41] Connexins were absent in the epicardium, decreased in the midmyocardium, and completely normal in the endocardium, likely attributable to an epicardially centered inflammatory response. Administration of atorvastatin 1 week before the pericardiotomy lowered the CRP level, increased the ERP, abbreviated intra-atrial conduction time, and shortened AF duration in this model, likely through its anti-inflammatory properties.[42] In a recent work, prednisone also attenuated tissue inflammation and decreased CRP levels, which returned to baseline after 4 days, correlating with a virtual absence of sustained arrhythmia.[43]

Aging

Increased age is a well-known risk factor for AF.[3] Anyukhovsky and colleagues[44] compared various parameters in older dogs (>8 years old) with those in younger adult dogs (1–5 years old). They found significant morphologic differences of the action potential (AP), including a decrease in peak and plateau AP voltage, a decrease in the rate of cellular depolarization, a slight decrease in resting membrane potential (−70 in older dogs versus −75 in younger dogs), and an increased dispersion of APD across the tissue. The P wave duration was also increased in the older dogs. The CV of regularly timed beats was similar in adult and old dogs, but it decreased for premature beats in older dogs. These investigators also found significant fibrosis in the older animals. From these data, they speculated that the fibrosis, slowed conduction of premature beats, and increased heterogeneity of repolarization may be important determinants of the initiation and subsequent stabilization of AF in the elderly.[45]

Transgenic mice

Atrial electrophysiologic effects and AF have been reported in several transgenic mouse lines. The possibility that inflammation and fibrosis affect AF vulnerability was shown by transgenic mice overexpressing tumor necrosis factor-α,[46] transforming growth factor-β,[47] Rac1 guanosine triphosphatase (GTPase)[48] and angiotensin-converting enzyme.[49] Each of these proteins affects inflammation or fibrosis of the atria, and each mouse had an increased propensity to AF. The connection between repolarization and fibrillatory potential was confirmed by mice overexpressing Kir 2.1 (IK1)[50] and KCNQ1 (IKs).[51] Overexpression of Kir 2.1 accelerated and stabilized fibrillatory rotors (ventricular in this case; however, conceptually, the same principle holds in the atria). The KCNQ1-overexpressing mice had AF with adrenergic stimulation–mediated amplification of the IKs effects on repolarization. Several other transgenic lines have shown AF in conjunction with cardiomyopathies or structural heart disease, which confounds the connection between the transgene and AF. Although the direct applicability of mouse AF to the human condition is unclear, these models can be taken as interrogations about the functional effects of particular proteins or systems on fibrillatory potential.

SUMMARY

At first glance, with this wide array of pathophysiologic findings in varying animal models, it is difficult to see any commonalities. That may be the most important point of this review. Human AF is likely an end point of numerous disease states, structural alterations, or inherited defects. We need to keep this in mind when interpreting the animal data. The goat burst atrial pacing model has no underlying structural disease or atrial pathologic changes caused by repetitive burst stimulation from an atrial point source, similar to the reported situation of paroxysmal AFn emanating from the PVs. The dog tachypacing cardiomyopathy without primary atrial disease is potentially analogous to AF in patients who have idiopathic ventricular myopathies (with the caveat that any

primary atrial or noncardiac manifestations of the underlying disease process would not be a part of the tachypacing model). The poor rate control of the pig model could compare with the situation of primary AF with cardiomyopathy from similarly poor rate control. Although each of these situations has AF as a component, each is unique, and the corresponding animal model must likewise be individualized.

Common themes that emerge from this survey of animal models include the frequent implications across models that intra-atrial heterogeneity (of conduction, repolarization, or cellular architecture), alterations in repolarization (shortened or prolonged but almost always abnormal), and CV slowing (homogeneous or heterogeneous) play a role in the pathogenesis of AF. The frequency of these observations suggests that these findings may be common to the fibrillation process, and therefore that therapeutic alterations targeting these areas may bear fruit. Ultimately, any conclusions drawn from animal models, and any suggested therapies, must be tested for validity in humans. Still, the similarities between the various human diseases and their corresponding animal models provide an excellent starting point for these investigations.

REFERENCES

1. Nattel S. Therapeutic implications of atrial fibrillation mechanisms: can mechanistic insights be used to improve AF management? Cardiovasc Res 2002; 54:347–60.
2. Chen PS, Tan AY. Autonomic nerve activity and atrial fibrillation. Heart Rhythm 2007;4:S61–4.
3. Allessie MA, Boyden PA, Camm AJ, et al. Pathophysiology and prevention of atrial fibrillation. Circulation 2001;103:769–77.
4. Jaïs P, Haïssaguerre M, Shah DC, et al. A focal source of atrial fibrillation treated by discrete radiofrequency ablation. Circulation 1997;95:572–6.
5. Allessie MA, Bonke FI, Schopman FJ. Circus movement in rabbit atrial muscle as a mechanism of tachycardia. III. The "leading circle" concept: a new model of circus movement in cardiac tissue without the involvement of an anatomical obstacle. Circ Res 1977;41:9–18.
6. Chou CC, Chen PS. New concepts in atrial fibrillation: mechanism and remodeling. Med Clin North Am 2008;92:53–63, x.
7. Wijffels MC, Kirchhof CJ, Dorland R, et al. Atrial fibrillation begets atrial fibrillation—a study in awake chronically instrumented goats. Circulation 1995; 92:195468.

8. Yue LX, Melnyk P, Gaspo R, et al. Molecular mechanisms underlying ionic remodeling in a dog model of atrial fibrillation. Circ Res 1999;84:776–84.

9. Fareh S, Villemaire C, Nattel S. Importance of refractoriness heterogeneity in the enhanced vulnerability to atrial fibrillation induction caused by tachycardia-induced atrial electrical remodeling. Circulation 1998;98:2202–9.

10. Shi Y, Ducharme A, Li D, et al. Remodeling of atrial dimensions and emptying function in canine models of atrial fibrillation. Cardiovasc Res 2001; 52:217–25.

11. Li DS, Fareh S, Leung TK, et al. Promotion of atrial fibrillation by heart failure in dogs—atrial remodeling of a different sort. Circulation 1999;100:87–95.

12. Dispersyn GD, Ausma J, Thoné F, et al. Cardiomyocyte remodelling during myocardial hibernation and atrial fibrillation: prelude to apoptosis. Cardiovasc Radiol 1999;43:947–57.

13. Ausma J, Litjens N, Lenders MH, et al. Time course of atrial fibrillation-induced cellular structural remodeling in atria of the goat. J Mol Cell Cardiol 2001;33: 2083–94.

14. van der Velden HM, Ausma J, Rook MB, et al. Gap junctional remodeling in relation to stabilization of atrial fibrillation in the goat. Cardiovasc Res 2000; 46:476–86.

15. Rothberger C, Winterberg H. Ueber Vorhofflimmern und Vorhofflattern. Archiv Ges Physiol 1914;160: 42–90.

16. Goldberger AL, Pavelec RS. Vagally-mediated atrial fibrillation in dogs: conversion with bretylium tosylate. Int J Cardiol 1986;13:47–55.

17. Sharifov OF, Fedorov VV, Beloshapko GG, et al. Roles of adrenergic and cholinergic stimulation in spontaneous atrial fibrillation in dogs. J Am Coll Cardiol 2004;43:483–90.

18. Olgin JE, Sih HJ, Hanish S, et al. Heterogeneous atrial denervation creates substrate for sustained atrial fibrillation. Circulation 1998;98:2608–14.

19. Hashimoto N, Yamashita T, Tsuruzoe N. Characterization of in vivo and in vitro electrophysiological and antiarrhythmic effects of a novel IKACh blocker, NIP-151: a comparison with an IKr-blocker dofetilide. J Cardiovasc Pharmacol 2008;51:162–9.

20. Liu L, Nattel S. Differing sympathetic and vagal effects on atrial fibrillation in dog: role of refractoriness heterogeneity. Am J Phys 1997;273:H805–16.

21. Ausma J, van der Velden HM, Lenders MH, et al. Reverse structural and gap-junctional remodeling after prolonged atrial fibrillation in the goat. Circulation 2003;107:2051–8.

22. Ausma J, Wijffels M, Thoné F, et al. Structural changes of atrial myocardium due to sustained atrial fibrillation in the goat. Circulation 1997;96:3157–63.

23. Duytschaever M, Blaauw Y, Allessie M. Consequences of atrial electrical remodeling for the anti-arrhythmic action of class IC and class III drugs. Cardiovasc Res 2005;67:69–76.

24. Blaauw Y, Schotten U, van Hunnik A, et al. Cardioversion of persistent atrial fibrillation by a combination of atrial specific and non-specific class III drugs in the goat. Cardiovasc Res 2007;75:89–98.

25. Verheule S, Wilson E, Banthia S, et al. Direction-dependent conduction abnormalities in a canine model of atrial fibrillation due to chronic atrial dilatation. Am J Physiol Heart Circ Physiol 2004;287: H634–44.

26. Gaspo R, Bosch RF, Talajic M, et al. Functional mechanisms underlying tachycardia-induced sustained atrial fibrillation in a chronic dog model. Circulation 1997;96:4027–35.

27. Voigt N, Maguy A, Yeh YH, et al. Changes in I K, ACh single-channel activity with atrial tachycardia remodelling in canine atrial cardiomyocytes. Cardiovasc Res 2008;77:35–43.

28. Shiroshita-Takeshita A, Brundel BJ, Lavoie J, et al. Prednisone prevents atrial fibrillation promotion by atrial tachycardia remodeling in dogs. Cardiovasc Res 2006;69:865–75.

29. Brundel BJ, Shiroshita-Takeshita A, Qi X, et al. Induction of heat shock response protects the heart against atrial fibrillation. Circ Res 2006;99: 1394–402.

30. Li D, Melnyk P, Feng J, et al. Effects of experimental heart failure on atrial cellular and ionic electrophysiology. Circulation 2000;101:2631–8.

31. Cha TJ, Ehrlich JR, Zhang L, et al. Dissociation between ionic remodeling and ability to sustain atrial fibrillation during recovery from experimental congestive heart failure. Circulation 2004;109: 412–8.

32. Cardin S, Libby E, Pelletier P, et al. Contrasting gene expression profiles in two canine models of atrial fibrillation. Circ Res 2007;100:425–33.

33. Shinagawa K, Shi YF, Tardif JC, et al. Dynamic nature of atrial fibrillation substrate during development and reversal of heart failure in dogs. Circulation 2002;105:2672–8.

34. Cha TJ, Ehrlich JR, Zhang L, et al. Atrial ionic remodeling induced by atrial tachycardia in the presence of congestive heart failure. Circulation 2004;110: 1520–6.

35. Bauer A, McDonald AD, Donahue JK. Pathophysiological findings in a model of persistent atrial fibrillation and severe congestive heart failure. Cardiovasc Res 2004;61:764–70.

36. Lin CS, Lai LP, Lin JL, et al. Increased expression of extracellular matrix proteins in rapid atrial pacing-induced atrial fibrillation. Heart Rhythm 2007;4: 938–49.

37. Lai LP, Lin JL, Lin CS, et al. Functional genomic study on atrial fibrillation using cDNA microarray and two-dimensional protein electrophoresis

techniques and identification of the myosin regu-latory light chain isoform reprogramming in atrial fibrillation. J Cardiovasc Electrophysiol 2004;15: 214–23.

38. Page PL, Plumb VJ, Okumura K, et al. A new model of atrial flutter. J Am Coll Cardiol 1986;8:872–9.

39. Kumagai K, Khrestian C, Waldo AL. Simultaneous multisite mapping studies during induced atrial fi-brillation in the sterile pericarditis model—insights into the mechanism of its maintenance. Circulation 1997;95:511–21.

40. Kumagai K, Uno K, Khrestian C, et al. Single site ra-diofrequency catheter ablation of atrial fibrillation: studies guided by simultaneous multisite mapping in the canine sterile pericarditis model. J Am Coll Cardiol 2000;36:917–23.

41. Ryu K, Li L, Khrestian CM, et al. Effects of sterile pericarditis on connexins 40 and 43 in the atria: cor-relation with abnormal conduction and atrial arrhyth-mias. Am J Physiol Heart Circ Physiol 2007;293: H1231–41.

42. Kumagai K, Nakashima H, Saku K. The HMG-CoA reductase inhibitor atorvastatin prevents atrial fibril-lation by inhibiting inflammation in a canine sterile pericarditis model. Cardiovasc Res 2004;62:105–11.

43. Goldstein RN, Ryu K, Khrestian C, et al. Prednisone prevents inducible atrial flutter in the canine sterile pericarditis model. J Cardiovasc Electrophysiol 2008;19:74–81.

44. Anyukhovsky EP, Sosunov EA, Plotnikov A, et al. Cel-lular electrophysiologic properties of old canine atria

provide a substrate for arrhythmogenesis. Cardio-vasc Res 2002;54:462–9.

45. Anyukhovsky EP, Sosunov EA, Chandra P, et al. Age-associated changes in electrophysiologic re-modeling: a potential contributor to initiation of atrial fibrillation. Cardiovasc Res 2005;66:353–63.

46. Saba S, Janczewski AM, Baker LC, et al. Atrial con-tractile dysfunction, fibrosis, and arrhythmias in a mouse model of cardiomyopathy secondary to cardiac-specific overexpression of tumor necrosis factor-α. Am J Physiol Heart Circ Physiol 2005;289: H1456–67.

47. Verheule S, Sato T, Everett T 4th, et al. Increased vul-nerability to atrial fibrillation in transgenic mice with selective atrial fibrosis caused by overexpression of TGF-beta1. Circ Res 2004;94:1458–65.

48. Adam O, Frost G, Custodis F, et al. Role of Rac1 GTPase activation in atrial fibrillation. J Am Coll Car-diol 2007;50:359–67.

49. Xiao HD, Fuchs S, Campbell DJ, et al. Mice with car-diac-restricted angiotensin-converting enzyme (ACE) have atrial enlargement, cardiac arrhythmia, and sudden death. Am J Pathol 2004;165:1019–32.

50. Noujaim SF, Pandit SV, Berenfeld O, et al. Up-regu-lation of the inward rectifier K+ current (I K1) in the mouse heart accelerates and stabilizes rotors. J Physiol 2007;578:315–26.

51. Sampson KJ, Terrenoire C, Cervantes DO, et al. Ad-renergic regulation of a key cardiac potassium chan-nel can contribute to atrial fibrillation: evidence from an I Ks transgenic mouse. J Physiol 2008;586:627–37.

Diagnosis and Management of Typical Atrial Flutter

Navinder S. Sawhney, MD[a], Ramtin Anousheh, MD, MPH[b],
Wei-Chung Chen, MPH[c], Gregory K. Feld, MD[c],*

KEYWORDS

• Atrial flutter • Cavo-tricuspid isthmus • Ablation

Type 1 atrial flutter (AFL) is a common atrial arrhythmia that may cause significant symptoms and serious adverse effects including embolic stroke, myocardial ischemia and infarction, and rarely a tachycardia-induced cardiomyopathy as a result of rapid atrioventricular conduction. The electrophysiologic substrate underlying type 1 AFL has been shown to be a combination of slow conduction velocity in the cavo-tricuspid isthmus (CTI), plus anatomic and/or functional conduction block along the crista terminalis and Eustachian ridge (**Fig. 1**). This electrophysiologic milleu allows for a long enough reentrant path length relative to the average tissue wavelength around the tricuspid valve annulus to allow for sustained reentry.

Type 1 AFL is relatively resistant to pharmacologic suppression. As a result of the well-defined anatomic substrate and the pharmacologic resistance of type 1 AFL, radiofrequency catheter ablation has emerged in the past decade as a safe and effective first-line treatment. Although several techniques have been described for ablating type 1 AFL, the most widely accepted and successful technique is an anatomically guided approach targeting the CTI. Recent technological developments, including three-dimensional electro-anatomic contact and noncontact mapping, and the use of irrigated tip and large-tip ablation electrode catheters with high-power generators,

have produced nearly uniform efficacy without increased risk. This article reviews the electrophysiology of human type 1 AFL, techniques currently used for its diagnosis and management, and emerging technologies.

ATRIAL FLUTTER TERMINOLOGY

Because of the variety of terms used to describe atrial flutter in humans, including type 1 AFL and type 2 AFL, typical and atypical atrial flutter, counterclockwise and clockwise atrial flutter, and isthmus and non-isthmus dependent flutter, the Working Group of Arrhythmias of the European Society of Cardiology and the North American Society of Pacing and Electrophysiology convened and published a consensus document in 2001 in an attempt to develop a generally accepted standardized terminology for atrial flutter.[1] The consensus terminology derived from this working group to describe CTI-dependent, right atrial macroreentry tachycardia, in the counterclockwise or clockwise direction around the tricuspid valve annulus, was "typical" or "reverse typical" AFL respectively.[1] For the purposes of this article, these two arrhythmias will be referred to specifically as typical and reverse typical AFL when being individually described, but as type 1 AFL when being referred to jointly.

A version of this article originally appeared in *Medical Clinics of North America*, volume 92, issue 1.
[a] Cardiac Electrophysiology Program, Division of Cardiology, University of California San Diego Medical Center, 4169 Front Street, San Diego, CA 92103-8648, USA
[b] Loma Linda University Medical Center, 11234 Anderson Street, Loma Linda, CA, USA
[c] Electrophysiology Laboratory, Cardiac Electrophysiology Program, Division of Cardiology University of California Sand Diego Medical Center, 4168 Front Street, San Diego, CA 92103-8649, USA
* Corresponding author.
E-mail address: gfeld@ucsd.edu (G.K. Feld).

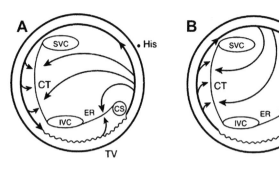

Fig. 1. Schematic diagrams demonstrating the activation patterns in the typical (*A*) and reverse typical (*B*) forms of human type 1 AFL, as viewed from below the tricuspid valve annulus (TV) looking up into the right atrium. In the typical form of AFL, the reentrant wavefront rotates counterclockwise in the right atrium, whereas in the reverse typical form reentry is clockwise. Note that the Eustachian ridge (ER) and crista terminalis (CT) form lines of block, and that an area of slow conduction (*wavy line*) is present in the isthmus between the inferior vena cava (IVC) and Eustachian ridge and the tricuspid valve annulus. CS, coronary sinus ostium; His, His bundle; SVC, superior vena cava.

PATHOPHYSIOLOGIC MECHANISMS OF TYPE 1 ATRIAL FLUTTER

The development of successful radiofrequency catheter ablation techniques for human type 1 AFL was largely dependent on the delineation of its electrophysiologic mechanism. Through the use of advanced electrophysiologic techniques, including intraoperative and transcatheter activation mapping,[2–7] type 1 AFL was determined to be attributable to a macro-reentrant circuit rotating in either a counter-clockwise (typical) or clockwise (reverse typical) direction in the right atrium around the tricuspid valve annulus, with an area of relatively slow conduction velocity in the low posterior right atrium (see **Fig. 1**A, B). The predominate area of slow conduction in the AFL reentry circuit has been shown to be in the CTI, through which conduction times may reach 80 to 100 msec, accounting for one third to one half of the AFL cycle length.[8–10] The CTI is anatomically bounded by the inferior vena cava and Eustachian ridge posteriorly and the tricuspid valve annulus anteriorly (see **Fig. 1**A, B), both of which form lines of conduction block or barriers delineating a protected zone of slow conduction in the reentry circuit.[5,11–13] The presence of conduction block along the Eustachian ridge has been confirmed by demonstrating double potentials along its length during AFL. Double potentials have also been recorded along the crista terminalis suggesting that it also forms a line of block separating the smooth septal right atrium from the trabeculated right atrial free wall. Such lines of block, which may be either functional or anatomic, are necessary to create an adequate path-length for reentry to be sustained and to prevent short circuiting of the reentrant wavefront.[12–14] The medial CTI is contiguous with the interatrial septum near the coronary sinus ostium, and the lateral CTI is contiguous with the low lateral right atrium near the inferior vena cava (**Fig. 1**A, B). These areas correspond electrophysiologically to the exit and entrance to the zone of slow conduction, depending on whether the direction of reentry is counterclockwise (CCW) or clockwise (CW) in the right atrium. The path of the reentrant circuit outside the confines of the CTI consists of a broad activation wavefront in the interatrial septum and right atrial free wall around the crista terminalis and the tricuspid valve annulus.[11–14]

The slower conduction velocity in the CTI, relative to the interatrial septum and right atrial free wall, may be caused by anisotropic fiber orientation in the CTI.[2,8–10,15,16] This may also predispose to development of unidirectional block during rapid atrial pacing, and account for the observation that typical (CCW) AFL is more likely to be induced when pacing is performed from the coronary sinus ostium. Conversely, reverse typical (CW) AFL is more likely to be induced when pacing from the low lateral right atrium.[17,18] This hypothesis is further supported by direct mapping in animal studies demonstrating that the direction of rotation of the reentrant wavefront during AFL is dependent on the direction of the paced wavefront producing unidirectional block at the time of its induction.[19] In humans, the predominate clinical presentation of type 1 AFL is the typical variety, likely because the trigger(s) for AFL commonly arise from the left atrium in the form of premature atrial contractions or nonsustained atrial fibrillation.[20] Triggers arising from the left atrium or pulmonary veins usually conduct to the right atrium via the coronary sinus or interatrial septum, thus entering the CTI from medial to lateral, which results in clockwise unidirectional block in the CTI with resultant initiation of counterclockwise typical AFL.

The development of abnormal dispersion or shortening of atrial refractoriness as a result of atrial electrical remodeling may increase the likelihood of developing regional conduction block and abnormal shortening of tissue wavelength responsible for initiating and sustaining reentry in AFL.[21,22]

ECG DIAGNOSIS OF TYPE 1 ATRIAL FLUTTER

The surface 12-lead ECG is helpful in establishing a diagnosis of type 1 AFL, particularly the typical form (**Box 1**). In typical AFL, an inverted saw-tooth flutter (F) wave pattern is observed in the inferior ECG leads II, III, and aVF, with a low amplitude biphasic F waves in leads I and aVL, an upright F wave in precordial lead V1, and an inverted F wave in lead V6. In contrast, in reverse typical AFL, the F wave pattern on the 12-lead ECG is less specific, often with a sine wave pattern in the inferior ECG leads (**Fig. 2**A, B). The determinants of F wave pattern on ECG are largely dependent on the activation pattern of the left atrium resulting from reentry in the right atrium, with inverted F waves inscribed in the inferior ECG leads in typical AFL as a result of activation of the left atrium initially posterior near the coronary sinus, and upright F waves inscribed in the inferior ECG leads in reverse typical AFL as a result of activation of the left atrium initially anterior near Bachman's bundle[23,24] Because the typical and reverse typical forms of type 1 AFL use the same reentry circuit, but in opposite directions, their rates are usually similar.

Box 1
Diagnostic criteria for typical and reverse typical AFL

1. Demonstration of a saw-tooth F wave pattern in the inferior ECG leads (typical AFL) or a sine wave or upright F wave pattern in the inferior ECG leads (reverse typical AFL), with atrial rate between 240 and 350 beats per minute, and 2:1 or variable AV conduction
2. Demonstration of counterclockwise (typical) or clockwise (reverse typical) macroreentrant circuit around tricuspid valve annulus by standard multi-electrode catheter mapping or 3-D computerized mapping
3. Demonstration of concealed entrainment criteria during pacing from the cavotricuspid isthmus, including acceleration of the tachycardia to the paced cycle length, first post-pacing interval equal to the tachycardia cycle length, and stimulus-to-F wave interval equal to electrogram-to-F wave interval on the pacing catheter

---

MEDICAL THERAPY VERSUS CATHETER ABLATION

Class III antiarrhythmic drugs, by selectively lengthening the cardiac action potential, have shown efficacy in converting atrial flutter to normal sinus rhythm.[25] However, despite an 80% initial success rate with the Class III agent Ibutilide,[26] recurrence rates are extremely high (70% to 90%) despite maintenance on antiarrhythmic drugs.[27,28] Therefore, catheter ablation is considered a first-line approach for many patients with atrial flutter given the high acute and chronic efficacy of the procedure (>90%) and relatively low complication rates.[29] Prospective trials that have randomized patients to medical therapy versus first-line catheter ablation have shown that patients who received ablation as a first-line strategy had significantly better maintenance of sinus rhythm, fewer hospitalizations, better quality of life, and fewer overall complications when compared with patients who received antiarrhythmic drug therapy.[28,30]

Despite the excellent acute results and long-term outcome after radiofrequency catheter ablation for freedom from type 1 atrial flutter, one must keep in mind that development of atrial fibrillation is high in this population of patients; 30% of these patients may develop atrial fibrillation over a 5-year period, especially if there is a history of atrial fibrillation or underlying heart disease.[28,30–32] However, ablation of the CTI may reduce or in rare cases may eliminate recurrences of atrial fibrillation, and CTI ablation is also effective in patients undergoing pharmacologic treatment for atrial fibrillation with antiarrhythmic drug–induced type 1 atrial flutter (the so-called "hybrid approach"). Ablation of the CTI may also be required in patients undergoing ablation for atrial fibrillation who also have a history of type 1 atrial flutter.[33]

ELECTROPHYSIOLOGIC MAPPING OF TYPE 1 ATRIAL FLUTTER

Despite the utility of the 12-lead ECG in making a presumptive diagnosis of typical AFL, an electrophysiologic study with mapping and entrainment must be performed to confirm the underlying mechanism if radiofrequency catheter ablation is to be successfully performed (see **Box 1**). This is particularly true in the case of reverse typical AFL, which is much more difficult to diagnose on 12-lead ECG. For the electrophysiologic study of AFL, activation mapping may be performed using standard multi-electrode catheters, or one of the currently available three-dimensional computerized activation mapping systems. For standard multi-electrode catheter mapping, catheters are

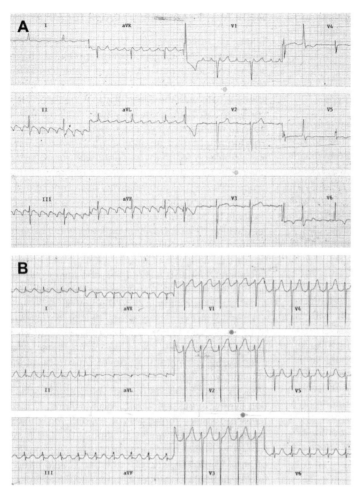

Fig. 2. (*A*) A 12-lead electrocardiogram recorded from a patient with typical AFL. Note the typical sawtoothed pattern of inverted F waves in the inferior leads II, III, aVF. Typical AFL is also characterized by flat to biphasic F waves in I and aVL respectively, an upright F wave in V1 and an inverted F wave in V6. (*B*) A 12-lead electrocardiogram recorded from a patient with the reverse typical AFL. The F wave in the reverse typical form of AFL has a less distinct sine wave pattern in the inferior leads. In this case, the F waves are upright in the inferior leads II, III, and aVF; biphasic in leads I, aVL, and V1; and upright in V6.

positioned in the right atrium, His bundle region, and coronary sinus. To most precisely elucidate the endocardial activation sequence, a Halo 20-electrode mapping catheter (Cordis-Webster, Inc., Diamond Bar, CA) is most commonly used in the right atrium positioned around the tricuspid valve annulus (**Fig. 3**). Recordings obtained during AFL from all electrodes are then analyzed to determine the right atrial activation sequence. In patients presenting to the laboratory in sinus rhythm it is necessary to induce AFL to confirm its mechanism. Induction of AFL is accomplished by atrial programmed stimulation or burst pacing. Preferred pacing sites are the coronary sinus ostium or low lateral right atrium. Burst pacing is the preferred method to induce AFL, with pacing cycle lengths between 180 and 240 msec typically effective in producing unidirectional CTI block and inducing AFL. Induction of atrial flutter typically occurs immediately following the onset of unidirectional CTI isthmus block.[17,18]

During electrophysiologic study, a diagnosis of either typical or reverse typical AFL is suggested by observing a counterclockwise or clockwise activation pattern in the right atrium and around the tricuspid valve annulus. For example, as seen in **Fig. 4**A in a patient with typical AFL, the atrial electrogram recorded at the coronary sinus ostium is timed with the initial down stroke of the F wave in the inferior surface ECG leads, followed by caudal-to-cranial activation in the interatrial septum to the His bundle atrial electrogram, and then cranial-to-caudal activation in the right atrial free wall from proximal to distal on the Halo catheter, and finally to the ablation catheter in the CTI, indicating that the underlying mechanism is a counter-clockwise macro-reentry circuit with electrical activity encompassing the entire tachycardia cycle length. In a patient with reverse typical AFL, the mirror image of this activation pattern is seen, as shown in **Fig. 4**B.

RADIOFREQUENCY CATHETER ABLATION OF TYPE 1 ATRIAL FLUTTER

Radiofrequency catheter ablation of type 1 AFL is performed with a steerable mapping/ablation

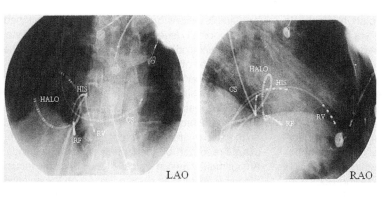

Fig. 3. Left anterior oblique (LAO) and right anterior oblique (RAO) fluoroscopic projections showing the intracardiac positions of the right ventricular (RV), His bundle (HIS), coronary sinus (CS), Halo (HALO), and mapping/ablation catheter (RF). Note that the Halo catheter is positioned around the tricuspid valve annulus, with the proximal electrode pair at 1 o'clock and the distal electrode pair at 7 o'clock in the LAO view. The mapping/ablation catheter is positioned in the sub-Eustachian isthmus, midway between the interatrial septum and low lateral right atrium, with the distal 8-mm ablation electrode near the tricuspid valve annulus.

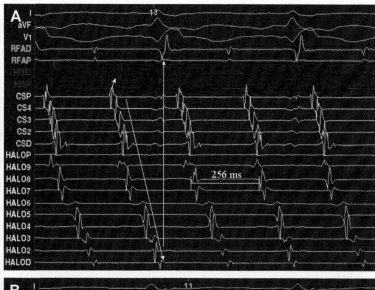

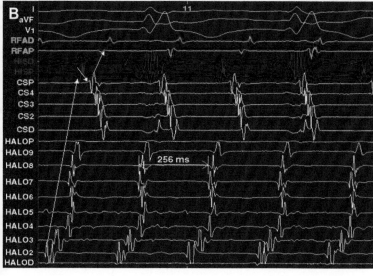

Fig. 4. Endocardial electrograms from the mapping/ablation, Halo, CS, and His bundle catheters and surface ECG leads I, aVF, and V1 demonstrating a counterclockwise (CCW) rotation of activation in the right atrium in a patient with typical AFL (*A*) and a clockwise (CW) rotation of activation in the right atrium in a patient with reverse typical AFL (*B*). The AFL cycle length was 256 msec for both CCW and CW forms. Arrows demonstrate activation sequence. Halo D - Halo P tracings are 10 bipolar electrograms recorded from the distal (low lateral right atrium) to proximal (high right atrium) poles of the 20-pole Halo catheter positioned around the tricuspid valve annulus with the proximal electrode pair at 1 o'clock and the distal electrode pair at 7 o'clock. CSP, electrograms recorded from the coronary sinus catheter proximal electrode pair positioned at the ostium of the coronary sinus; HISP, electrograms recorded from the proximal electrode pair of the His bundle catheter; RF, electrograms recorded from the mapping/ablation catheter positioned with the distal electrode pair in the cavo-tricuspid isthmus.

catheter with a large distal ablation electrode positioned in the right atrium via the femoral vein.[3,5–7,34–36] The typical radiofrequency generator used by most laboratories is capable of automatically adjusting applied power to achieve an operator programmable tissue-electrode interface temperature. Tissue temperature is monitored via a thermistor or thermocouple embedded in the distal ablation electrode. Programmable temperature with automatic power control is important because successful ablation requires a stable temperature of at least 50 to 60°C and occasionally 70°C. Temperatures in excess of 70°C may cause tissue vaporization (steam pops), tissue charring, and formation of blood coagulum on the ablation electrode resulting in a rise in impedance, which limits energy delivery and lesion formation, and may lead to complications such as cardiac perforation or embolization. A variety of mapping/ablation catheters with different shapes and curve lengths are currently available from several commercial manufacturers. We prefer to use a larger curve catheter (K2 or mid-distal large curve, EP Technologies, San Jose, CA), with or without a preshaped guiding sheath such as an SR 0, SL1, or ramp sheath (Daig, Minnetonka, MN), to ensure that the ablation electrode will reach the tricuspid valve annulus.

Recently, radiofrequency ablation catheters with either saline-cooled ablation electrodes or large distal ablation electrodes (ie, 8–10 mm) have been approved by the Food and Drug Administration (FDA) for ablation of type 1 atrial flutter (EP Technologies, Inc., Biosense-Webster, Inc., Medtronic, Inc.). During ablation with saline-cooled catheters, the use of lower power and temperature settings is recommended to avoid steam pops, because higher intramyocardial tissue temperatures are produced than measured at the tissue-electrode interface owing to the electrode cooling effect of saline perfusion.[37–39] Although studies have reported use of up to 50 W and 60°C for ablation of AFL without higher than expected complication rates, a maximum power of 35 to 40 watts and temperature of 43 to 45°C should be used initially.[37–40] In contrast, the large-tip (8- to 10-mm) ablation catheters require a higher power, up to 100 watts, to achieve target temperatures of 50 to 70°C owing to the greater energy dispersive effects of the larger ablation electrode. This also requires the use of two grounding pads applied to the patient's skin to avoid skin burns.[29,39,41,42]

The preferred target for type 1 AFL ablation is the CTI, which when using standard multipolar electrode catheters for mapping and ablation, is localized with a combined fluoroscopically and electrophysiologically guided approach.[3,5–7,29,34–40,42] Initially,

a steerable mapping/ablation catheter is positioned fluoroscopically (see **Fig. 3**) in the CTI with the distal ablation electrode on or near the TV annulus in the right anterior oblique (RAO) view, and midway between the septum and low right atrial free wall (6 or 7 o'clock position) in the left anterior oblique view (LAO). The distal ablation electrode position is then adjusted toward or away from the TV annulus based on the ratio of atrial and ventricular electrogram amplitude recorded by the bipolar ablation electrode. An optimal AV ratio is typically 1:2 or 1:4 at the tricuspid valve annulus as seen in **Fig. 4**A on the ablation electrode (RFAD). After positioning the ablation catheter on or near the tricuspid valve annulus, it is very slowly withdrawn a few millimeters at a time (usually the length of the distal ablation electrode) pausing for 30 to 60 seconds at each location during a continuous or interrupted energy application. Electrogram recordings may be used in addition to fluoroscopy to ensure that the ablation electrode is in contact with viable tissue in the CTI throughout each energy application. Ablation of the entire CTI may require several sequential 30- to 60-second energy applications during a stepwise catheter pullback, or a prolonged energy application of up to 120 seconds, or more during a continuous catheter pullback. The catheter should be gradually withdrawn until the distal ablation electrode records no atrial electrogram indicating it has reached the inferior vena cava or until the ablation electrode is noted to abruptly slip off the Eustachian ridge fluoroscopically. Radiofrequency energy application should be immediately interrupted when the catheter has reached the inferior vena cava, because ablation in the venous structures is known to cause significant pain to the patient.

PROCEDURE END POINTS FOR RADIOFREQUENCY CATHETER ABLATION OF TYPE 1 ATRIAL FLUTTER

Ablation may be performed during sustained AFL or during sinus rhythm. If performed during AFL, the first end point is its termination during energy application. Despite termination of AFL, it is common to find that CTI conduction persists. After the entire CTI ablation is completed, electrophysiologic testing should then be performed. Pacing should be done at a cycle length of 600 msec (or greater depending on sinus cycle length) to determine if there is bidirectional conduction block in the CTI (**Fig. 5**A, B and **Fig. 6**A, B). Bidirectional conduction block in the CTI is confirmed by demonstrating a change from a bidirectional wavefront with collision in the right atrial free wall or interatrial septum before ablation to a strictly cranial to caudal activation sequence following ablation during

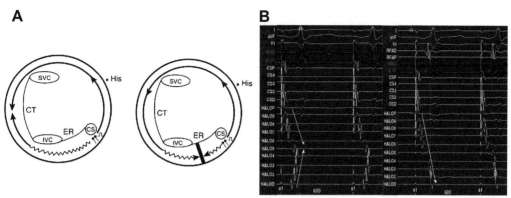

Fig. 5. (A) A schematic diagram of the expected right atrial activation sequence during pacing in sinus rhythm from the coronary sinus (CS) ostium before (*left panel*) and after (*right panel*) ablation of the cavo-tricuspid isthmus (CTI). Before ablation the activation pattern during coronary sinus pacing is caudal to cranial in the interatrial septum and low right atrium, with collision of the septal and right atrial wavefronts in the mid-lateral right atrium. Following ablation, the activation pattern during coronary sinus pacing is still caudal to cranial in the interatrial septum, but the lateral right atrium is now activated in a strictly cranial to caudal pattern (ie, counterclockwise), indicating complete clockwise conduction block in the CTI. CT, crista terminalis; ER, Eustachian ridge; His, His bundle; IVC, inferior vena cava; SVC, superior vena cava. (B) Surface ECG and right atrial endocardial electrograms recorded during pacing in sinus rhythm from the coronary sinus (CS) ostium before (*left panel*) and after (*right panel*) ablation of the cavo-tricuspid isthmus (CTI). Tracings include surface ECG leads I, aVF, and V1, and endocardial electrograms from the proximal coronary sinus (CSP), His bundle (HIS), tricuspid valve annulus at 1 o'clock (HaloP) to 7 o'clock (HaloD), and high right atrium (HRA or RFA). Before ablation, during coronary sinus pacing, there is collision of the cranial and caudal right atrial wavefronts in the mid-lateral right atrium (HALO5). Following ablation, the lateral right atrium is activated in a strictly cranial to caudal pattern (ie, counterclockwise), indicating complete medial to lateral conduction block in the CTI.

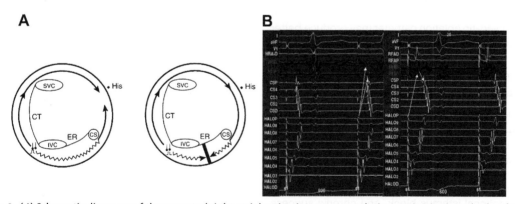

Fig. 6. (A) Schematic diagrams of the expected right atrial activation sequence during pacing in sinus rhythm from the low lateral right atrium before (*left panel*) and after (*right panel*) ablation of the cavo-tricuspid isthmus (CTI). Before ablation the activation pattern during coronary sinus pacing is caudal to cranial in the right atrial free wall, with collision of the cranial and caudal wavefronts in the mid-septum, with simultaneous activation at the His bundle (HISP) and proximal coronary sinus (CSP). Following ablation, the activation pattern during low lateral right atrial sinus pacing is still caudal to cranial in the right atrial free wall, but the septum is now activated in a strictly cranial to caudal pattern (ie, clockwise), indicating complete lateral to medial conduction block in the CTI. CT, crista terminalis; ER, Eustachian ridge; His, His bundle; SVC, superior vena cava; IVC, inferior vena cava. (B) Surface ECG and right atrial endocardial electrograms during pacing in sinus rhythm from the low lateral right atrium before (*left panel*) and after (*right panel*) ablation of the CTI. Tracings include surface ECG leads I, aVF, and V1, and endocardial electrograms from the proximal coronary sinus (CSP), His bundle (HIS), tricuspid valve annulus at 1 o'clock (HaloP) to 7 o'clock (HaloD), and high right atrium (HRA or RFA). Before ablation, during low lateral right atrial pacing, there is collision of the cranial and caudal right atrial wavefronts in the mid-septum (HIS and CSP). Following ablation, the septum is activated in a strictly cranial to caudal pattern (ie, clockwise), indicating complete lateral to medial conduction block in the CTI.

pacing from the coronary sinus ostium or low lateral right atrium respectively.[43-45] The presence of bidirectional conduction block in the CTI is also strongly supported by recording widely spaced double potentials at the site of linear ablation during pacing from the low lateral right atrium or coronary sinus ostium.[46,47] If ablation is done during sinus rhythm, pacing can be also done during energy application to monitor for the development of conduction block in the CTI. The use of this end point for ablation may be associated with a significantly lower recurrence rate of type 1 AFL during long-term follow-up.[43-45,48] Programmed stimulation and burst pacing should be repeated over the course of at least 30 minutes to ensure that bidirectional CTI block has been achieved, and that neither typical nor reverse typical AFL can be reinduced.[3,5-7,29,34-38,40-42,49]

If AFL is not terminated during the first attempt at CTI ablation, the activation sequence and isthmus dependence of the AFL should be reconfirmed, and then ablation should be repeated. During repeat ablation, it may be necessary to use a slightly higher power and/or ablation temperature, or to rotate the ablation catheter away from the initial line of energy application, either medially or laterally in the CTI, to create new or additional lines of block. In addition, if ablation is initially attempted using a standard 4- to 5-mm tip electrode and is not successful, repeat ablation with a larger-tip 8- to 10-mm electrode catheter or cooled-tip ablation catheter may produce better result.[29,37-42]

OUTCOMES AND COMPLICATIONS OF CATHETER ABLATION OF TYPE 1 ATRIAL FLUTTER

Early reports[3-6] of radiofrequency catheter ablation of AFL revealed high initial success rates but with recurrence rates up to 20% to 45% (**Table 1**). However, as experience with radiofrequency catheter ablation of AFL has increased, both acute success rates, defined as termination of AFL and bidirectional isthmus block, and chronic success rates, defined as no recurrence of type 1 atrial flutter, have risen to 85% to 95%. Contributing in large degree to these improved results has been the introduction of bidirectional conduction block in the CTI as an end point for successful radiofrequency catheter ablation of AFL.[29,34-42] In the most recent studies using either large-tip (8- to 10-mm) electrode ablation catheters with high-power radiofrequency generators, or cooled-tip electrode ablation catheters with standard radiofrequency generators, acute success rates as high as 100% and chronic success rates as high as 98% have been reported.[29,39,42] Randomized

comparisons of internally cooled, externally cooled, and large-tip ablation catheters suggest a slightly better acute and chronic success rate with the externally cooled ablation catheters, compared with internally cooled ablation catheters or large-tip ablation catheters.[37,38,40,42,49]

In nearly all the large-scale studies where CTI ablation has successfully eliminated recurrence of type 1 AFL, and where quality-of-life scores (QOL) have been assessed, there have been statistically significant improvements in QOL as a result of reduced symptoms and antiarrhythmic medication use.[28,29,49]

Radiofrequency catheter ablation of the CTI for type 1 AFL is relatively safe, but serious complications can occur including heart block, cardiac perforation and tamponade, and thromboembolic events, which include pulmonary embolism and stroke. In recent large-scale studies, major complications have been observed in approximately 2.5% to 3.0% of patients.[29,42,49] In the studies of large-tip ablation electrode catheters there did not appear to be any relationship between complication rates and the use of higher power (ie, >50 W) for ablation of the CTI. Anticoagulation with warfarin before ablation must be considered in patients with chronic type 1 AFL to help decrease the risk of thromboembolic complications such as stroke.[50] This may be particularly important in those patients with depressed left ventricular function, mitral valve disease, and left atrial enlargement with spontaneous contrast (ie, smoke) on echocardiography. As an alternative, the use of transesophageal echocardiography to rule out left atrial clot before ablation may be acceptable, but subsequent anticoagulation with warfarin is still recommended, as atrial stunning may occur after conversion of AFL, as it does with atrial fibrillation.[50]

ROLE OF COMPUTERIZED THREE-DIMENSIONAL MAPPING IN DIAGNOSIS AND ABLATION OF TYPE 1 ATRIAL FLUTTER

While not required for successful ablation of type I atrial flutter, the three-dimensional (3-D) electroanatomical Carto (BioSense-Webster, Baldwin Park, CA) or noncontact Ensite (Endocardial Solutions, St. Paul, MN) activation mapping systems have specific advantages that have made them a widely used and accepted technology. Although it is not within the scope of this article to describe the technological basis of these systems in detail, there are unique characteristics of each system that make them more or less suitable for mapping and ablation of atrial flutter.

Table 1
Success rates for radiofrequency catheter ablation of atrial flutter

Author, Year, Reference No.	N	Electrode Length	% Acute Success	Follow-up, Mo	% Chronic Success
Feld 1992[5]	16	4	100	4 ± 2	83
Cosio 1993[6]	9	4	100	2–18	56
Kirkorian 1994[35]	22	4	86	8 ± 13	84
Fischer 1995[34]	80	4	73	20 ± 8	81
Poty 1995[44]	12	6/8	100	9 ± 3	92
Schwartzman 1996[45]	35	8	100	1–21	92
Chauchemez 1996[48]	20	4	100	8 ± 2	80
Tsai 1999[41]	50	8	92	10 ± 5	100
Atiga 2002[40]	59	4 versus cooled	88	13 ± 4	93
Scavee 2004[38]	80	8 versus cooled	80	15	98
Feld 2004[29]	169	8 or 10	93	6	97
Calkins 2004[49]	150	8	88	6	87
Ventura 2004[42]	130	8 versus cooled	100	14 ± 2	98
Feld 2008[53]	160	Cryoablation	87.5	6	80.3

Acute and chronic success rates are reported as overall results in randomized or comparison studies.
Abbreviations: N, number of patients studied, % acute success, termination of atrial flutter during ablation and/or demonstration of isthmus block following ablation; % chronic success, % of patients in whom type 1 atrial flutter did not recur during follow-up.

The Ensite system uses a saline inflated balloon catheter on which is mounted a wire mesh containing electrodes that are capable of sensing the voltage potential of surrounding atrial endocardium, without actual electrode-tissue contact, from which the computerized mapping system can generate up to 3000 virtual endocardial electrograms and create a propagation map of the macro-reentrant circuit. In addition, a low-amplitude high-frequency electrical current emitted from the ablation catheter can be sensed and tracked in 3-D space by the mapping balloon. A 3-D anatomy can be created by roving the mapping catheter around the right atrial endocardium, upon which the propagation map demonstrating the atrial flutter reentrant circuit is superimposed. The appropriate ablation target can then be localized, and the ablation catheter can be positioned and tracked while ablation is performed. Following ablation, the mapping system can then be used to assess for bidirectional CTI conduction block during pacing from the low lateral right atrium and coronary sinus ostium. The advantages of the Ensite system include the ability to map the entire AFL activation sequence in one beat, precise anatomic representation of the right atrium including the CTI and adjacent structures, precise localization of the ablation catheter within the right atrium, and propagation maps of endocardial activation during atrial flutter and pacing after ablation to assess for CTI conduction block. In addition, any ablation catheter system can be used with the Ensite system. The major disadvantages of the Ensite system are the need to use the balloon mapping catheter, with its large 10-Fr introducer sheath, and the need for full anticoagulation during the mapping procedure.

The Carto uses a magnetic sensor in the ablation catheter, a magnetic field generated by a grid placed under the patient, and a reference pad on the skin to track the ablation catheter in 3-D space. The computer system sequentially records anatomic location and electrograms for on-line analysis of activation time and computation of isochronal patterns that are then superimposed on the endocardial geometry (**Fig. 7**A). A propagation map can also be produced. The advantages of the Carto include precise anatomic representation of the right atrium including the CTI and adjacent structures, precise localization of the ablation catheter within the right atrium, and static activation and propagation maps of endocardial activation can be constructed during atrial flutter and during pacing after ablation to assess for CTI conduction block (**Fig. 7**B). The disadvantages of the Carto system include the need to use the proprietary catheters and ablation generator and the need for sustained tachycardia to map the entire endocardial activation sequence.

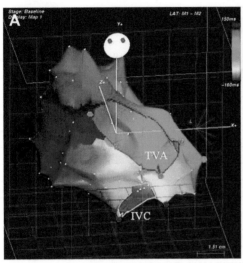
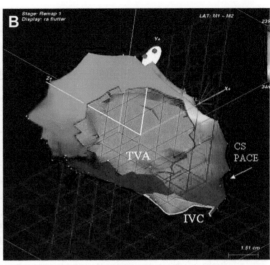

Fig. 7. A 3-D electroanatomical (Carto, Biosense Webster) map of the right atrium in a patient with typical AFL, before (*A*) and after (*B*) CTI ablation. Note the counterclockwise activation pattern around the tricuspid valve during AFL (*A*), which is based on color scheme indicating activation time from orange (early) to purple (late). Following ablation of the CTI (*B*), during pacing from the coronary sinus ostium, there is evidence of medial to lateral isthmus block as indicated by juxtaposition of orange and purple color in the CTI, indicating early and late activation, respectively. A 3-D propagation map can also be produced using the Carto system, which in some cases allows better visualization of the atrial activation sequence during AFL. IVC, inferior vena cava; TVA, tricuspid valve annulus.

The 3-D computerized mapping systems may be particularly useful in difficult cases such as those where prior ablation has failed, or in those where complex anatomy may be involved including idiopathic or postoperative scarring, or unoperated or surgically corrected congenital heart disease.

ALTERNATIVE ENERGY SOURCES FOR ABLATION OF TYPE 1 ATRIAL FLUTTER

The development of new energy sources for ablation of cardiac arrhythmias is an ongoing effort because of the disadvantages of radiofrequency energy for ablation, including the risk of coagulum formation, tissue charring, subendocardial steam pops, embolization, failure to achieve transmural ablation, and long procedure and fluoroscopy times required to ablate large areas of myocardium. Many of these disadvantages have been overcome in the case of ablation of type 1 AFL in the past decade. Nonetheless, several clinical and preclinical studies have recently been published on the use of catheter cryoablation and microwave ablation for treatment of atrial flutter and other arrhythmias.[51–57] Recent studies have been reported demonstrating that catheter cryoablation of type 1 AFL can be achieved with similar results to that achieved with radiofrequency ablation.[51–53] The potential advantages of cryoablation include

the lack of pain associated with ablation, the ability to produce a large transmural ablation lesion, and the lack of tissue charring or coagulum formation. In addition, early work has begun on the use of a linear microwave ablation catheter system (Medwaves, San Diego, CA) with antenna lengths up to 4 cm.[54–57] These studies have shown the feasibility of linear microwave ablation, which may have the advantage of very rapid ablation of the CTI with a single energy application over the entire length of the ablation electrode.

SUMMARY

Radiofrequency catheter ablation has become a first-line treatment for type 1 AFL with nearly uniform acute and chronic success and low complication rates. The most effective approach preferred by most laboratories is combined anatomically and electrophysiologically guided ablation of the CTI, with procedure end points of arrhythmia noninducibility and bidirectional CTI conduction block. Currently, the use of a large-tip 8- to 10-mm ablation catheter with a high output radiofrequency generator (ie, up to 100 W) or a cooled-tip ablation catheter is recommended for optimal success rates. Computerized 3-D activation mapping is an adjunctive method, which while not mandatory, may have significant advantages in some cases resulting in improved overall success rates. New alternate energy sources including cryoablation and microwave ablation are under investigation with the hope of further improving procedure times and success rates and potentially reducing the risk of complications during AFL ablation.

REFERENCES

1. Saoudi N, Cosio F, Waldo A, et al. Classification of atrial flutter and regular atrial tachycardia according to electrophysiologic mechanism and anatomic bases: a statement from a joint expert group from the Working Group of Arrhythmias of the European Society of Cardiology and the North American Society of Pacing and Electrophysiology. J Cardiovasc Electrophysiol 2001;12(7):852–66.
2. Olshansky B, Okumura K, Hess PG, et al. Demonstration of an area of slow conduction in human atrial flutter. J Am Coll Cardiol 1990;16(7):1639–48.
3. Lesh MD, Van Hare GF, Epstein LM, et al. Radiofrequency catheter ablation of atrial arrhythmias. Results and mechanisms. Circulation 1994;89(3):1074–89.
4. Cosio FG, Goicolea A, Lopez-Gil M, et al. Atrial endocardial mapping in the rare form of atrial flutter. Am J Cardiol 1990;66(7):715–20.
5. Feld GK, Fleck RP, Chen PS, et al. Radiofrequency catheter ablation for the treatment of human type 1 atrial flutter. Identification of a critical zone in the reentrant circuit by endocardial mapping techniques. Circulation 1992;86(4):1233–40.
6. Cosio FG, Lopez-Gil M, Goicolea A, et al. Radiofrequency ablation of the inferior vena cava-tricuspid valve isthmus in common atrial flutter. Am J Cardiol 1993;71(8):705–9.
7. Tai CT, Chen SA, Chiang CE, et al. Electrophysiologic characteristics and radiofrequency catheter ablation in patients with clockwise atrial flutter. J Cardiovasc Electrophysiol 1997;8(1):24–34.
8. Feld GK, Mollerus M, Birgersdotter-Green U, et al. Conduction velocity in the tricuspid valve-inferior vena cava isthmus is slower in patients with type I atrial flutter compared to those without a history of atrial flutter. J Cardiovasc Electrophysiol 1997;8(12):1338–48.
9. Kinder C, Kall J, Kopp D, et al. Conduction properties of the inferior vena cava-tricuspid annular isthmus in patients with typical atrial flutter. J Cardiovasc Electrophysiol 1997;8(7):727–37.
10. Da Costa A, Mourot S, Romeyer-Bouchard C, et al. Anatomic and electrophysiological differences between chronic and paroxysmal forms of common atrial flutter and comparison with controls. Pacing Clin Electrophysiol 2004;27(9):1202–11.
11. Kalman JM, Olgin JE, Saxon LA, et al. Activation and entrainment mapping defines the tricuspid annulus as the anterior barrier in typical atrial flutter. Circulation 1996;94(3):398–406.
12. Olgin JE, Kalman JM, Lesh MD. Conduction barriers in human atrial flutter: correlation of electrophysiology and anatomy. J Cardiovasc Electrophysiol 1996;7(11):1112–26.
13. Olgin JE, Kalman JM, Fitzpatrick AP, et al. Role of right atrial endocardial structures as barriers to conduction during human type I atrial flutter. Activation and entrainment mapping guided by intracardiac echocardiography. Circulation 1995;92(7):1839–48.
14. Tai CT, Huang JL, Lee PC, et al. High-resolution mapping around the crista terminalis during typical atrial flutter: new insights into mechanisms. J Cardiovasc Electrophysiol 2004;15(4):406–14.
15. Spach MS, Dolber PC, Heidlage JF. Influence of the passive anisotropic properties on directional differences in propagation following modification of the sodium conductance in human atrial muscle. A model of reentry based on anisotropic discontinuous propagation. Circ Res 1988;62(4):811–32.
16. Spach MS, Miller WT III, Dolber PC, et al. The functional role of structural complexities in the propagation of depolarization in the atrium of the dog. Cardiac conduction disturbances due to discontinuities of effective axial resistivity. Circ Res 1982;50(2):175–91.
17. Olgin JE, Kalman JM, Saxon LA, et al. Mechanism of initiation of atrial flutter in humans: site of unidirectional block and direction of rotation. J Am Coll Cardiol 1997;29(2):376–84.
18. Suzuki F, Toshida N, Nawata H, et al. Coronary sinus pacing initiates counterclockwise atrial flutter while pacing from the low lateral right atrium initiates clockwise atrial flutter. Analysis of episodes of direct initiation of atrial flutter. J Electrocardiol 1998;31(4):345–61.
19. Feld GK, Shahandeh-Rad F. Activation patterns in experimental canine atrial flutter produced by right atrial crush injury. J Am Coll Cardiol 1992;20(2):441–51.
20. Haissaguerre M, Sanders P, Hocini M, et al. Pulmonary veins in the substrate for atrial fibrillation: the "venous wave" hypothesis. J Am Coll Cardiol 2004;43(12):2290–2.
21. Sparks PB, Jayaprakash S, Vohra JK, et al. Electrical remodeling of the atria associated with paroxysmal and chronic atrial flutter. Circulation 2000;102(15)):1807–13.
22. Cha Y, Wales A, Wolf P, et al. Electrophysiologic effects of the new class III antiarrhythmic drug dofetilide compared to the class IA antiarrhythmic drug quinidine in experimental canine atrial flutter: role of dispersion of refractoriness in antiarrhythmic efficacy. J Cardiovasc Electrophysiol 1996;7(9):809–27.

23. Oshikawa N, Watanabe I, Masaki R, et al. Relationship between polarity of the flutter wave in the surface ECG and endocardial atrial activation sequence in patients with typical counterclockwise and clockwise atrial flutter. J Interv Card Electrophysiol 2002;7(3):215–23.

24. Okumura K, Plumb VJ, Page PL, et al. Atrial activation sequence during atrial flutter in the canine pericarditis model and its effects on the polarity of the flutter wave in the electrocardiogram. J Am Coll Cardiol 1991;17(2):509–18.

25. Singh BN, Feld G, Nademanee K. Arrhythmia control by selective lengthening of cardiac repolarization: role of N-acetylprocainamide, active metabolite of procainamide. Angiology 1986;37(12 Pt 2):930–8.

26. Kafkas NV, Patsilinakos SP, Mertzanos GA, et al. Conversion efficacy of intravenous ibutilide compared with intravenous amiodarone in patients with recent-onset atrial fibrillation and atrial flutter. Int J Cardiol 2007;118:321–5.

27. Babaev A, Suma V, Tita C, et al. Recurrence rate of atrial flutter after initial presentation in patients on drug treatment. Am J Cardiol 2003;92(9):1122–4.

28. Natale A, Newby KH, Pisano E, et al. Prospective randomized comparison of antiarrhythmic therapy versus first-line radiofrequency ablation in patients with atrial flutter. J Am Coll Cardiol 2000;35(7):1898–904.

29. Feld G, Wharton M, Plumb V, et al. Radiofrequency catheter ablation of type 1 atrial flutter using large-tip 8- or 10-mm electrode catheters and a high-output radiofrequency energy generator: results of a multicenter safety and efficacy study. J Am Coll Cardiol 2004;43(8):1466–72.

30. Da Costa A, Thevenin J, Roche F, et al. Results from the Loire-Ardeche-Drome-Isere-Puy-de-Dome (LADIP) trial on atrial flutter, a multicentric prospective randomized study comparing amiodarone and radiofrequency ablation after the first episode of symptomatic atrial flutter. Circulation 2006;114(16):1676–81.

31. Gilligan DM, Zakaib JS, Fuller I, et al. Long-term outcome of patients after successful radiofrequency ablation for typical atrial flutter. Pacing Clin Electrophysiol 2003;26(1 Pt 1):53–8.

32. Tai CT, Chen SA, Chiang CE, et al. Long-term outcome of radiofrequency catheter ablation for typical atrial flutter: risk prediction of recurrent arrhythmias. J Cardiovasc Electrophysiol 1998;9(2):115–21.

33. Scharf C, Veerareddy S, Ozaydin M, et al. Clinical significance of inducible atrial flutter during pulmonary vein isolation in patients with atrial fibrillation. J Am Coll Cardiol 2004;43(11):2057–62.

34. Fischer B, Haissaguerre M, Garrigues S, et al. Radiofrequency catheter ablation of common atrial flutter in 80 patients. J Am Coll Cardiol 1995;25(6):1365–72.

35. Kirkorian G, Moncada E, Chevalier P, et al. Radiofrequency ablation of atrial flutter. Efficacy of an anatomically guided approach. Circulation 1994;90(6):2804–14.

36. Calkins H, Leon AR, Deam AG, et al. Catheter ablation of atrial flutter using radiofrequency energy. Am J Cardiol 1994;73(5):353–6.

37. Jais P, Haissaguerre M, Shah DC, et al. Successful irrigated-tip catheter ablation of atrial flutter resistant to conventional radiofrequency ablation. Circulation 1998;98(9):835–8.

38. Scavee C, Jais P, Hsu LF, et al. Prospective randomised comparison of irrigated-tip and large-tip catheter ablation of cavotricuspid isthmus-dependent atrial flutter. Eur Heart J 2004;25(11):963–9.

39. Calkins H. Catheter ablation of atrial flutter: do outcomes of catheter ablation with "large-tip" versus "cooled-tip" catheters really differ? J Cardiovasc Electrophysiol 2004;15(10):1131–2.

40. Atiga WL, Worley SJ, Hummel J, et al. Prospective randomized comparison of cooled radiofrequency versus standard radiofrequency energy for ablation of typical atrial flutter. Pacing Clin Electrophysiol 2002;25(8):1172–8.

41. Tsai CF, Tai CT, Yu WC, et al. Is 8-mm more effective than 4-mm tip electrode catheter for ablation of typical atrial flutter? Circulation 1999;100(7):768–71.

42. Ventura R, Klemm H, Lutomsky B, et al. Pattern of isthmus conduction recovery using open cooled and solid large-tip catheters for radiofrequency ablation of typical atrial flutter. J Cardiovasc Electrophysiol 2004;15(10):1126–30.

43. Mangat I, Tschopp DR Jr, Yang Y, et al. Optimizing the detection of bidirectional block across the flutter isthmus for patients with typical isthmus-dependent atrial flutter. Am J Cardiol 2003;91(5):559–64.

44. Poty H, Saoudi N, Abdel Aziz A, et al. Radiofrequency catheter ablation of type 1 atrial flutter. Prediction of late success by electrophysiological criteria. Circulation 1995;92(6):1389–92.

45. Schwartzman D, Callans DJ, Gottlieb CD, et al. Conduction block in the inferior vena caval-tricuspid valve isthmus: association with outcome of radiofrequency ablation of type I atrial flutter. J Am Coll Cardiol 1996;28(6):1519–31.

46. Tada H, Oral H, Sticherling C, et al. Double potentials along the ablation line as a guide to radiofrequency ablation of typical atrial flutter. J Am Coll Cardiol 2001;38(3):750–5.

47. Tai CT, Haque A, Lin YK, et al. Double potential interval and transisthmus conduction time for prediction of cavotricuspid isthmus block after ablation of typical atrial flutter. J Interv Card Electrophysiol 2002;7(1):77–82.

48. Cauchemez B, Haissaguerre M, Fischer B, et al. Electrophysiological effects of catheter ablation of inferior vena cava-tricuspid annulus isthmus in common atrial flutter. Circulation 1996;93(2):284–94.

49. Calkins H, Canby R, Weiss R, et al. Results of catheter ablation of typical atrial flutter. Am J Cardiol 2004;94(4):437–42.

50. Gronefeld GC, Wegener F, Israel CW, et al. Thromboembolic risk of patients referred for radiofrequency catheter ablation of typical atrial flutter without prior appropriate anticoagulation therapy. Pacing Clin Electrophysiol 2003;26(1 Pt 2):323–7.

51. Manusama R, Timmermans C, Limon F, et al. Catheter-based cryoablation permanently cures patients with common atrial flutter. Circulation 2004;109(13):1636–9.

52. Timmermans C, Ayers GM, Crijns HJ, et al. Randomized study comparing radiofrequency ablation with cryoablation for the treatment of atrial flutter with emphasis on pain perception. Circulation 2003;107(9): 1250–2.

53. Feld GK, Daubert JP, Weiss R, et al. Cryoablation Atrial Flutter Efficacy (CAFÉ). Trial Investigators. Acute and long-term efficacy and safety of catheter cryoablation of the cavotricuspid isthmus for treatment of type 1 atrial flutter. Heart Rhythm 2008; 5(7):1009–14.

54. Adragao P, Parreira L, Morgado F, et al. Microwave ablation of atrial flutter. Pacing Clin Electrophysiol 1999;22(11):1692–5.

55. Liem LB, Mead RH. Microwave linear ablation of the isthmus between the inferior vena cava and tricuspid annulus. Pacing Clin Electrophysiol 1998;21(11 Pt 1):2079–86.

56. Iwasa A, Storey J, Yao B, et al. Efficacy of a microwave antenna for ablation of the tricuspid valve–inferior vena cava isthmus in dogs as a treatment for type 1 atrial flutter. J Interv Card Electrophysiol 2004;10(3):191–8.

57. Chan JY, Fung JW, Yu CM, et al. Preliminary results with percutaneous transcatheter microwave ablation of typical atrial flutter. J Cardiovasc Electrophysiol 2007;18(3):286–9.

Postoperative Atrial Fibrillation

Krit Jongnarangsin, MD, Hakan Oral, MD*

KEYWORDS

- Atrial fibrillation • Arrhythmia
- Postoperative • Antiarrhythmic • Surgery

The incidence of atrial fibrillation (AF) in the general population is estimated as 0.4% in patients younger than 70 years, and 2% to 4% in older patients.[1] The incidence of AF is higher in patients with cardiovascular disease. The Cardiovascular Health Study demonstrated that the prevalence of AF was 9.1%, 4.6%, and 1.6% in patients with clinical, subclinical and no cardiovascular disease, respectively.[2] Atrial arrhythmias occur frequently after major cardiothoracic surgery and result in increased morbidity and length of hospital stay.[3–6] The prevalence of atrial arrhythmias after cardiac surgery has been reported to vary between 10% and 65%,[4,7–27] depending on type and technique of surgery, patient characteristics, method of arrhythmia surveillance, and definition of arrhythmia. Postoperative AF may occur in up to 40% of patients undergoing coronary artery bypass surgery,[28–31] 35% to 40% after valvular surgery,[13,28,32] 60% after combined coronary artery bypass graft (CABG) and valve surgery, and 11% to 24% after cardiac transplantation.[13,33] In a large, multicenter, international cohort study, the majority of the initial episodes of AF occurred within the first few (2–5) days after CABG surgery (**Fig. 1**).[29]

PATHOGENESIS

The electrophysiologic mechanisms of AF after cardiac surgery are not yet well understood. However, preexisting atrial substrate, such as atrial fibrosis or dilatation may predispose to atrial fibrillation.[34] Perioperative factors, such as atrial injury or ischemia, inflammation, increase in adrenergic tone, catecholamines, atrial stretch from volume overload, or electrolyte disturbances, may trigger postoperative AF in patients who are susceptible to AF through dispersion of atrial refractoriness,[35,36] nonuniform atrial conduction,[37] or increased premature atrial complexes.[38]

Expression of proinflammatory cytokines and activation of oxidases with an increase in oxidative stress have also been implicated in the genesis of postoperative AF.[39–46] Oxidative stress may decrease atrial effective refractory period and may also promote progressive fibrosis.[47] Consistent with these mechanisms, steroids and statins have been shown to attenuate profibrillatory effects of oxidative stress.[48,49]

CLINICAL IMPLICATIONS

Postoperative AF is associated with increased incidence of postoperative complications and longer length of hospital stay.[7,8,13,29,30] Patients with postoperative AF are more likely to develop hypotension, pulmonary edema,[19] and cerebrovascular accident.[7,8,13,50,51] The incidence of stroke is significantly higher in patients who developed AF after cardiac surgery (3.3% versus 1.4%).[13] The incidence of a composite outcome, including encephalopthy, decline in Mini-Mental State Examination score, increase in National Institutes of Health Stroke Scale score, renal dysfunction, renal failure, pneumonia, mediastinitis or deep sternal wound infection, sepsis, harvest site infection, vascular catheter infection, and genitourinary infection is also higher in patients with postoperative AF (22.6% versus 15.4%).[29] The cost of care on patients who developed postoperative AF was increased by approximately $10,000 per patient.[30]

A version of this article originally appeared in *Medical Clinics of North America*, volume 92, issue 1.
Division of Cardiovascular Medicine, Cardiovascular Center, University of Michigan, Room 2556, 1500 East Medical Center Drive, Ann Arbor, MI 48109-5853, USA
* Corresponding author.
E-mail address: oralh@umich.edu (H. Oral).

Cardiol Clin 27 (2009) 69–78
doi:10.1016/j.ccl.2008.09.011

cardiology.theclinics.com

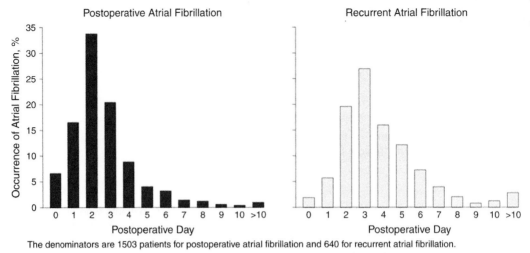

The denominators are 1503 patients for postoperative atrial fibrillation and 640 for recurrent atrial fibrillation.

Fig. 1. Postoperative atrial fibrillation after CABG surgery was most common on postoperative day 2 (*left graph*) and recurrence was most common on postoperative day 3 (*right graph*). More than 60% of initial recurrence occurred within 2 days of first onset. (*Reproduced from* Mathew JP, Fontes ML, Tudor, IC, et al. A multicenter risk index for atrial fibrillation after cardiac surgery. JAMA 2004;291:1720; with permission.)

Postoperative AF is also associated with lower in-hospital and long-term survival. A retrospective cohort study found that patients who developed AF after CABG surgery had higher in-hospital mortality (odds ratio or OR 1.7, P = .0001) and a decrease in survival at 4 to 5 years (74% versus 87%, P<.0001).[30]

PREDICTORS OF ATRIAL FIBRILLATION AFTER CARDIAC SURGERY

Several clinical factors have been shown to be associated with an increased incidence of AF following cardiac surgery.[28,29] These include age, gender, hypertension, prior history of AF, obesity, chronic obstructive pulmonary disease (COPD), left atrial size, and left ventricular ejection fraction.[52]

Older age has been consistently shown in multiple studies as a predictor for postoperative AF. Every 10-year increase in age is associated with a 75% increase in the odds of developing AF and age greater than 70-years old alone is considered to be high risk.[29] The increase in postoperative AF in older age is likely related to degenerative changes in atrial myocardium, dilatation, and nonuniform anisotropic conduction.[53]

Men are more likely to develop AF after CABG surgery than women.[7-9,21,27] Previous history of AF also increases the risk of postoperative AF.[4,11] Hypertension is a predictor of AF in the general population as well as after cardiac surgery.[7,8] Higher body mass index has been shown to be an independent predictor for new-onset AF after cardiac surgery.[52] There is a strong correlation between body mass index and left atrial

enlargement.[54-56] Patients with COPD have been reported to have a 43% increase in the probability of developing postoperative AF,[29] likely because of an increase in P-wave dispersion and heterogeneity of conduction.[57]

PREVENTION

The incidence of AF after cardiac surgery is high, especially in patients with multiple risk factors described above. Although it is often transient, postoperative AF often is associated with increased morbidity and prolonged intensive care unit and hospital stay. Therefore, prophylactic therapy should be considered in all patients, particularly high risk, who are considered for cardiac surgery. Pharmacologic therapy and cardiac pacing have been evaluated in several trials.

Pharmacologic Prophylaxis

β-adrenergic receptor antagonists
β-adrenergic receptor antagonists alone or combined with other antiarrhythmic drugs, such as digitalis or calcium channel blockers, have been commonly used to prevent postoperative AF. Beta-blockers attenuate the effects of beta-adrenergic stimulation, which facilitates vulnerability to AF after cardiac surgery. The efficacy of beta-blockers in reducing the incidence of postoperative AF has been demonstrated in several trials. Therefore, beta-blockers should be administered perioperatively in patients without contraindications as the standard therapy to reduce the incidence of AF after CABG.[58]

Sotalol

Sotalol, a combined β-receptor and potassium channel-blocking agent, has been shown to decrease postoperative AF by 41% to 93% in comparison to placebo.[59–66] Although sotalol was well tolerated, ventricular arrhythmias were reported in two patients among the six trials.[60,61,63–66] However, it is not clear whether sotalol provides an incremental antiarrhythmic effect for postoperative AF prophylaxis compared with regular beta-blockers. Sotalol is considered a class IIb indication for postoperative arrhythmia prevention in the American College of Cardiology/American Heart Association (ACC/AHA) 2004 guideline for CABG surgery, and low-dose sotalol should be considered in patients who are not candidates for traditional beta-blockers.[58]

Amiodarone

Amiodarone is a class III antiarrhythmic agent that inhibits multiple ion channels and α- and β-adrenergic receptors. The efficacy of amiodarone in preventing postoperative AF has been evaluated in multiple randomized trials using various regimens. Overall, it has been shown that amiodarone significantly reduces the incidence of postoperative AF, whether it is administered orally,[67–71] intravenously,[72–75] or both.[76–79] A meta-analysis of 10 trials confirms that amiodarone therapy is associated with a significant reduction in the incidence of postoperative AF or atrial flutter (relative risk or RR 0.64; 95% confidence interval or CI, 0.55–0.75).[80]

In the largest double-blind, randomized, controlled trial of prophylactic oral amiodarone for the prevention of arrhythmias (PAPABEAR),[70] postoperative atrial tachyarrhythmias were reduced by 48% in patients who received oral amiodarone (10 mg/kg daily) 6 days before surgery through 6 days after surgery, in comparison to placebo, as shown in **Fig. 2.** A reduction in postoperative AF was also observed across subgroups predefined according to age, type of cardiac surgery, and concomitant beta-blocker therapy. Although oral amiodarone has been shown to be effective in postoperative AF prophylaxis, it should be administered several days before the surgery. A single-day loading dose of oral amiodarone given 1 day before the cardiac surgery has been shown to be ineffective in preventing postoperative AF.[81] However, intravenous formulation acts more rapidly than oral preparation. The Amiodarone Reduction in Coronary Heart trial[73] demonstrated that low dose intravenous amiodarone (1 g/day for 2 days) administered immediately after cardiac surgery was safe and effective in reducing the incidence of postoperative AF.

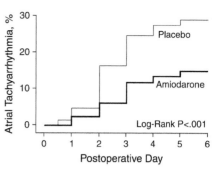

Fig. 2. Posoperative atrial tachyarrhythmia occurred in 48 of 299 (16.1%) patients who were on amiodarone and 89 of 302 (29.5%) patients who were on placebo (hazard ratio or HR, 0.52; 95% CI 0.34–0.69; P<.001). (*Reproduced from* Mitchell LB, Exner DV, Wyse DG, et al. Prophylactic oral amiodarone for the prevention of arrhythmias that begin early after revascularzation valve replacement, or repair; PAPABEAR: A randomized controlled trial. JAMA 2005;294:3093; with permission.)

The efficacy of amiodarone to prevent postoperative AF was shown to be similar to that of beta-blockers in the meta-analysis of prophylactic therapies against postoperative AF.[82] Side effects of amiodarone therapy were uncommon in clinical trials. Amiodarone was discontinued mainly because of bradycardia. Amiodarone is considered a class IIa indication in ACC/AHA 2004 guidelines for CABG surgery. Preoperative administration of amiodarone is an appropriate prophylactic therapy for patients at high risk for postoperative AF who have contraindications to therapy with beta-blockers.[58]

Calcium channel antagonists

Prior studies have demonstrated that verapamil does not have a significant effect on the incidence of postoperative AF.[15,23,24,83] A meta-analysis of randomized, controlled trials also confirmed that verapamil does not reduce the probability of developing supraventricular arrhythmias after CABG (OR 0.91, CI 0.57–1.46).[84] Similar to verapamil, diltiazem was not effective in preventing postoperative AF when compared with placebo.[85] Therefore, nondihydropyridine calcium channel blockers are considered a class IIa indication primarily for ventricular rate control during AF. However, calcium channel blockers have no role in prophylaxis of postoperative AF.[58]

Digitalis

The efficacy of digitalis for postoperative AF prophylaxis has been previously evaluated in randomized, controlled trials. However, results have been conflicting about the potential benefits of digitalis for postoperative AF prophylaxis. Two meta-analyses[84,86] showed no significant reduction in the incidence of supraventricular arrhythmias after CABG in patients receiving digitalis in comparison to controls. However, digitalis may be helpful when administered with beta-blockers. Similar to calcium channel blockers, digitalis has a class IIa indication primarily for ventricular rate control. There is no indication to use digitalis for prevention of postoperative AF.

Magnesium

Hypomagnesemia is common after cardiac surgery and may predispose patients to postoperative arrhythmias. The efficacy of prophylactic magnesium administration on postoperative arrhythmias have been evaluated previously. However, the results have been variable. A meta-analysis of randomized, controlled trials suggested that prophylactic treatment with magnesium reduces postoperative supraventricular arrhythmias by 23% (AF by 29%).[87] Because of conflicting results, prophylactic magnesium therapy is not routinely recommended. However, serum magnesium levels should be maintained in patients undergoing cardiac surgery.[88]

Statins

Statin therapy has been shown to reduce the incidence of postoperative AF after noncardiac thoracic[89] and CABG surgery.[90] Statin therapy was associated with a reduction of postoperative AF regardless of the C-reactive protein levels. A recent randomized, controlled trial demonstrated that atorvastatin (40 mg/d) starting 7 days before cardiac surgery significantly reduced the incidence of postoperative AF in comparison to placebo (OR 0.39, 95% CI 0.18–0.85).[91] Because benefits of statins, besides prevention of postoperative AF, have been well established in patients with coronary artery disease, all patients without contraindications for statin therapy should receive it before CABG surgery.

Corticosteroids

Corticosteroid treatment has been shown to reduce the incidence of postoperative AF after cardiac surgery in previous randomized, controlled trials.[92,93] A prospective, double-blind, randomized multicenter study found that intravenous hydrocortisone reduced the relative risk of postoperative AF by 37% compared with placebo. Corticosteroids may decrease the incidence of postoperative AF by reducing inflammatory response after the surgery. No significant adverse events related to corticosteroid treatment were reported in these trials.[92,94]

Atrial Pacing

The efficacy of temporary atrial overdrive pacing on postoperative AF prevention has been evaluated in a number of studies. Algorithm and site of pacing varied among these studies. Although the results of postoperative AF reduction with right atrial pacing are conflicting,[95–101] most studies showed no significant reduction in postoperative AF.[96–100] In contrast, bi-atrial overdrive pacing has been shown to be effective in preventing postoperative AF.[99,100,102] Postoperative atrial pacing at the Bachmann's bundle was also evaluated in a prior study.[101] Although pacing at the Bachmann's bundle was associated with better pacing thresholds, it did not reduce the incidence of postoperative AF.

Therapy

Although prophylactic therapy can reduce the incidence of postoperative AF, some patients will still develop AF after cardiac surgery. Spontaneous conversion of AF may occur within 2 hours in 15% to 30% and within 24 hours in 25% to 80% of the patients. If AF persists or recurs, two therapeutic strategies of rate and rhythm control may be considered.

Rate control

Rate control is a reasonable option in patients who are asymptomatic and hemodynamically stable. A prior study showed that patients with postoperative AF could be safely discharged home in AF after ventricular rate had been controlled and anticoagulation initiated.[103] Medications that slow atrioventricular nodal conduction, such as beta-blockers, nondihydropyridine calcium-channel blockers (verapamil or diltiazem), or digoxin can be used for rate control. However, beta-blockers seem to be the most effective agent for patients with postoperative AF with rapid ventricular response because of augmented postoperative sympathetic tone. Digoxin alone may control ventricular rate at rest but rarely is adequate when sympathetic tone is high in the postoperative period. Combined therapy may be required to achieve adequate heart rate control. In patients who cannot tolerate beta-blockers or calcium-blockers, intravenous amiodarone is an alternative option for ventricular rate control.[104] Because amiodarone has both sympatholytic and calcium channel blocker action, it is effective in slowing atrioventricular nodal conduction in patients with AF and rapid ventricular response rates.

Rhythm control

Rhythm control is preferred in patients who are highly symptomatic or hemodynamically unstable or when anticoagulation is contraindicated. Sinus rhythm can be restored by either electrical or pharmacologic cardioversion. Direct-current cardioversion should be considered in patients who are hemodynamically unstable because of hypotension or heart failure. In patients with unsuccessful electrical cardioversion or early recurrence of AF, direct-current cardioversion may be repeated after administration of antiarrhythmic drugs, such as ibutilide[105] or amiodarone. Electrical cardioversion using a rectilinear biphasic waveform is more effective than a monophasic sinusoidal waveform.[106]

Pharmacologic conversion can be achieved by class IA (quinidine, procainamide, and disopyramide), class IC (flecanide and propafenone), and class III (amiodarone, sotalol, ibulitide, and dofetilide) agents. Although intravenous administration of class IA and IC agents in patients with AF after CABG surgery results in conversion to sinus rhythm in 40% to 75% of patients within 1 hour,[107–110] and in 50% to 90% of patients within 12 hours,[16,111–114] class IA agents are not available in the United States and can be proarrhythmic in patients with ischemia or impaired left ventricular systolic function. The efficacy of intravenous class III agents for the acute conversion of postoperative AF appears comparable to class IA and IC drugs. However, amiodarone is preferable over the other antiarrhythmic drugs because it also provides ventricular rate control and is less proarrhythmic, particularly in patients with a reduced ejection fraction.

ANTICOAGULATION

Atrial fibrillation is associated with a higher risk of thromboembolic events. There are no specific guidelines for antithrombotic therapy in patients postoperative AF. Antithrombotic therapy is recommended for all patients with AF that persists more than 48 hours to prevent thromboembolic events.[34] The type and intensity of antithrombotic therapy is based upon the risk of thromboembolism. Warfarin with a target international normalized ratio of 2 to 3 is recommended for patients with prior thromboembolism or more than 1 moderate risk factor (age >75, hypertension, heart failure, impaired left ventricular systolic function, and diabetes mellitus). Aspirin 81 mg to 325 mg daily is recommended as an alternative to warfarin in low-risk patients or in those with contraindications to warfarin. Routine anticoagulation with heparin to prevent thrombus formation in patients with postoperative AF is generally not advised because of

---

Box 1
Current recommendations for management of postoperative AF

Class I

Unless contraindicated, treatment with an oral beta-blocker to prevent postoperative AF is recommended for patients undergoing cardiac surgery. (Level of evidence: A)

Administration of AV nodal blocking agents is recommended to achieve rate control in patients who develop postoperative AF. (Level of evidence: B)

Class IIa

Preoperative administration of amiodarone reduces the incidence of AF in patients undergoing cardiac surgery and represents appropriate prophylactic therapy for patients at high risk for postoperative AF. (Level of evidence: A)

It is reasonable to restore sinus rhythm by pharmacologic cardioversion with ibutilide or direct-current cardioversion in patients who develop postoperative AF as advised for nonsurgical patients. (Level of evidence: B)

It is reasonable to administer antiarrhythmic medications in an attempt to maintain sinus rhythm in patients with recurrent or refractory postoperative AF, as recommended for other patients who develop AF. (Level of evidence: B)

It is reasonable to administer antithrombotic medication in patients who develop postoperative AF, as recommended for nonsurgical patients. (Level of evidence: B)

Class IIb

Prophylactic administration of sotalol may be considered for patients at risk of developing AF following cardiac surgery. (Level of evidence: B)

Adapted from Fuster V, Rydén LE, Cannom DS, et al. ACC/AHA/ESC 2006 guidelines for the management of patients with atrial fibrillation—executive summary: a report of the American College of Cardiology/American Heart Association Task Force and the European Society of Cardiology Committee for Practice Guidelines (Writing Committee to Revise the 2001 Guidelines for the Management of Patients With Atrial Fibrillation). J Am Coll Cardiol 2006; 48:854–906; with permission.

---

the risk for postoperative bleeding.[28] Although the incidence of large pericardial effusions and cardiac tamponade was found to be higher in patients receiving warfarin,[115,116] it still can be administered in the immediate after-CABG period with only a minimal risk of bleeding[116] in most patients.

Current recommendations for management of postoperative AF according to the ACC/AHA and European Society of Cardiology 2006 guidelines for the management of patients with atrial fibrillation[34] are summarized in **Box 1**.

SUMMARY

Atrial fibrillation is a common arrhythmia that occurs after cardiac surgery. It is associated with an increase in morbidity, length of hospital stay, and mortality. Patients who are at higher risk of postoperative atrial fibrillation should receive prophylactic treatment. Atrial fibrillation usually resolves spontaneously after heart rate is controlled; however, if patients are highly symptomatic or hemodynamically unstable, sinus rhythm should be restored by electrical or pharmacologic cardioversion. Patients with atrial fibrillation of more than 48 hours should receive antithrombotic therapy for thromboembolism prevention.

REFERENCES

1. Alpert JS, Petersen P, Godtfredsen J. Atrial fibrillation: natural history, complications, and management. Annu Rev Med. 1988;39:41–52.
2. Furberg CD, Psaty BM, Manolio TA, et al. Prevalence of atrial fibrillation in elderly subjects (the Cardiovascular Health Study). Am J Cardiol 1994;74: 236–41.
3. Hravnak M, Hoffman LA, Saul MI, et al. Predictors and impact of atrial fibrillation after isolated coronary artery bypass grafting. Crit Care Med 2002; 30:330–7.
4. Mathew JP, Parks R, Savino JS, et al. Atrial fibrillation following coronary artery bypass graft surgery: predictors, outcomes, and resource utilization. Multicenter study of perioperative ischemia research group. JAMA 1996;276:300–6.
5. Borzak S, Tisdale JE, Amin NB, et al. Atrial fibrillation after bypass surgery: does the arrhythmia or the characteristics of the patients prolong hospital stay? Chest 1998;113:1489–91.
6. Nickerson NJ, Murphy SF, Davila-Roman VG, et al. Obstacles to early discharge after cardiac surgery. Am J Manag Care 1999;5:29–34.
7. Aranki SF, Shaw DP, Adams DH, et al. Predictors of atrial fibrillation after coronary artery surgery. Current trends and impact on hospital resources. Circulation 1996;94:390–7.
8. Almassi GH, Schowalter T, Nicolosi AC, et al. Atrial fibrillation after cardiac surgery: a major morbid event? Ann Surg 1997;226:501–11 [discussion: 511–3].
9. Mendes LA, Connelly GP, McKenney PA, et al. Right coronary artery stenosis: an independent predictor of atrial fibrillation after coronary artery bypass surgery. J Am Coll Cardiol 1995;25: 198–202.
10. Crosby LH, Pifalo WB, Woll KR, et al. Risk factors for atrial fibrillation after coronary artery bypass grafting. Am J Cardiol 1990;66:1520–2.
11. Hashimoto K, Ilstrup DM, Schaff HV. Influence of clinical and hemodynamic variables on risk of supraventricular tachycardia after coronary artery bypass. J Thorac Cardiovasc Surg 1991;101:56–65.
12. Leitch JW, Thomson D, Baird DK, et al. The importance of age as a predictor of atrial fibrillation and flutter after coronary artery bypass grafting. J Thorac Cardiovasc Surg. 1990;100:338–42.
13. Creswell LL, Schuessler RB, Rosenbloom M, et al. Hazards of postoperative atrial arrhythmias. Ann Thorac Surg 1993;56:539–49.
14. Kalman JM, Munawar M, Howes LG, et al. Atrial fibrillation after coronary artery bypass grafting is associated with sympathetic activation. Ann Thorac Surg 1995;60:1709–15.
15. Ferraris VA, Ferraris SP, Gilliam H, et al. Verapamil prophylaxis for postoperative atrial dysrhythmias: a prospective, randomized, double-blind study using drug level monitoring. Ann Thorac Surg 1987; 43:530–3.
16. Gavaghan TP, Feneley MP, Campbell TJ, et al. Atrial tachyarrhythmias after cardiac surgery: results of disopyramide therapy. Aust N Z J Med 1985;15:27–32.
17. Caretta Q, Mercanti CA, De Nardo D, et al. Ventricular conduction defects and atrial fibrillation after coronary artery bypass grafting. Multivariate analysis of preoperative, intraoperative and postoperative variables. Eur Heart J 1991;12:1107–11.
18. Frost L, Molgaard H, Christiansen EH, et al. Atrial ectopic activity and atrial fibrillation/flutter after coronary artery bypass surgery. A case-base study controlling for confounding from age, beta-blocker treatment, and time distance from operation. Int J Cardiol 1995;50:153–62.
19. Yousif H, Davies G, Oakley CM. Peri-operative supraventricular arrhythmias in coronary bypass surgery. Int J Cardiol 1990;26:313–8.
20. Rubin DA, Nieminski KE, Reed GE, et al. Predictors, prevention, and long-term prognosis of atrial fibrillation after coronary artery bypass graft operations. J Thorac Cardiovasc Surg 1987;94:331–5.
21. Fuller JA, Adams GG, Buxton B. Atrial fibrillation after coronary artery bypass grafting. Is it a disorder of the elderly? J Thorac Cardiovasc Surg 1989;97:821–5.
22. Roffman JA, Fieldman A. Digoxin and propranolol in the prophylaxis of supraventricular

tachydysrhythmias after coronary artery bypass surgery. Ann Thorac Surg 1981;31:496–501.

23. Williams DB, Misbach GA, Kruse AP, et al. Oral verapamil for prophylaxis of supraventricular tachycardia after myocardial revascularization. A randomized trial. J Thorac Cardiovasc Surg 1985;90: 592–6.

24. Davison R, Hartz R, Kaplan K, et al. Prophylaxis of supraventricular tachyarrhythmia after coronary bypass surgery with oral verapamil: a randomized, double-blind trial. Ann Thorac Surg 1985;39: 336–9.

25. Tyras DH, Stothert JC Jr, Kaiser GC, et al. Supraventricular tachyarrhythmias after myocardial revascularization: a randomized trial of prophylactic digitalization. J Thorac Cardiovasc Surg 1979; 77:310–4.

26. Ommen SR, Odell JA, Stanton MS. Atrial arrhythmias after cardiothoracic surgery. N Engl J Med 1997;336:1429–34.

27. Zaman AG, Archbold RA, Helft G, et al. Atrial fibrillation after coronary artery bypass surgery: a model for preoperative risk stratification. Circulation 2000; 101:1403–8.

28. Maisel WH, Rawn JD, Stevenson WG. Atrial fibrillation after cardiac surgery. Ann Intern Med 2001; 135:1061–73.

29. Mathew JP, Fontes ML, Tudor IC, et al. A multicenter risk index for atrial fibrillation after cardiac surgery. JAMA 2004;291:1720–9.

30. Villareal RP, Hariharan R, Liu BC, et al. Postoperative atrial fibrillation and mortality after coronary artery bypass surgery. J Am Coll Cardiol 2004;43: 742–8.

31. Lauer MS, Eagle KA, Buckley MJ, et al. Atrial fibrillation following coronary artery bypass surgery. Prog Cardiovasc Dis 1989;31:367–78.

32. Asher CR, Miller DP, Grimm RA, et al. Analysis of risk factors for development of atrial fibrillation early after cardiac valvular surgery. Am J Cardiol 1998; 82:892–5.

33. Pavri BB, O'Nunain SS, Newell JB, et al. Prevalence and prognostic significance of atrial arrhythmias after orthotopic cardiac transplantation. J Am Coll Cardiol 1995;25:1673–80.

34. Fuster V, Ryden LE, Cannom DS, et al. ACC/AHA/ ESC 2006 Guidelines for the management of patients with atrial fibrillation: a report of the American college of cardiology/American heart association task force on practice guidelines and the European society of cardiology committee for practice guidelines (Writing committee to revise the 2001 Guidelines for the management of patients with atrial fibrillation): developed in collaboration with the European heart rhythm association and the heart rhythm Society. Circulation 2006;114: e257–354.

35. Cox JL. A perspective of postoperative atrial fibrillation in cardiac operations. Ann Thorac Surg 1993; 56:405–9.

36. Sato S, Yamauchi S, Schuessler RB, et al. The effect of augmented atrial hypothermia on atrial refractory period, conduction, and atrial flutter/ fibrillation in the canine heart. J Thorac Cardiovasc Surg 1992;104:297–306.

37. Tsikouris JP, Kluger J, Song J, et al. Changes in P-wave dispersion and P-wave duration after open heart surgery are associated with the peak incidence of atrial fibrillation. Heart Lung 2001;30: 466–71.

38. Frost L, Christiansen EH, Molgaard H, et al. Premature atrial beat eliciting atrial fibrillation after coronary artery bypass grafting. J Electrocardiol 1995; 28:297–305.

39. Kim YM, Guzik TJ, Zhang YH, et al. A myocardial Nox2 containing NAD(P)H oxidase contributes to oxidative stress in human atrial fibrillation. Circ Res 2005;97:629–36.

40. Clermont G, Vergely C, Jazayeri S, et al. Systemic free radical activation is a major event involved in myocardial oxidative stress related to cardiopulmonary bypass. Anesthesiology 2002;96:80–7.

41. Levy JH, Tanaka KA. Inflammatory response to cardiopulmonary bypass. Ann Thorac Surg 2003;75: S715–20.

42. Ochoa JJ, Vilchez MJ, Ibanez S, et al. Oxidative stress is evident in erythrocytes as well as plasma in patients undergoing heart surgery involving cardiopulmonary bypass. Free Radic Res 2003;37: 11–7.

43. Gaudino M, Andreotti F, Zamparelli R, et al. The -174G/C interleukin-6 polymorphism influences postoperative interleukin-6 levels and postoperative atrial fibrillation. Is atrial fibrillation an inflammatory complication? Circulation 2003;108(Suppl 1): II195–9.

44. Mihm MJ, Yu F, Carnes CA, et al. Impaired myofibrillar energetics and oxidative injury during human atrial fibrillation. Circulation 2001;104:174–80.

45. Carnes CA, Chung MK, Nakayama T, et al. Ascorbate attenuates atrial pacing-induced peroxynitrite formation and electrical remodeling and decreases the incidence of postoperative atrial fibrillation. Circ Res 2001;89:E32–8.

46. Allessie M, Ausma J, Schotten U. Electrical, contractile and structural remodeling during atrial fibrillation. Cardiovasc Res 2002;54:230–46.

47. Griendling KK, Sorescu D, Ushio-Fukai M. NAD(P)H oxidase: role in cardiovascular biology and disease. Circ Res 2000;86:494–501.

48. Shiroshita-Takeshita A, Schram G, Lavoie J, et al. Effect of simvastatin and antioxidant vitamins on atrial fibrillation promotion by atrial-tachycardia remodeling in dogs. Circulation 2004;110:2313–9.

49. Shiroshita-Takeshita A, Brundel BJ, Lavoie J, et al. Prednisone prevents atrial fibrillation promotion by atrial tachycardia remodeling in dogs. Cardiovasc Res 2006;69:865–75.

50. Reed GL 3rd, Singer DE, Picard EH, et al. Stroke following coronary-artery bypass surgery. A case-control estimate of the risk from carotid bruits. N Engl J Med 1988;319:1246–50.

51. Taylor GJ, Malik SA, Colliver JA, et al. Usefulness of atrial fibrillation as a predictor of stroke after isolated coronary artery bypass grafting. Am J Cardiol 1987;60:905–7.

52. Zacharias A, Schwann TA, Riordan CJ, et al. Obesity and risk of new-onset atrial fibrillation after cardiac surgery. Circulation 2005;112:3247–55.

53. Spach MS, Dolber PC. Relating extracellular potentials and their derivatives to anisotropic propagation at a microscopic level in human cardiac muscle. Evidence for electrical uncoupling of side-to-side fiber connections with increasing age. Circ Res 1986;58:356–71.

54. Pritchett AM, Jacobsen SJ, Mahoney DW, et al. Left atrial volume as an index of left atrial size: a population-based study. J Am Coll Cardiol 2003;41:1036–43.

55. Vaziri SM, Larson MG, Lauer MS, et al. Influence of blood pressure on left atrial size. The Framingham Heart Study. Hypertension 1995;25:1155–60.

56. Gerdts E, Oikarinen L, Palmieri V, et al. Correlates of left atrial size in hypertensive patients with left ventricular hypertrophy: the Losartan Intervention For Endpoint Reduction in Hypertension (LIFE) Study. Hypertension 2002;39:739–43.

57. Tukek T, Yildiz P, Akkaya V, et al. Factors associated with the development of atrial fibrillation in COPD patients: the role of P-wave dispersion. Ann Noninvasive Electrocardiol 2002;7:222–7.

58. Eagle KA, Guyton RA, Davidoff R, et al. ACC/AHA 2004 guideline update for coronary artery bypass graft surgery: summary article. A report of the American college of cardiology/American heart association task force on practice guidelines (Committee to update the 1999 Guidelines for coronary artery bypass graft surgery). J Am Coll Cardiol 2004;44:e213–310.

59. Evrard P, Gonzalez M, Jamart J, et al. Prophylaxis of supraventricular and ventricular arrhythmias after coronary artery bypass grafting with low-dose sotalol. Ann Thorac Surg 2000;70:151–6.

60. Gomes JA, Ip J, Santoni-Rugiu F, et al. Oral d,l sotalol reduces the incidence of postoperative atrial fibrillation in coronary artery bypass surgery patients: a randomized, double-blind, placebo-controlled study. J Am Coll Cardiol 1999;34:334–9.

61. Jacquet L, Evenepoel M, Marenne F, et al. Hemodynamic effects and safety of sotalol in the prevention of supraventricular arrhythmias after coronary artery bypass surgery. J Cardiothorac Vasc Anesth. 1994;8:431–6.

62. Janssen J, Loomans L, Harink J, et al. Prevention and treatment of supraventricular tachycardia shortly after coronary artery bypass grafting: a randomized open trial. Angiology 1986;37:601–9.

63. Matsuura K, Takahara Y, Sudo Y, et al. Effect of sotalol in the prevention of atrial fibrillation following coronary artery bypass grafting. Jpn J Thorac Cardiovasc Surg 2001;49:614–7.

64. Pfisterer ME, Kloter-Weber UC, Huber M, et al. Prevention of supraventricular tachyarrhythmias after open heart operation by low-dose sotalol: a prospective, double-blind, randomized, placebo-controlled study. Ann Thorac Surg 1997;64:1113–9.

65. Suttorp MJ, Kingma JH, Peels HO, et al. Effectiveness of sotalol in preventing supraventricular tachyarrhythmias shortly after coronary artery bypass grafting. Am J Cardiol 1991;68:1163–9.

66. Weber UK, Osswald S, Buser P, et al. Significance of supraventricular tachyarrhythmias after coronary artery bypass graft surgery and their prevention by low-dose sotalol: a prospective double-blind randomized placebo-controlled study. J Cardiovasc Pharmacol Ther 1998;3:209–16.

67. Giri S, White CM, Dunn AB, et al. Oral amiodarone for prevention of atrial fibrillation after open heart surgery, the Atrial Fibrillation Suppression Trial (AFIST): a randomised placebo-controlled trial. Lancet 2001;357:830–6.

68. Daoud EG, Strickberger SA, Man KC, et al. Preoperative amiodarone as prophylaxis against atrial fibrillation after heart surgery. N Engl J Med 1997;337:1785–91.

69. White CM, Giri S, Tsikouris JP, et al. A comparison of two individual amiodarone regimens to placebo in open heart surgery patients. Ann Thorac Surg 2002;74:69–74.

70. Mitchell LB, Exner DV, Wyse DG, et al. Prophylactic oral amiodarone for the prevention of arrhythmias that begin early after revascularization, valve replacement, or repair: PAPABEAR: a randomized controlled trial. JAMA 2005;294:3093–100.

71. Yazigi A, Rahbani P, Zeid HA, et al. Postoperative oral amiodarone as prophylaxis against atrial fibrillation after coronary artery surgery. J Cardiothorac Vasc Anesth 2002;16:603–6.

72. Lee SH, Chang CM, Lu MJ, et al. Intravenous amiodarone for prevention of atrial fibrillation after coronary artery bypass grafting. Ann Thorac Surg 2000;70:157–61.

73. Guarnieri T, Nolan S, Gottlieb SO, et al. Intravenous amiodarone for the prevention of atrial fibrillation after open heart surgery: the Amiodarone Reduction in Coronary Heart (ARCH) trial. J Am Coll Cardiol 1999;34:343–7.

Roy N, et al. Comparison of the acute

...ger TV, et al. ...gnesium sulphate is ...ylaxis for atrial fibrillation ...ery bypass surgery. Br J Anaesth ...00–5.

...te CM, Caron MF, Kalus JS, et al. Intravenous plus oral amiodarone, atrial septal pacing, or both strategies to prevent post-cardiothoracic surgery atrial fibrillation: the Atrial Fibrillation Suppression Trial II (AFIST II). Circulation 2003;108(Suppl 1): II200–6.

77. Yagdi T, Nalbantgil S, Ayik F, et al. Amiodarone reduces the incidence of atrial fibrillation after coronary artery bypass grafting. J Thorac Cardiovasc Surg 2003;125:1420–5.

78. Tokmakoglu H, Kandemir O, Gunaydin S, et al. Amiodarone versus digoxin and metoprolol combination for the prevention of postcoronary bypass atrial fibrillation. Eur J Cardiothorac Surg 2002;21: 401–5.

79. Butler J, Harriss DR, Sinclair M, et al. Amiodarone prophylaxis for tachycardias after coronary artery surgery: a randomised, double blind, placebo controlled trial. Br Heart J 1993;70:56–60.

80. Aasbo JD, Lawrence AT, Krishnan K, et al. Amiodarone prophylaxis reduces major cardiovascular morbidity and length of stay after cardiac surgery: a meta-analysis. Ann Intern Med 2005;143:327–36.

81. Maras D, Boskovic SD, Popovic Z, et al. Single-day loading dose of oral amiodarone for the prevention of new-onset atrial fibrillation after coronary artery bypass surgery. Am Heart J 2001;141:E8.

82. Crystal E, Connolly SJ, Sleik K, et al. Interventions on prevention of postoperative atrial fibrillation in patients undergoing heart surgery: a meta-analysis. Circulation 2002;106:75–80.

83. Smith EE, Shore DF, Monro JL, et al. Oral verapamil fails to prevent supraventricular tachycardia following coronary artery surgery. Int J Cardiol 1985;9: 37–44.

84. Andrews TC, Reimold SC, Berlin JA, et al. Prevention of supraventricular arrhythmias after coronary artery bypass surgery. A meta-analysis of randomized control trials. Circulation 1991;84:III236–44.

85. Babin-Ebell J, Keith PR, Elert O. Efficacy and safety of low-dose propranolol versus diltiazem in the prophylaxis of supraventricular tachyarrhythmia after coronary artery bypass grafting. Eur J Cardiothorac Surg 1996;10:412–6.

86. Kowey PR, Taylor JE, Rials SJ, et al. Meta-analysis of the effectiveness of prophylactic drug therapy in preventing supraventricular arrhythmia early after

artery bypass grafting. Am J Cardiol ...2;69:963–5.

87. Shiga T, Wajima Z, Inoue T, et al. Magnesium prophylaxis for arrhythmias after cardiac surgery: a meta-analysis of randomized controlled trials. Am J Med 2004;117:325–33.

88. Bradley D, Creswell LL, Hogue CW Jr, et al. Pharmacologic prophylaxis: American College of Chest Physicians guidelines for the prevention and management of postoperative atrial fibrillation after cardiac surgery. Chest 2005;128:39S–47S.

89. Amar D, Zhang H, Heerdt PM, et al. Statin use is associated with a reduction in atrial fibrillation after noncardiac thoracic surgery independent of C-reactive protein. Chest 2005;128:3421–7.

90. Hazelrigg SR, Boley TM, Cetindag IB, et al. The efficacy of supplemental magnesium in reducing atrial fibrillation after coronary artery bypass grafting. Ann Thorac Surg 2004;77:824–30.

91. Patti G, Chello M, Candura D, et al. Randomized trial of atorvastatin for reduction of postoperative atrial fibrillation in patients undergoing cardiac surgery: results of the ARMYDA-3 (Atorvastatin for Reduction of MYocardial Dysrhythmia After cardiac surgery) study. Circulation 2006;114: 1455–61.

92. Prasongsukarn K, Abel JG, Jamieson WR, et al. The effects of steroids on the occurrence of postoperative atrial fibrillation after coronary artery bypass grafting surgery: a prospective randomized trial. J Thorac Cardiovasc Surg 2005;130:93–8.

93. Halvorsen P, Raeder J, White PF, et al. The effect of dexamethasone on side effects after coronary revascularization procedures. Anesth Analg 2003; 96:1578–83, table of contents.

94. Halonen J, Halonen P, Jarvinen O, et al. Corticosteroids for the prevention of atrial fibrillation after cardiac surgery: a randomized controlled trial. JAMA 2007;297:1562–7.

95. Blommaert D, Gonzalez M, Mucumbitsi J, et al. Effective prevention of atrial fibrillation by continuous atrial overdrive pacing after coronary artery bypass surgery. J Am Coll Cardiol 2000;35:1411–5.

96. Gerstenfeld EP, Hill MR, French SN, et al. Evaluation of right atrial and biatrial temporary pacing for the prevention of atrial fibrillation after coronary artery bypass surgery. J Am Coll Cardiol 1999;33: 1981–8.

97. Chung MK, Augostini RS, Asher CR, et al. Ineffectiveness and potential proarrhythmia of atrial pacing for atrial fibrillation prevention after coronary artery bypass grafting. Ann Thorac Surg 2000;69: 1057–63.

98. Greenberg MD, Katz NM, Iuliano S, et al. Atrial pacing for the prevention of atrial fibrillation after cardiovascular surgery. J Am Coll Cardiol 2000;35: 1416–22.

99. Fan K, Lee KL, Chiu CS, et al. Effects of biatrial pacing in prevention of postoperative atrial fibrillation after coronary artery bypass surgery. Circulation 2000;102:755–60.

100. Daoud EG, Dabir R, Archambeau M, et al. Randomized, double-blind trial of simultaneous right and left atrial epicardial pacing for prevention of post-open heart surgery atrial fibrillation. Circulation 2000;102:761–5.

101. Goette A, Mittag J, Friedl A, et al. Pacing of Bachmann's bundle after coronary artery bypass grafting. Pacing Clin Electrophysiol 2002;25:1072–8.

102. Levy T, Fotopoulos G, Walker S, et al. Randomized controlled study investigating the effect of biatrial pacing in prevention of atrial fibrillation after coronary artery bypass grafting. Circulation 2000;102:1382–7.

103. Solomon AJ, Kouretas PC, Hopkins RA, et al. Early discharge of patients with new-onset atrial fibrillation after cardiovascular surgery. Am Heart J 1998;135:557–63.

104. Clemo HF, Wood MA, Gilligan DM, et al. Intravenous amiodarone for acute heart rate control in the critically ill patient with atrial tachyarrhythmias. Am J Cardiol 1998;81:594–8.

105. Oral H, Souza JJ, Michaud GF, et al. Facilitating transthoracic cardioversion of atrial fibrillation with ibutilide pretreatment. N Engl J Med 1999;340:1849–54.

106. Wozakowska-Kaplon B, Janion M, Sielski J, et al. Efficacy of biphasic shock for transthoracic cardioversion of persistent atrial fibrillation: can we predict energy requirements? Pacing Clin Electrophysiol 2004;27:764–8.

107. Gentili C, Giordano F, Alois A, et al. Efficacy of intravenous propafenone in acute atrial fibrillation complicating open-heart surgery. Am Heart J 1992;123:1225–8.

108. Geelen P, O'Hara GE, propafenone versus procainamide treatment of atrial fibrillation after cardiac surgery. Am J Cardiol 1999;84:345–7, A8–9.

109. Connolly SJ, Mulji AS, Hoffert DL, et al. Randomized placebo-controlled trial of propafenone for treatment of atrial tachyarrhythmias after cardiac surgery. J Am Coll Cardiol 1987;10:1145–8.

110. Wafa SS, Ward DE, Parker DJ, et al. Efficacy of flecainide acetate for atrial arrhythmias following coronary artery bypass grafting. Am J Cardiol 1989;63:1058–64.

111. Delfaut P, Saksena S, Prakash A, et al. Long-term outcome of patients with drug-refractory atrial flutter and fibrillation after single- and dual-site right atrial pacing for arrhythmia prevention. J Am Coll Cardiol 1998;32:1900–8.

112. Campbell TJ, Morgan JJ. Treatment of atrial arrhythmias after cardiac surgery with intravenous disopyramide. Aust N Z J Med 1980;10:644–9.

113. Campbell TJ, Gavaghan TP, Morgan JJ. Intravenous sotalol for the treatment of atrial fibrillation and flutter after cardiopulmonary bypass. Comparison with disopyramide and digoxin in a randomised trial. Br Heart J 1985;54:86–90.

114. Gavaghan TP, Koegh AM, Kelly RP, et al. Flecainide compared with a combination of digoxin and disopyramide for acute atrial arrhythmias after cardiopulmonary bypass. Br Heart J 1988;60:497–501.

115. Malouf JF, Alam S, Gharzeddine W, et al. The role of anticoagulation in the development of pericardial effusion and late tamponade after cardiac surgery. Eur Heart J 1993;14:1451–7.

116. Weber MA, Hasford J, Taillens C, et al. Low-dose aspirin versus anticoagulants for prevention of coronary graft occlusion. Am J Cardiol 1990;66:1464–8.

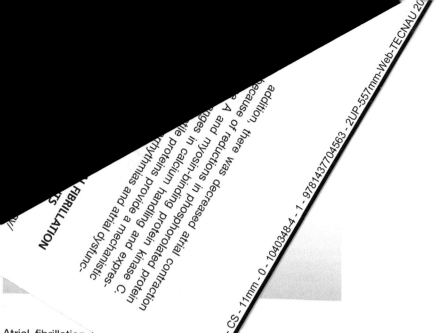

Atrial fibrillation (A...   Failure (CHF) are two co...   conditions and have been a...   modern
"epidemics" in cardiovascu... ...ease by
Braunwald[1] in the New England Journal of Medicine in 1997. Both conditions are increasingly
common with age, with an estimated prevalence
of 5.3 million people over age 20 years with
CHF[2] and 2.2 million adults with AF in the
United States.[3]

In the population-based Framingham Heart
Study, each condition is associated with and
increased risk of developing the other and each increases the mortality risk associated with the
other. The cumulative incidence of first CHF in patients with AF was 15% at 5 years, whereas in patients with CHF, the cumulative incidence of AF
was approximately 25% at 5 years.[4] The
prevalence of AF is related to the extent of the
left ventricular (LV) dysfunction, with AF occurring
in about 10% of New York Heart Association
(NYHA) functional class I/II heart failure and in
to up to 50% of NYHA functional class IV patients
in the large CHF trials.[5] In the Atrial fibrillation
Follow-up and Investigation of Rhythm
Management (AFFIRM) trial, which evaluated the
management of AF in a general population of older
patients with AF, 23% of patients had a history of
CHF.[6]

MECHANISMS

There is a complex interplay between AF and CHF
with heart failure predisposing to AF through atrial
stretch and neurohormonal activation and AF promoting heart failure via fast irregular ventricular
rates and loss atrio-ventricular (AV) synchrony
(Fig. 1). AF results in loss of AV synchrony and
a rapid and irregular ventricular response, which
contribute to the development of CHF. In CHF,
atrial volume and pressure overload contribute to
the development of atrial enlargement, altered
atrial refractory properties, and interstitial fibrosis,
which then predispose to AF development.[5]

AF results in electrical, contractile, and structural remodeling of the atria (Fig. 2).[7] Both rapid
atrial pacing and episodes of AF shorten the atrial
refractory period, resulting in shorter wavelength,
which allows more wavelets to coexist in the
atrium supporting AF. This was the basis of the
concept introduced by Allessie and coworkers
that "atrial fibrillation begets atrial fibrillation."
The ionic mechanisms underlying this process
include reductions in the L-type calcium current
and the transient outward potassium currents occurring over 1 to 2 days, resulting in shortening of
the action potential and in contractile dysfunction.
Within 1 week, signs of structural remodeling
appear with changes in nuclear chromatin, and

Dr. Kalyanam Shivkumar is supported by grants from American Heart Association and the NHLBI
(R01HL084261).
UCLA Cardiac Arrhythmia Center, Division of Cardiology, Department of Medicine, BH 407 CHS, David Geffen
School of Medicine at UCLA, 10833 Le Conte Avenue, Los Angeles, CA 90095-1679, USA
* Corresponding author.
E-mail address: nboyle@mednet.ucla.edu (N.G. Boyle).

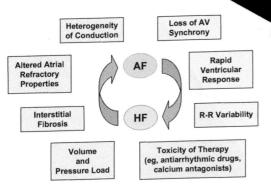

Fig. 1. Mechanisms involved in the interaction of AF and CHF. (*From* Maisel WH, Stevenson LW. Atrial fibrillation in heart failure: epidemiology, pathophysiology, and rationale for therapy. Am J Cardiol 2003;91(6A):2D–8D; with permission.)

by week 4, there is deceased connexin-40, sarcomere distortion, and accumulation of glycogen.

The work of Nattel and colleagues[8–10] has provided significant insights into the mechanisms of CHF-related AF. Using a model of ventricular high-rate pacing-induced CHF (240 beats per minute × 2 weeks in dogs), there was recovery of the ionic remodeling and contractile dysfunction in 4 weeks, but not of the structural remodeling or the ability to maintain AF.[11] This suggests that anatomic remodeling could be the primary factor contributing to AF in CHF. Angiotensin-converting enzyme (ACE) inhibitors can reduce CHF-associated atrial angiotensin II levels and attenuate this anatomic remodeling including atrial fibrosis and conduction abnormalities.[12] CHF-induced AF also resulted in atrial sarcoplasmic reticulum calcium overload and increased triggered activity.[13] The underlying mechanism was a reduction in ryanodine receptor and calsequestrin expression. In

kinas̸͟...
These cha̸...
sion of contrac̸...
link between atrial a̸...
tion seen in CHF.

CLINICAL MANAGEMENT OF ATRIA̸ IN CONGESTIVE HEART FAILURE PATIEN̸

The most recent American College of Cardiology̸ American Heart Association/European Society of Cardiology (ACC/AHA/ESC) guidelines on the management of AF were published in 2006 and provide an extensive referenced document on the management of AF (**Fig. 3**).[14] When AF is initially suspected clinically, the diagnosis should be confirmed by electrocardiogram, Holter, or an event monitor. It is helpful, both in terms of treatment and prognosis, to classify it as paroxysmal (self-terminating episodes lasting <48 hours), persistent (not self-terminating and lasting from 48 hours to 6 months), and permanent or chronic (>6 months for which cardioversion has failed or has not been attempted). Often the clinical group to which a patient belongs will not be clear for a period of time, especially until cardioversion is attempted.

Optimal heart failure management with current state-of-the-art evidence-based therapy forms the basis of treatment in all heart failure patients with AF.[15] This includes ACE inhibitor or an angiotensin-receptor blocker (ARB) for all patients with maximum-tolerated doses of beta blockers. Diuretics, aldosterone antagonists, digoxin, and cardiac resynchronization therapy should be used as appropriate. It is noteworthy that these optimal heart failure therapies may also be beneficial in the treatment of AF as discussed below.

THERAPEUTIC APPROACH

The initial treatment approach to AF involves the standard approach targeting three different aspects of the condition: (1) risk assessment for thromboembolism and anticoagulation as appropriate, (2) ventricular rate control, and (3) assessment for conversion to and maintenance of sinus rhythm.

Anticoagulation

Although we do not have specific trials on anticoagulation in patients with AF and CHF, the major clinical trials on anticoagulation reported in the 1990s[16] included many patients with CHF—approximately 25% overall and 50% in the Danish

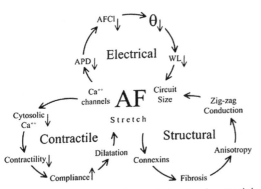

Fig. 2. Electrical, contractile, and structural remodeling in atrial fibrillation. (*From* Allessie M, Ausma J, Schotten U. Electrical, contractile and structural remodeling during atrial fibrillation. Cardiovasc Res 2002;54(2):230–46; with permission).

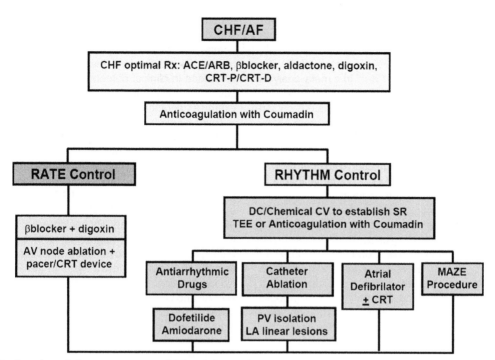

Fig. 3. Overview of the management of AF and CHF patients.

Atrial Fibrillation, Aspirin and Anticoagulant Therapy (AFASAK) trial. In the CHADS$_2$ (CHF, Hypertension, Age >75 years, Diabetes [each 1 point] and Stroke [2 points]) scoring system for stroke risk evaluation,[17] heart failure is assigned one point with an associated annual stroke risk of 2.8%; if the common associated conditions of hypertension and diabetes are added to CHF, yielding a total score of three, then the annual stroke rate is 5.9% (**Table 1**). The CHADS$_2$ score is

Table 1
Stroke risk in patients with nonvalvular atrial fibrillation not treated with anticoagulation according to CHADS$_2$ index

CHADS$_2$ Risk Criteria		Score
Prior stroke or transient ischemic attack		2
Age >75 yr		1
Hypertension		1
Diabetes mellitus		1
Heart failure		1
Patients (N = 1733)	Adjusted Stroke Rate (%/yr)* (95% CI)	CHADS$_2$ Score
120	1.9 (1.2 to 3.0)	0
463	2.8 (2.0 to 3.8)	1
523	4.0 (3.1 to 5.1)	2
337	5.9 (4.6 to 7.3)	3
220	8.5 (6.3 to 11.1)	4
65	12.5 (8.2 to 17.5)	5
5	18.2 (10.5 to 27.4)	6

Data from Fuster V, Ryden LE, Cannom DS, et al. ACC/AHA/ESC 2006 Guidelines for the Management of Patients with Atrial Fibrillation. Circulation 2006;114(7):e257–354.

a good predictor of stroke risk in clinical practice.[18] In an analysis of the Sudden Cardiac Death in Heart Failure trial population (class II or III CHF, ejection fraction (EF) $\leq$35%; no history of VT), the annual stroke rate was 1.7%.[19] In a meta-analysis of five major trials, Coumadin was associated with a 68% reduction in the stroke risk, whereas aspirin results in only a 21% reduction. The current American College of Chest Physicians guidelines classify CHF as a major risk factor for stroke and also recommend anticoagulation with coumadin.[20] Multiple clinical trials looking at other inhibitors of thrombin or factor Xa are ongoing.[21]

Nonpharmacologic approaches, such as left atrial appendage occluder devices ("watchman") currently are undergoing clinical trials for use in patients who cannot take Coumadin because of bleeding risks;[22] however, serious complications may also be associated with these devices.[23] It is worth remembering that only 65% of embolic strokes in patients with AF are thought to originate in the left atrial appendage, with the remainder caused by other mechanisms.[24]

Rate control

For acute rate control in a patient presenting with AF and rapid ventricular rate, in the setting of CHF, either an intravenous beta blocker or a calcium channel blocker such as diltiazem can be used to achieve short-term rate control.[25] In the chronic AF setting, the most effective drug therapy for rate control is a combination of a beta blocker and digoxin, already appropriate therapy in the heart failure setting. Carvedilol in combination with digoxin has also been shown to be superior to either carvedilol or digoxin alone.[26] In the AFFIRM and AF-CHF trials, effective rate control, defined as a heart rate less than 80 beats per minute at rest and less than 110 beats per minute with moderate exercise such as the 6-minute walk was achieved in more than 80% of patients assigned to this strategy by year 5 of follow-up.[27]

In approximately 5% of patients in the AFFIRM trial, rate control drug therapy was deemed ineffective, and AV node ablation and pacing was needed. Two trials have compared rate control drug therapy with AV node ablation and pacing. In an Australian trial of patients with chronic AF without CHF, there was no difference in exercise duration or ejection fraction at 12 months of follow-up; however, better rate control with exercise and quality-of-life measurements were found in the AV node ablation and pacer group.[28] In an Italian trial of patients with chronic AF with CHF (mean EF, 40%), there was no difference in exercise tolerance or measured EF at 1 year of follow-up, but the AV node ablation and pacer group

experience decreased symptoms of palpitations and dyspnea. In a meta-analysis of all six trials comparing AV junction ablation and pacer with pharmacologic therapy, there was no statistical difference in clinical outcomes including survival, stroke, hospitalization, functional class, EF, or exercise tolerance.[29]

There is much debate on whether chronic right ventricular pacing in itself can promote right ventricle (RV) dyssynchrony and possible worsen CHF.[30] Cardiac resynchronization therapy may provide improved outcomes when compared with RV pacing alone in the setting of AF and CHF.[31] In a nonrandomized trial of patients with permanent AF, AV node ablation, and RV pacing in whom class III-IV CHF developed, upgrading to biventricular pacing resulted in improvement in functional status and EF at 6 months' follow-up.[32] In the Post AV Nodal Ablation Evaluation (PAVE) trial, patients with AF and CHF (class II–III, mean EF 46%) undergoing AV nodal ablation were randomly assigned to either biventricular or right ventricular pacing.[33] At 6 months' follow-up, the biventricular pacing group has improved 6-minute walk and ejection fraction compared with the right ventricular pacing group, with most improvement seen in those with lower EF. In a meta-analysis looking at three available randomized trials of patients with AF treated with AV node ablation and randomly assigned to cardiac resynchronization therapy (CRT) versus RV pacing, the investigators found that CRT was associated with a statistically significant improvement in EF in two of the three trials and a trend toward reduced all-cause mortality.[29] Large-scale randomized trials are still needed to answer this question. Permanent para-Hisian pacing may offer another option to prevent development of ventricular dyssynchrony after AV node ablation in patients with permanent AF.[34]

Rhythm control—acute conversion

Direct current cardioversion with a biphasic shock is the most effective method to acutely establish sinus rhythm in a patient with AF, with initial success rates greater than 90%.[35] For pharmacologic cardioversion, digoxin is no better than placebo,[36] and although ibutilide is approximately 50% successful for acute conversion of AF, it is associated with a 5% risk of torsades de pointes in patients with CHF and is probably best avoided in this group except for possibly cardiac care unit settings.[37] Oral class I drugs, propafenone and flecainaide, used as a "pill in the pocket approach" are highly effective in acutely restoring sinus rhythm in a paroxysmal AF population without structural heart disease;[38] however, the use of class I drugs is contraindicated in CHF patients because of the risks of pro-arrhythmia.[39] Although amiodarone is not usually considered a first choice drug for restoring sinus rhythm, when loaded intravenously and followed by a high-dose orally, it is approximately 60% effective in restoring sinus rhythm in 24 hours in a mixed group of paroxysmal and persistent patients with AF.[40] However, the efficacy of any drug used for chemical cardioversion will decrease depending on the duration of the AF.

Current guidelines indicate that chemical or electrical cardioversion may be undertaken after anticoagulation with Coumadin and a therapeutic International Normalized Ratio (INR) for approximately 1 month or after a negative transesophageal echocardiogram (TEE).[14] In the Assessment of Cardioversion using Transesophageal Echocardiography trial, 1222 patients were randomly assigned to either standard approach of anticoagulation with Coumadin for 1 month followed by cardioversion versus TEE and early cardioversion if negative for thrombus; at 8 weeks of follow-up, clinical outcomes for embolic events, and for restoration and maintenance of sinus rhythm were equivalent.[41] Approximately one quarter of the patients in this trial had a history of CHF and 15% were NYHA class III or IV. The *approach* of TEE followed by early cardioversion may be particularly useful for patients with AF and worsening CHF.

Rhythm control—maintenance of sinus rhythm
There are multiple studies in the literature comparing antiarrhythmic drug therapies for maintenance of sinus rhythm in patients with AF.[42] Three major trials reported in this decade make the overall findings clear. In the Canadian Trial of Atrial Fibrillation, Amiodarone was superior to sotalol or propafenone in the maintenance of sinus rhythm over a 5-year follow-up.[43] In the antiarrhythmic drug substudy of the AFFIRM trial[44] and the SAFE –T trial,[45] the results were similar. Overall amiodarone was approximately 70% effective in maintaining sinus rhythm and Sotalol or class I drugs approximately 40% effective at 1 year for patients with persistent AF. Amiodarone has also been shown not to increase mortality in patients with heart failure in the Grupo de Estudio de la Sobrevida en la Insuficienca Cardica en Argentina (GESICA) Trial[46] and Congestive Heart Failure—Survival Trial of Antiarrhythmic Therapy (CHF-STAT)[47] studies. The proarrhythmic effects of Sotalol and the class I drugs and the well-known organ toxic side effects of Amiodarone have propelled the search for new antiarrhythmic drugs.[39]

Dofetilide is a newer class III antiarrhythmic agent for the approved for the maintenance of sinus rhythm by the US Food and Drug Administration (FDA) in 1999. Dofetilide was evaluated specifically in heart failure patients (predominantly class II–III) in the Danish Investigators of Arrhythmia and Mortality on Dofetilide (DIAMOND)-CHF trial.[48] In a 3-year follow-up, there was no difference in survival rate between the dofetilide and placebo groups. Although dofetilide was poor at achieving chemical cardioversion (12% at 1 month), it was effective at maintaining sinus rhythm (approximately 75% at 1 year). There was a 3.3% incidence of torsades in the dofetilide group. This has led to the FDA current "black box" warning with dofetilide and the mandatory in hospital initiation by the manufacturer, limiting its utility compared with amiodarone. Interestingly dofetilide may be more effective in patients with persistent AF compared with those with paroxysmal AF.[49]

Dronedarone currently is an investigational drug for the treatment of AF. It has received much attention because it is a noniodinated derivative of amiodarone developed with the aim of reducing adverse effects while maintaining the efficacy of amiodarone. In addition, in a report of combined US (African American Trial of Dronedarone in Atrial Fibrillation) and European (European Trial of Dronedarone in Atrial Fibrillation) trials for non–heart failure patients with AF, dronedarone more than doubled the median time to recurrence of AF compared with placebo and was not associated with any increase in pulmonary, thyroid, or liver dysfunction at 12 months of follow-up.[50] In the A Trial of Dronedarone For Prevention Of Hospitalization in Patients with AF (ATHENA) trial, 4628 patients with paroxysmal AF were randomly assigned to dronedarone, 400 mg versus placebo; of note, 20% of patients had a history of class II or III CHF. The primary outcome of death or cardiovascular hospitalization was reduced by 24% and all-cause mortality by 16% with a mean follow-up of 1 year.[51] However, when used prophylactically in patients with class II–III heart failure in the Antiarrhythmic Trial in Heart Failure in the Antiarrhythmic Trial in Heart Failure (ANDROMEDA) study, dronedarone was associated with increased mortality primarily caused by worsening heart failure.[52] There was also an increase in renal insufficiency in the dronedarone group. The results of this trial have been widely debated—it has been suggested that the decrease or discontinuation of ACE inhibitors in patients who had worsening renal function may explain the increase in mortality rate from CHF in the treated group.[53]

RATE CONTROL VERSUS RHYTHM CONTROL
The AFFIRM and AF-CHF Trials

The definite AFFIRM trial compared rate control drug therapy with rhythm control drug therapy (reflecting the standard drug therapy of the mid 1990s).[6] There was no difference in mortality or thromboembolic events between the two treatment groups. Four smaller rate control versus rhythm control trials—Pharmacologic Intervention in Atrial Fibrillation (PIAF),[54] Rate Control versus Electrical Cardioversion of Persistent Atrial Fibrillation (RACE),[55] Strategies of Treatment of Atrial Fibrillation (STAF),[56] and How to Treat Chronic Atrial Fibrillation (HOT CAFE)[57] looked at clinical endpoints only, and all showed no statistical difference between the defined clinical endpoints (**Table 2**).[58] It was notable in AFFIRM that at 5 years, 63% of the "rhythm control" group and 35% of the "rate control" group were in sinus rhythm; conversely, rate control as defined in the trial (heart rate, <80 at rest and <110 with moderate exercise), was successfully achieved in 70% to 80% of those assigned to this group.[27] This highlights a fundamental problem with all these studies—antiarrhythmic drugs are ineffective at actually achieving rhythm control, whereas AV nodal blocking drugs are relatively effective at achieving rate control. Hence, the trials are really comparing a rhythm control strategy with a rate control strategy, with the available drug therapy. Interestingly, only two variables in an AFFIRM subset analysis were possibly associated with a better outcome for rhythm control: age <65 years and CHF.

The Atrial Fibrillation and Congestive Heart Failure (AF-CHF) trial is a multicenter randomized trial comparing medical therapies for rhythm control versus rate control in a population with AF, EF less than 35%, and congestive heart failure (NYHA class II-IV) (**Fig. 4**).[59] A total of 1376 patients were randomly assigned to rate control (n = 694; beta blocker or digoxin or both) or rhythm control (n = 682; overwhelmingly, amiodarone was used), and followed up for a mean of 37 months. The average age was 67 years, 18% were women, 31% were NYHA class III or IV, and the mean EF was 27%. Fifty percent had been hospitalized previously for CHF, 31% had paroxysmal AF, 71% had persistent AF, and approximately 90% of patients in both groups received oral anticoagulation. A flow chart showing the design and outcomes of the trial is shown in **Fig. 4**. At follow-up visits, the prevalence of AF was approximately 60% in the rate control group and 20% to 30% in the rhythm control group over 4 years. In the rate control group, the target heart rate of less than 80 at rest and less than 110 during a 6-minute walk was achieved in approximately 85% of the patients studied during 3 years of follow-up.

The primary outcome—cardiovascular mortality—was 27% in the rhythm control group and 25% in the rate control group (hazard ratio [HR], 1.06; confidence interval [CI]: 0.86–1.30; P value

Table 2
Rate Control versus Rhythm Control Trials

	PIAF	STAF	RACE	AFFIRM
No.	252	200	522	4060
Follow-up (range)	1 yr	19.6 mo (0-36)	2.3 yr	3.5 yr (3.5–6)
Mean age (yr)	61.5	65.8	68	69.7
Duration of AF	<360 d	<2 yr	<1 yr	<6 mo
Important inclusion criteria	Symptomatic patients	Moderate risk of AF recurrence	1–2 previous DCC within 2 years	High risk of AF recurrence
Primary endpoint	Symptom improvement	Composite[a]	Composite[b]	Overall mortality
Rhythm control	55.1%	10%	22.6%	23.8% (at 5 yr)
Rate control	60.8%	9%	17.2%	21.8% (at 5 yr)
P (primary end point)	0.317	0.99	0.11	0.08

[a] Combination death, stroke, or transient ischemic attack, cardiopulmonary resuscitation, or systemic embolism.
[b] Death from cardiovascular causes, heart failure, thromboembolic complications, bleeding, implantation of a pacemaker, or severe adverse effects of anti-arrhythmic drugs.
    Abbreviation: DCC, direct current cardioversion.
    Data from Fuster V, Ryden LE, Cannom DS, et al. ACC/AHA/ESC 2006 Guidelines for Management of Patients with Atrial Fibrillation. Circulation 2006:114(7):e257–354; and Chung MK. Randomized trials of rate control versus rhythm control for atrial fibrillation. Journal of Interventional Cardiac Electrophysiology 2004;10:45–53.

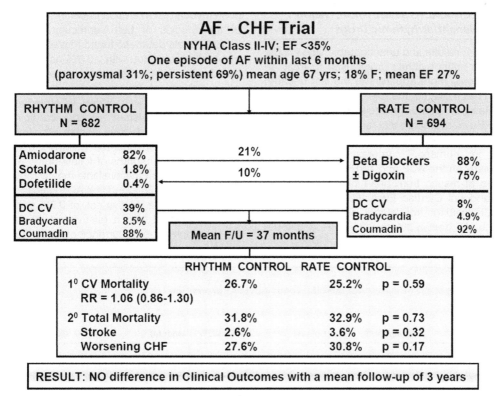

Fig. 4. Flow chart shows design and results of AF-CHF trial.

not significant). Secondary outcomes including all-cause mortality, stroke, and worsening heart failure were the same in both groups. This result mirrors the findings of the main AFFIRM trial;[6] an analysis of AFFIRM stratified by ejection fraction (<30%, 30%–39%, 40%–49%)[60] and other rate-versus-rhythm control trials, showed no survival or clinical advantage for a rhythm control strategy.

Several explanations have been suggested for these findings.[59,61] First antiarrhythmic drugs, even amiodarone, are ineffective at maintaining sinus rhythm (0 ~ 30% relapse rate), and up to 40% of patients in the rate control group were in sinus rhythm at some time during the follow-up; hence, a greater difference in the prevalence of sinus rhythm between the two groups may have been necessary to show a reduction in mortality with rhythm control. Second, it is possible that any benefit achieved in maintaining sinus rhythm was counterbalanced by the harmful effect of antiarrhythmic drugs. Third, radiofrequency (RF) ablation was not used in this trial as a treatment option for AF, which offers the possibility of achieving sinus rhythm without the toxicities of antiarrhythmic drugs. Fourth, at the end of the trial recruitment in June 2005, only 16% of the patients had received an implantable cardioverter defibrillator (ICD) implant, based on standard care

approached in that period; this could have influenced outcomes because approximately one third of all deaths in the trial were presumed associated with arrhythmia. It is also possible that AF may be a marker of an overall poor prognosis and not independently associated with survival.

SINUS RHYTHM AND SURVIVAL

There are some intriguing pointers that sinus rhythm, if achievable without drug toxicity or procedure or device complications, is a marker for improved survival. An analysis of the CHF-STAT study found that patients with AF and CHF treated with Amiodarone who converted to and remained in sinus rhythm had an improved survival rate.[62] In a substudy of the DIAMOND trials, for patients with ejection fraction less than 35%, the maintenance of sinus rhythm at 1 year was associated with a significant reduction in mortality, either with dofetilide or placebo (relative risk [RR] = 0.44).[63] An analysis of the AFFIRM trial outcomes found that sinus rhythm (HR = 0.54) and warfarin use (HR = 0.47) were associated with increased survival.[64] It remains to be confirmed in future randomized trials if newer therapies that can maintain sinus rhythm without toxicities will prove superior to rate control therapy.

FROM ELECTRICAL TO STRUCTURAL THERAPY
Role of Nonantiarrhythmic Drugs

As the poor results and unacceptable side effects of current antiarrhythmic drugs used to treat AF have become more apparent in the last decade, interest has moved to the role of other drug therapies. Basic studies on the role of ACE inhibitors and ARBs in reversing atrial remodeling have provided a basis to evaluate these drugs as AF therapies in humans.[65] Interest has focused particularly on the ACE and ARB drugs based on analysis of results from heart failure studies. In the Trandopril Cardiac Evaluation (TRACE) trial, the ACE inhibitor trandolapril reduced the incidence of AF from 5.3% to 2.8% (RR = 0.45) in post–myocardial infarction patients.[66] An analysis of the Studies of Left Ventricular Dysfunction (SOLVD) trials database found that enalapril treatment was associated with a 5.4% risk of AF compared with a 24% risk in the treatment group (HR = 0.22).[67]

When enalapril was added to amiodarone in patients with persistent AF after cardioversion, the maintenance of sinus rhythm was improved compared with amiodarone therapy alone (74% versus 57% at 9 months of follow-up).[68] A meta-analysis looking at the available mostly retrospective studies to 2005 found that ACE inhibitors were associated with a relative risk of 0.78, and ARBs were associated with a relative risk of 0.71 for the development or recurrence of AF (**Table 3**).[69]

Table 3
Meta-analysis of the effects of ACE inhibitors and ARBs in AF prevention

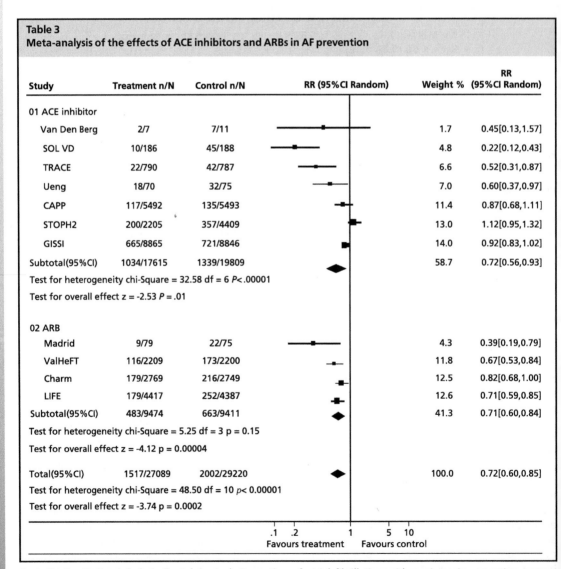

Study	Treatment n/N	Control n/N	RR (95%CI Random)	Weight %	RR (95%CI Random)
01 ACE inhibitor					
Van Den Berg	2/7	7/11		1.7	0.45[0.13,1.57]
SOL VD	10/186	45/188		4.8	0.22[0.12,0.43]
TRACE	22/790	42/787		6.6	0.52[0.31,0.87]
Ueng	18/70	32/75		7.0	0.60[0.37,0.97]
CAPP	117/5492	135/5493		11.4	0.87[0.68,1.11]
STOPH2	200/2205	357/4409		13.0	1.12[0.95,1.32]
GISSI	665/8865	721/8846		14.0	0.92[0.83,1.02]
Subtotal(95%CI)	1034/17615	1339/19809		58.7	0.72[0.56,0.93]
Test for heterogeneity chi-Square = 32.58 df = 6 P<.00001					
Test for overall effect z = -2.53 P = .01					
02 ARB					
Madrid	9/79	22/75		4.3	0.39[0.19,0.79]
ValHeFT	116/2209	173/2200		11.8	0.67[0.53,0.84]
Charm	179/2769	216/2749		12.5	0.82[0.68,1.00]
LIFE	179/4417	252/4387		12.6	0.71[0.59,0.85]
Subtotal(95%CI)	483/9474	663/9411		41.3	0.71[0.60,0.84]
Test for heterogeneity chi-Square = 5.25 df = 3 p = 0.15					
Test for overall effect z = -4.12 p = 0.00004					
Total(95%CI)	1517/27089	2002/29220		100.0	0.72[0.60,0.85]
Test for heterogeneity chi-Square = 48.50 df = 10 p< 0.00001					
Test for overall effect z = -3.74 p = 0.0002					

.1 .2   1   5 10
Favours treatment   Favours control

From Healey JS, Baranchuk A, Crystal E, et al. Prevention of atrial fibrillation with angiotensin-converting enzyme inhibitors and angiotensin receptor blockers a meta-analysis. J Am Coll Cardiol 2005;45(11):1832–9; with permission.

More recent studies, however, have shown less impressive results. In the Heart Outcomes Prevention Trial (HOPE), use of the ACE inhibitor ramipril was not associated with any reduction in the incidence of AF in patients without systolic dysfunction, although the incidence of AF was low at 5%.[70] In a single-center, double-blind randomized study, treatment with the ARB candesartan for 6 weeks before and 6 months after electrical cardioversion of persistent AF had no effect on the recurrence of AF.[71] Large ongoing randomized trials such as the ACTIVE-I trial[72] should provide more reliable information on the role of ACE and ARBs in AF treatment. The role of nonantiarrhythmic drugs such as statins, fish oil, and anti-inflammatory agents continues to be investigated actively.[73,74] This represents a paradigm shift in the treatment of AF from electrical to structural therapy (**Fig. 5**);[75,76] however, the precise role of these therapies in clinical practice remains to be established.

NONPHARMACOLOGIC THERAPY
Cardiac Resynchronization Therapy

Biventricular pacing has emerged in the last decade as an additional treatment for patients with advanced CHF, left bundle branch block (LBBB), and EF less than 35% refractory to medical therapy. Large clinical trials in patients with sinus rhythm have shown clinical benefit in approximately two thirds of patients implanted.[77,78]

Although there are randomized trials specifically for CHF patients with AF, information is available from several smaller trials and substudies. In the Multisite Stimulation in Cardiomyopathy (MUSTIC) trial, a crossover substudy of patients with chronic AF (n = 45) and class III CHF, biventricular pacing resulted in improved clinical outcomes and decreased hospitalizations.[79] Approximately 60% of the patients required AV node ablation to ensure ventricular pacing. In a prospective multicenter study comparing permanent AF patients (n = 1620) with sinus rhythm patients treated with CRT (n = 511), both groups had significant improvement in clinical parameters.[80] However, within the AF group, only those who underwent AV node ablation (n = 114) had a significant increase in ejection fraction and exercise tolerance. The authors of the study emphasized the importance of AV node ablation for optimal results in patients with permanent AF and CHF undergoing a CRT device implant in this study as well as in a recent study in which they also showed improved survival CHF patients with AF treated with CRT.[81] However, another single-center, prospective study comparing CRT in patients with AF (n = 86) and sinus rhythm (n = 209) showed significant and comparable clinical endpoint improvements in both groups, without the need for AV node ablation in the AF patients.[82] A randomized trial is again awaited.[83]

Conversely, it is of interest to ask if CRT prevents development of AF in patients with CHF. In

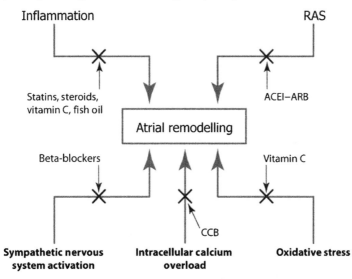

Multiple pathways leading to atrial remodelling that predisposes the atria to atrial fibrillation

Dorian, P. et al. Eur Heart J Suppl 2008 10:H11-31; doi:10.1093/eurheartj/sun033

Fig. 5. Proposed mechanisms for nonantiarrhythmic drugs in AF (*From* Dorian P, Singh BN. Upstream therapies to prevent atrial fibrillation. European Heart Journal Supplements 2008; 10(Supplement H):H11–H31; with permission.)

Table 4
RF ablation of AF in CHF studies

Study (Yr)	n	Baseline, EF (%)	Paroxysmal or Persistent AF, %	Procedure (Second Procedure)	Complications Rate	Follow-Up (mo)	Increase in EF	%SR at 1 yr (+AAD)
Chen et al.[91] (2004)	94	<40	67	PVI, LA abl. (22%)	3.1%			69% (78%)
Hsu et al.[92] (2004)	58	35	15	PVI, LA abl. (50%)	3%	12	+21%	69% (78%)
PABA-CHF (2006)	39	28	55	PVI	—	6	+8%	72% (90%)
Gentlesk et al.[93] (2007)	67	42	100	PVI (60%)	—	20	+14%	57% (86%)
Efremidis et al.[94] (2008)	13	35	77	PVI, LA abl.	0	9	+22.5	62% (—)
Lutomsky et al.[95] (2008)	18	41	100	PVI	—	6	+10%	50% (—)

Abbreviations: abl, ablation; LA, left atrial ablation; PVI, pulmonary vein isolation.

the Cardiac Resynchronization in Heart Failure Study (CARE-HF) trial[78] (n = 813), CRT did not result in any difference in the incidence of AF (approx. 15%) at 30 months of follow-up. CRT improved the clinical outcomes regardless of whether AF occurred.[84] We[85] and others[86] have found that patients with CHF who respond to CRT have shorter duration of AF, a lower likelihood of persistent AF, and evidence of reverse atrial remodeling. In the first reported randomized trial of an algorithm for AF prevention with atrial overdrive pacing in patients receiving CRT, no benefit was seen.[87]

Catheter Ablation

Since it was first described in 1998,[88] catheter ablation targeting pulmonary vein isolation for the treatment of AF has developed at a rapid rate.[89] Currently reported success rates average 70% to 90% at 1 year in maintaining sinus rhythm for persistent and paroxysmal AF; however, serious complications can arise.[90] A total of 6 nonrandomized studies (Table 4) have been reported. Five studies[91–95] have compared the outcomes of RF ablation in patients with AF, decreased EF, and history of CHF with those in non-CHF control patients. Although these are single-center studies with only small numbers of patients, the percentage of patients in SR at 1 year and the complication rates are consistent with the results for AF ablation in non-CHF patients. There was a consistent improvement in EF and decrease in the need for antiarrhythmic drugs. In one study,[92] patients with inadequate rate control before ablation had the most marked improvement in EF (86% of patients classified as inadequate rate control had an increase of >20% in EF), suggesting the role of tachycardia-mediated cardiomyopathy in CHF patients with AF may be much more significant than previously appreciated. One study, the Pulmonary Vein Antral Isolation versus Atrioventricular Node Ablation with Biventricular Pacing for the Treatment of AF in patients with CHF (PABA-CHF) trial, reported in abstract form,[96] compared pulmonary vein isolation (PVI) with atrioventricular node (AVN) node ablation and biventricular pacing in patients with AF and CHF (EF < 40%). The PVI approach resulted in significant improvement in EF and 6-minute walk test not seen in the AVN ablation and pacing group.

It remains to be shown in a multicenter, randomized trial that RF ablation is truly superior to antiarrhythmic drug (AAD) therapy as some single center studies have found.[97] In a recent meta-analysis of six trails, mostly single center, RF ablation reduced the risk of recurrence of AF at 1 year by 65% compared with antiarrhythmic drugs.[98] This would

suggest that the next "AFFIRM" type study should use RF ablation as the rhythm control approach, although the ablation techniques need to be refined and standardized further before a large-scale multicenter trial could be undertaken.

SUMMARY

AF and CHF are common conditions, and each predisposes to the development of the other. Basic research using animal models of the two conditions continues to yield insights that may improve therapies. The AFFIRM and AF-CHF trials have shown no clinical benefits from the use of antiarrhythmic drugs to achieve sinus rhythm. Only dofetilide and amiodarone have been shown to be mortality neutral in CHF patients with AF. The role of medical therapies aimed at the underlying structural changes in AF continues to be a subject of ongoing studies. CRT is an effective therapy in appropriately selected patients with both SR and AF. Catheter ablation is now emerging as a potential alternative to antiarrhythmic drug therapy, but large randomized trials will be needed to assess its role.

REFERENCES

1. Braunwald E. Shattuck lecture–cardiovascular medicine at the turn of the millennium: triumphs, concerns, and opportunities. N Engl J Med 1997; 337(19):1360–9.
2. Heart and stroke facts 2008.
3. Go AS, Hylek EM, Phillips KA, et al. Prevalence of diagnosed atrial fibrillation in adults: national implications for rhythm management and stroke prevention: the AnTicoagulation and Risk Factors in Atrial Fibrillation (ATRIA) Study. JAMA 2001; 285(18):2370–5.
4. Wang TJ, Larson MG, Levy D, et al. Temporal relations of atrial fibrillation and congestive heart failure and their joint influence on mortality: the Framingham Heart study. Circulation 2003;107(23):2920–5.
5. Maisel WH, Stevenson LW. Atrial fibrillation in heart failure: epidemiology, pathophysiology, and rationale for therapy. Am J Cardiol 2003;91(6A):2D–8D.
6. Wyse DG, Waldo AL, DiMarco JP, et al. A comparison of rate control and rhythm control in patients with atrial fibrillation. N Engl J Med 2002;347(23): 1825–33.
7. Allessie M, Ausma J, Schotten U. Electrical, contractile and structural remodeling during atrial fibrillation. Cardiovasc Res 2002;54(2):230–46.
8. Nattel S. New ideas about atrial fibrillation 50 years on. Nature 2002;415(6868):219–26.

9. Nattel S, Shiroshita-Takeshita A, Brundel BJ, et al. Mechanisms of atrial fibrillation: lessons from animal models. Prog Cardiovasc Dis;48(1):9–28.

10. Nattel S, Opie LH. Controversies in atrial fibrillation. Lancet 2006;367(9506):262–72.

11. Cha TJ, Ehrlich JR, Zhang L, et al. Dissociation between ionic remodeling and ability to sustain atrial fibrillation during recovery from experimental congestive heart failure. Circulation 2004;109(3): 412–8.

12. Li D, Shinagawa K, Pang L, et al. Effects of angiotensin-converting enzyme inhibition on the development of the atrial fibrillation substrate in dogs with ventricular tachypacing-induced congestive heart failure. Circulation 2001;104(21):2608–14.

13. Yeh Y-H, Wakili R, Qi X-Y, et al. Calcium handling abnormalities underlying atrial arrhythmogenesis and contractile dysfunction in dogs with congestive heart failure. Circ Arrhythm Electrophysiol 2008;1(2): 93–102.

14. Fuster V, Ryden LE, Cannom DS, et al. ACC/AHA/ESC 2006 Guidelines for the management of patients with atrial fibrillation: a report of the American College of Cardiology/American Heart Association Task Force on Practice Guidelines and the European Society of Cardiology Committee for Practice Guidelines (Writing Committee to Revise the 2001 Guidelines for the management of patients with atrial fibrillation): developed in collaboration with the European Heart Rhythm Association and the Heart Rhythm Society. Circulation 2006;114(7):e257–354.

15. Hunt SA, Abraham WT, Chin MH, et al. ACC/AHA 2005 Guideline update for the diagnosis and management of chronic heart failure in the adult: a report of the American College of Cardiology/American Heart Association Task Force on Practice Guidelines (Writing Committee to Update the 2001 Guidelines for the evaluation and management of heart failure): developed in collaboration with the American College of Chest Physicians and the International Society for Heart and Lung Transplantation: endorsed by the Heart Rhythm Society. Circulation 2005;112(12): e154–235.

16. Hart RG, Benavente O, McBride R, et al. Antithrombotic therapy to prevent stroke in patients with atrial fibrillation: a meta-analysis. Ann Intern Med 1999; 131(7):492–501.

17. van Walraven C, Hart RG, Wells GA, et al. A clinical prediction rule to identify patients with atrial fibrillation and a low risk for stroke while taking aspirin. Arch Intern Med 2003;163(8):936–43.

18. Rietbrock S, Heeley E, Plumb J, et al. Chronic atrial fibrillation: incidence, prevalence, and prediction of stroke using the Congestive heart failure, Hypertension, Age > 75, Diabetes mellitus, and prior Stroke or transient ischemic attack (CHADS2) risk stratification scheme. Am Heart J 2008;156(1):57–64.

19. Freudenberger RS, Hellkamp AS, Halperin JL, et al. Risk of thromboembolism in heart failure: an analysis from the Sudden Cardiac Death in Heart Failure Trial (SCD-HeFT). Circulation 2007;115(20):2637–41.

20. Singer DE, Albers GW, Dalen JE, et al. Antithrombotic therapy in atrial fibrillation: American College of Chest Physicians Evidence-Based Clinical Practice Guidelines (8th edition). Chest 2008; 133(6 Suppl):546S–92S.

21. Connolly SJ, Eikelboom J, O'Donnell M, et al. Challenges of establishing new antithrombotic therapies in atrial fibrillation. Circulation 2007; 116(4):449–55.

22. Sick PB, Schuler G, Hauptmann KE, et al. Initial worldwide experience with the WATCHMAN left atrial appendage system for stroke prevention in atrial fibrillation. J Am Coll Cardiol 2007;49(13):1490–5.

23. Stollberger C, Schneider B, Finsterer J. Serious complications from dislocation of a Watchman left atrial appendage occluder. J Cardiovasc Electrophysiol 2007;18(8):880–1.

24. Hart RG, Halperin JL. Atrial fibrillation and stroke: concepts and controversies. Stroke 2001;32(3): 803–8.

25. Demircan C, Cikriklar HI, Engindeniz Z, et al. Comparison of the effectiveness of intravenous diltiazem and metoprolol in the management of rapid ventricular rate in atrial fibrillation. Emerg Med J 2005; 22(6):411–4.

26. Khand AU, Rankin AC, Martin W, et al. Carvedilol alone or in combination with digoxin for the management of atrial fibrillation in patients with heart failure? J Am Coll Cardiol 2003;42(11):1944–51.

27. Olshansky B, Rosenfeld LE, Warner AL, et al. The Atrial Fibrillation Follow-up Investigation of Rhythm Management (AFFIRM) study: approaches to control rate in atrial fibrillation. J Am Coll Cardiol 2004; 43(7):1201–8.

28. Weerasooriya R, Davis M, Powell A, et al. The Australian Intervention Randomized Control of Rate in Atrial Fibrillation Trial (AIRCRAFT). J Am Coll Cardiol 2003;41(10):1697–702.

29. Bradley DJ, Shen WK. Atrioventricular junction ablation combined with either right ventricular pacing or cardiac resynchronization therapy for atrial fibrillation: the need for large-scale randomized trials. Heart Rhythm 2007;4(2):224–32.

30. McGavigan AD, Mond HG. Selective site ventricular pacing. Curr Opin Cardiol 2006;21(1):7–14.

31. Koneru JN, Steinberg JS. Cardiac resynchronization therapy in the setting of permanent atrial fibrillation and heart failure. Curr Opin Cardiol 2008;23(1): 9–15.

32. Valls-Bertault V, Fatemi M, Gilard M, et al. Assessment of upgrading to biventricular pacing in patients with right ventricular pacing and congestive heart failure after atrioventricular junctional ablation for

chronic atrial fibrillation. Europace 2004;6(5): 438–43.

33. Doshi RN, Daoud EG, Fellows C, et al. Left ventricular-based cardiac stimulation post AV nodal ablation evaluation (the PAVE study). J Cardiovasc Electrophysiol 2005;16(11):1160–5.

34. Occhetta E, Bortnik M, Magnani A, et al. Prevention of ventricular desynchronization by permanent para-Hisian pacing after atrioventricular node ablation in chronic atrial fibrillation: a crossover, blinded, randomized study versus apical right ventricular pacing. J Am Coll Cardiol 2006;47(10):1938–45.

35. Mittal S, Ayati S, Stein KM, et al. Transthoracic cardioversion of atrial fibrillation: comparison of rectilinear biphasic versus damped sine wave monophasic shocks. Circulation 2000;101(11):1282–7.

36. Intravenous digoxin in acute atrial fibrillation. Results of a randomized, placebo-controlled multicentre trial in 239 patients. The Digitalis in Acute Atrial Fibrillation (DAAF) Trial Group. Eur Heart J 1997;18(4): 649–54.

37. Volgman AS, Carberry PA, Stambler B, et al. Conversion efficacy and safety of intravenous ibutilide compared with intravenous procainamide in patients with atrial flutter or fibrillation. J Am Coll Cardiol 1998;31(6):1414–9.

38. Alboni P, Botto GL, Baldi N, et al. Outpatient treatment of recent-onset atrial fibrillation with the "pill-in-the-pocket" approach. N Engl J Med 2004; 351(23):2384–91.

39. Camm AJ. Safety considerations in the pharmacological management of atrial fibrillation. Int J Cardiol 2008;127(3):299–306.

40. Vardas PE, Kochiadakis GE, Igoumenidis NE, et al. Amiodarone as a first-choice drug for restoring sinus rhythm in patients with atrial fibrillation: a randomized, controlled study. Chest 2000;117(6):1538–45.

41. Klein AL, Grimm RA, Murray RD, et al. Use of transesophageal echocardiography to guide cardioversion in patients with atrial fibrillation. N Engl J Med 2001;344(19):1411–20.

42. Khand AU, Rankin AC, Kaye GC, et al. Systematic review of the management of atrial fibrillation in patients with heart failure. Eur Heart J 2000;21(8):614–32.

43. Roy D, Talajic M, Dorian P, et al. Amiodarone to prevent recurrence of atrial fibrillation. Canadian Trial of Atrial Fibrillation Investigators. N Engl J Med 2000; 342(13):913–20.

44. Maintenance of sinus rhythm in patients with atrial fibrillation: an AFFIRM substudy of the first antiarrhythmic drug. J Am Coll Cardiol 2003;42(1):20–9.

45. Singh BN, Singh SN, Reda DJ, et al. Amiodarone versus sotalol for atrial fibrillation. N Engl J Med 2005;352(18):1861–72.

46. Doval HC, Nul DR, Grancelli HO, et al. Randomised trial of low-dose amiodarone in severe congestive heart failure. Grupo de Estudio de la Sobrevida en la Insuficiencia Cardiaca en Argentina (GESICA). Lancet 1994;344(8921):493–8.

47. Singh SN, Fletcher RD, Fisher SG, et al. Amiodarone in patients with congestive heart failure and asymptomatic ventricular arrhythmia. Survival trial of antiarrhythmic therapy in congestive heart failure. N Engl J Med 1995;333(2):77–82.

48. Torp-Pedersen C, Moller M, Bloch-Thomsen PE, et al. Dofetilide in patients with congestive heart failure and left ventricular dysfunction. Danish Investigations of Arrhythmia and Mortality on Dofetilide Study Group. N Engl J Med. 1999;341(12): 857–65.

49. Banchs JE, Wolbrette DL, Samii SM, et al. Efficacy and safety of dofetilide in patients with atrial fibrillation and atrial flutter. J Interv Card Electrophysiol 2008;23:111–5.

50. Singh BN, Connolly SJ, Crijns HJ, et al. Dronedarone for maintenance of sinus rhythm in atrial fibrillation or flutter. N Engl J Med 2007;357(10):987–99.

51. Hohnloser SH, Connolly SJ, Crijns HJ, et al. Rationale and design of ATHENA: a placebo-controlled, double-blind, parallel arm trial to assess the efficacy of dronedarone 400 mg bid for the prevention of cardiovascular hospitalization or death from any cause in patients with atrial fibrillation/atrial flutter. J Cardiovasc Electrophysiol 2008;19(1):69–73.

52. Kober L, Torp-Pedersen C, McMurray JJ, et al. Increased mortality after dronedarone therapy for severe heart failure. N Engl J Med 2008;358(25):2678–87.

53. Ezekowitz MD. Maintaining sinus rhythm–making treatment better than the disease. N Engl J Med 2007;357(10):1039–41.

54. Hohnloser SH, Kuck KH, Lilienthal J. Rhythm or rate control in atrial fibrillation–Pharmacological Intervention in Atrial Fibrillation (PIAF): a randomised trial. Lancet 2000;356(9244):1789–94.

55. Van Gelder IC, Hagens VE, Bosker HA, et al. A comparison of rate control and rhythm control in patients with recurrent persistent atrial fibrillation. N Engl J Med 2002;347(23):1834–40.

56. Carlsson J, Miketic S, Windeler J, et al. Randomized trial of rate-control versus rhythm-control in persistent atrial fibrillation: the Strategies of Treatment of Atrial Fibrillation (STAF) study. J Am Coll Cardiol 2003;41(10):1690–6.

57. Opolski G, Torbicki A, Kosior DA, et al. Rate control vs rhythm control in patients with nonvalvular persistent atrial fibrillation: the results of the Polish How to Treat Chronic Atrial Fibrillation (HOT CAFE) study. Chest 2004;126(2):476–86.

58. Chung MK. Randomized trials of rate vs. rhythm control for atrial fibrillation. J Interv Card Electrophysiol 2004;10(Suppl 1):45–53.

59. Roy D, Talajic M, Nattel S, et al. Rhythm control versus rate control for atrial fibrillation and heart failure. N Engl J Med 2008;358(25):2667–77.

60. Freudenberger RS, Wilson AC, Kostis JB. Comparison of rate versus rhythm control for atrial fibrillation in patients with left ventricular dysfunction (from the AFFIRM Study). Am J Cardiol 2007;100(2):247–52.

61. Cain ME, Curtis AB. Rhythm control in atrial fibrillation–one setback after another. N Engl J Med 2008;358(25):2725–7.

62. Deedwania PC, Singh BN, Ellenbogen K, et al. Spontaneous conversion and maintenance of sinus rhythm by amiodarone in patients with heart failure and atrial fibrillation: observations from the veterans affairs Congestive Heart Failure Survival Trial of Antiarrhythmic Therapy (CHF-STAT). The Department of Veterans Affairs CHF-STAT Investigators. Circulation 1998;98(23):2574–9.

63. Pedersen OD, Brendorp B, Elming H, et al. Does conversion and prevention of atrial fibrillation enhance survival in patients with left ventricular dysfunction? Evidence from the Danish Investigations of Arrhythmia and Mortality ON Dofetilide/(DIAMOND) study. Card Electrophysiol Rev 2003;7(3):220–4.

64. Corley SD, Epstein AE, DiMarco JP, et al. Relationships between sinus rhythm, treatment, and survival in the Atrial Fibrillation Follow-Up Investigation of Rhythm Management (AFFIRM) study. Circulation 2004;109(12):1509–13.

65. Ehrlich JR, Hohnloser SH, Nattel S. Role of angiotensin system and effects of its inhibition in atrial fibrillation: clinical and experimental evidence. Eur Heart J 2006;27(5):512–8.

66. Pedersen OD, Bagger H, Kober L, et al. Trandolapril reduces the incidence of atrial fibrillation after acute myocardial infarction in patients with left ventricular dysfunction. Circulation 1999;100(4):376–80.

67. Vermes E, Tardif JC, Bourassa MG, et al. Enalapril decreases the incidence of atrial fibrillation in patients with left ventricular dysfunction: insight from the Studies of Left Ventricular Dysfunction (SOLVD) trials. Circulation 2003;107(23):2926–31.

68. Ueng KC, Tsai TP, Yu WC, et al. Use of enalapril to facilitate sinus rhythm maintenance after external cardioversion of long-standing persistent atrial fibrillation. Results of a prospective and controlled study. Eur Heart J 2003;24(23):2090–8.

69. Healey JS, Baranchuk A, Crystal E, et al. Prevention of atrial fibrillation with angiotensin-converting enzyme inhibitors and angiotensin receptor blockers: a meta-analysis. J Am Coll Cardiol 2005;45(11):1832–9.

70. Salehian O, Healey J, Stambler B, et al. Impact of ramipril on the incidence of atrial fibrillation: results of the Heart Outcomes Prevention Evaluation study. Am Heart J 2007;154(3):448–53.

71. Tveit A, Grundvold I, Olufsen M, et al. Candesartan in the prevention of relapsing atrial fibrillation. Int J Cardiol 2007;120(1):85–91.

72. Connolly S, Yusuf S, Budaj A, et al. Rationale and design of ACTIVE: the atrial fibrillation clopidogrel trial with irbesartan for prevention of vascular events. Am Heart J 2006;151(6):1187–93.

73. Murray KT, Mace LC, Yang Z. Nonantiarrhythmic drug therapy for atrial fibrillation. Heart Rhythm 2007;4(3 Suppl):S88–90.

74. Burstein B, Nattel S. Atrial structural remodeling as an antiarrhythmic target. J Cardiovasc Pharmacol 2008;52(1):4–10.

75. Heidbuchel H. A paradigm shift in treatment for atrial fibrillation: from electrical to structural therapy? Eur Heart J 2003;24(23):2077–8.

76. Dorian P, Singh BN. Upstream therapies to prevent atrial fibrillation. Eur Heart J Suppl 2008;10(Suppl H): H11–31.

77. Bristow MR, Saxon LA, Boehmer J, et al. Cardiac-resynchronization therapy with or without an implantable defibrillator in advanced chronic heart failure. N Engl J Med 2004;350(21):2140–50.

78. Cleland JG, Daubert JC, Erdmann E, et al. The effect of cardiac resynchronization on morbidity and mortality in heart failure. N Engl J Med 2005;352(15): 1539–49.

79. Leclercq C, Walker S, Linde C, et al. Comparative effects of permanent biventricular and right-univentricular pacing in heart failure patients with chronic atrial fibrillation. Eur Heart J 2002;23(22):1780–7.

80. Gasparini M, Auricchio A, Regoli F, et al. Four-year efficacy of cardiac resynchronization therapy on exercise tolerance and disease progression: the importance of performing atrioventricular junction ablation in patients with atrial fibrillation. J Am Coll Cardiol 2006;48(4):734–43.

81. Gasparini M, Auricchio A, Metra M, et al. Long-term survival in patients undergoing cardiac resynchronization therapy: the importance of performing atrioventricular junction ablation in patients with permanent atrial fibrillation. Eur Heart J 2008; 29(13):1644–52.

82. Khadjooi K, Foley PW, Chalil S, et al. Long-term effects of cardiac resynchronisation therapy in patients with atrial fibrillation. Heart 2008;94(7):879–83.

83. Steinberg JS. Desperately seeking a randomized clinical trial of resynchronization therapy for patients with heart failure and atrial fibrillation. J Am Coll Cardiol 2006;48(4):744–6.

84. Hoppe UC, Casares JM, Eiskjaer H, et al. Effect of cardiac resynchronization on the incidence of atrial fibrillation in patients with severe heart failure. Circulation 2006;114(1):18–25.

85. Lellouche N, De Diego C, Vaseghi M, et al. Cardiac resynchronization therapy response is associated with shorter duration of atrial fibrillation. Pacing Clin Electrophysiol 2007;30(11):1363–8.

86. Yannopoulos D, Lurie KG, Sakaguchi S, et al. Reduced atrial tachyarrhythmia susceptibility after

upgrade of conventional implanted pulse generator to cardiac resynchronization therapy in patients with heart failure. J Am Coll Cardiol 2007;50(13):1246–51.

87. Padeletti L, Muto C, Maounis T, et al. Atrial fibrillation in recipients of cardiac resynchronization therapy device: 1-year results of the randomized MASCOT trial. Am Heart J 2008;156(3):520–6.

88. Haissaguerre M, Jais P, Shah DC, et al. Spontaneous initiation of atrial fibrillation by ectopic beats originating in the pulmonary veins. N Engl J Med 1998;339(10):659–66.

89. Calkins H, Brugada J, Packer DL, et al. HRS/EHRA/ECAS expert consensus statement on catheter and surgical ablation of atrial fibrillation: recommendations for personnel, policy, procedures and follow-up. A report of the Heart Rhythm Society (HRS) task force on catheter and surgical ablation of atrial fibrillation. Heart Rhythm 2007;4(6):816–61.

90. Spragg DD, Dalal D, Cheema A, et al. Complications of catheter ablation for atrial fibrillation: incidence and predictors. J Cardiovasc Electrophysiol 2008; 19(6):627–31.

91. Chen MS, Marrouche NF, Khaykin Y, et al. Pulmonary vein isolation for the treatment of atrial fibrillation in patients with impaired systolic function. J Am Coll Cardiol 2004;43(6):1004–9.

92. Hsu LF, Jais P, Sanders P, et al. Catheter ablation for atrial fibrillation in congestive heart failure. N Engl J Med 2004;351(23):2373–83.

93. Gentlesk PJ, Sauer WH, Gerstenfeld EP, et al. Reversal of left ventricular dysfunction following ablation of atrial fibrillation. J Cardiovasc Electrophysiol 2007;18(1):9–14.

94. Efremidis M, Sideris A, Xydonas S, et al. Ablation of atrial fibrillation in patients with heart failure: reversal of atrial and ventricular remodelling. Hellenic J Cardiol 2008;49(1):19–25.

95. Lutomsky BA, Rostock T, Koops A, et al. Catheter ablation of paroxysmal atrial fibrillation improves cardiac function: a prospective study on the impact of atrial fibrillation ablation on left ventricular function assessed by magnetic resonance imaging. Europace 2008;10(5):593–9.

96. Cleland JG, Coletta AP, Abdellah AT, et al. Clinical trials update from the American Heart Association 2006: OAT, SALT 1 and 2, MAGIC, ABCD, PABA-CHF, IMPROVE-CHF, and percutaneous mitral annuloplasty. Eur J Heart Fail 2007;9(1):92–7.

97. Pappone C, Augello G, Sala S, et al. A randomized trial of circumferential pulmonary vein ablation versus antiarrhythmic drug therapy in paroxysmal atrial fibrillation: the APAF Study. J Am Coll Cardiol 2006; 48(11):2340–7.

98. Nair GM, Nery PB, Diwakaramenon S, et al. A systematic review of randomized trials comparing radiofrequency ablation with antiarrhythmic medications in patients with atrial fibrillation. J Cardiovasc Electrophysiol September 3, 2008 [Epub ahead of print].

Electrical and Pharmacologic Cardioversion for Atrial Fibrillation

Susan S. Kim, MD, Bradley P. Knight, MD*

KEYWORDS

• Atrial fibrillation • Cardioversion • Electrical

Cardioversion is a useful tool in managing patients who have atrial fibrillation (AF) when rhythm control is appropriate. It is used most frequently for those who are symptomatic or newly diagnosed. Transthoracic electrical cardioversion is the overwhelmingly preferred method because of its relative simplicity and efficacy, even in patients who have multiple comorbid conditions and significant structural heart disease. In selected circumstances, pharmacologic cardioversion is preferred. This article discusses indications for cardioversion and management of pericardioversion anticoagulation and describes electrical and pharmacologic cardioversion in detail. Finally, management strategies are offered for initial failure to convert or immediate recurrence of AF (IRAF).

PATTERNS OF ATRIAL FIBRILLATION

Before discussing the indications for cardioversion, it is useful to define the clinical patterns of the occurrence of AF. Generally, patients who have AF demonstrate one of three clinical patterns: paroxysmal, persistent, or permanent AF **(Fig. 1)**.[1] Paroxysmal AF consists of self-terminating episodes, each usually lasting fewer than 7 days and often less than 24 hours. Persistent AF consists of non–self-terminating episodes, each lasting more than 7 days, whereas permanent AF is defined as a long episode with failed or no attempt at cardioversion.

Given these definitions, cardioversion can be clinically useful in some patients who have paroxysmal AF and in many who have persistent AF. By definition, cardioversion is not used for patients who have permanent AF.

INDICATIONS FOR CARDIOVERSION

Broadly, cardioversion should be considered for two populations of patients: those who are symptomatic with AF and those who present with AF for the first time.

Patients who have symptomatic AF can have severe enough symptoms, such as severely decompensated heart failure, hypotension, uncontrolled ischemia, or angina, to mandate urgent cardioversion. Other patients who have AF may have less severe symptoms, such as palpitations, fatigue, lightheadedness, and exertional dyspnea. Regardless of the degree of severity, any symptoms caused by atrial fibrillation warrant consideration of cardioversion as a management option.

Restoration of sinus rhythm is a reasonable goal in patients who have a first-time diagnosis of AF, regardless of symptoms, unless some indication shows that the AF has been present for many years before identification. The purpose of cardioversion, even in patients who are asymptomatic or newly diagnosed, is to slow the progression of the clinical pattern of AF. Many lines of evidence support the principle that "atrial fibrillation begets

A version of this article originally appeared in *Medical Clinics of North America*, volume 92, issue 1.
Section of Cardiology, Department of Medicine, University of Chicago Medical Center, 5758 South Maryland Avenue MC9024, Chicago, IL 60637, USA
* Corresponding author.
E-mail address: bknight@medicine.bsd.uchicago.edu (B.P. Knight).

Cardiol Clin 27 (2009) 95–107
doi:10.1016/j.ccl.2008.09.008
0733-8651/08/$ – see front matter © 2009 Elsevier Inc. All rights reserved.

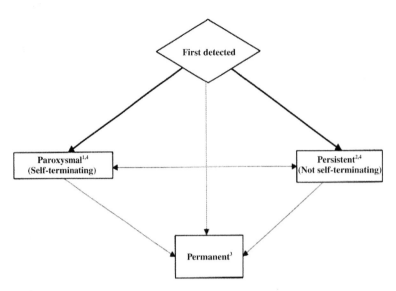

Fig. 1. Patterns of AF. (1) Episodes that last generally 7 days or fewer (most less than 24 hours); (2) episodes that last usually longer than 7 days; (3) cardioversion failed or not attempted; and (4) paroxysmal and persistent AF may be recurrent. (*From* Fuster V, Ryden LE, Cannom DS, et al. ACC/AHA/ESC 2006 guidelines for the management of patients with atrial fibrillation. Circulation 2006;114:e257–354, © 2006; with permission from the American Heart Association.)

atrial fibrillation".[2] Natural history studies show that AF can be a progressive disease: patients who have paroxysmal AF progress to persistent and permanent AF. Even those who have lone paroxysmal AF may progress,[3] and the tendency to progress seems to correlate with the duration of the paroxysmal AF episodes.[4]

In addition, many clinical trials show that pharmacologic and electrical cardioversion are more likely to succeed in patients experiencing shorter episodes.[5] A study comparing short- versus longer-duration episodes of AF in goat hearts showed that with longer-duration episodes, the rate, inducibility, and stability of AF increased significantly. In addition, a marked shortening of the atrial effective refractory period was seen.[2] These lines of evidence strongly support the principle that AF begets itself; this principle underlies the rationale for cardioverting patients who have newly diagnosed AF.

As evidenced in large-scale, randomized clinical trials, repeated cardioversion and other attempts to maintain sinus rhythm are unlikely to have a meaningful clinical impact on older patients who are asymptomatic. Also, by definition, cardioversion is not applied to patients who have permanent AF. Both populations of patients, however, should undergo therapeutic anticoagulation or antiplatelet therapy as dictated by their risk for a thromboembolic event versus the risks from this therapy.[6,7]

Another group of patients who may benefit from cardioversion are those who have postoperative AF. Postoperative AF occurs most commonly in the first few days after surgery, when anticoagulation may be undesirable. Many episodes of postoperative AF resolve spontaneously. Patients who do not experience spontaneous resolution may be cardioverted before an AF duration of 48 hours to avoid anticoagulation.

RATE OF SUCCESSFUL CARDIOVERSION

With electrical cardioversion and use of biphasic waveforms, cardioversion success rates are consistently at or greater than 90%.[8,9] These high rates of successful cardioversion apply even in populations of patients who have advanced age, multiple comorbid conditions, and significant structural heart disease. In one study of 1355 patients who had persistent AF (>7 days) undergoing electrical cardioversion,[8] 92% were successfully converted to sinus rhythm. With biphasic energy cardioversion, multivariate analysis showed that no patient characteristic, gender, age, comorbid condition, or cardiac structural abnormality (eg, reduced left ventricular ejection fraction, enlarged left atrium, other structural heart disease) was associated with failure to convert to sinus rhythm. Therefore, although these baseline characteristics should be considered with regard to successful maintenance of sinus rhythm, they should not necessarily deter attempts at cardioversion.

PERICARDIOVERSION ANTICOAGULATION

AF results in mechanical stasis in the atria and is associated with a proinflammatory and therefore potentially prothrombotic state.[10] Therefore, patients who have AF are at risk for developing intracardiac thrombi and subsequent embolization. The risk for a thromboembolic event is particularly high around cardioversion for two reasons. First, if an unstable thrombus is present precardioversion, the recovery of atrial contraction postcardioversion and the force of atrial contraction may cause fragmentation and embolization of the preexisting thrombus.[11,12] Second, in many patients, the recovery of atrial mechanical function can lag behind restoration of normal electrical function.[13] This period of atrial mechanical "stunning" after cardioversion can last up to 4 weeks postcardioversion. Thus, stasis in the atria and the risk for clot formation may endure for several weeks postcardioversion, even with persistent sinus rhythm. Therefore, the goals of pericardioversion anticoagulation for AF are twofold: (1) to minimize the likelihood of an unstable thrombus being present at cardioversion and (2) to prevent the formation of new thrombus in the postcardioversion phase. Without anticoagulation, the risk for a thromboembolic event postcardioversion can be as high as 5%.[14]

To minimize the likelihood of an unstable thrombus being present at cardioversion, one of two different strategies may be used: (1) empiric anticoagulation for 3 weeks or (2) short-term anticoagulation and transesophageal echocardiography (TEE)-guided cardioversion. Presuming that an unstable thrombus takes approximately 2 weeks to organize and adhere to the atrial wall, under the empiric anticoagulation strategy patients should be treated for a minimum of 3 weeks with warfarin (target international normalized ratio [INR], 2.5; range, 2.0–3.0) or enoxaparin before cardioversion.[1,12,15]

The 3 weeks' duration allows for organization and even potential resolution of preexisting thrombus in addition to minimizing the risk for new thrombus formation. When using warfarin, a therapeutic effect must be verified with weekly INR levels before cardioversion. One retrospective study examined 1435 patients who had AF greater than 48 hours' duration who were receiving warfarin and undergoing direct current cardioversion. In these patients, embolic events were significantly more likely when the INR was 1.5 to 2.4, compared with an INR greater than or equal to 2.5 (0.93% versus 0%; $P = .012$).[16]

Alternatively, patients may be therapeutically anticoagulated with heparin followed by TEE. If no thrombus is seen on TEE, cardioversion is performed. The advantage of TEE-guided cardioversion is a shorter time to cardioversion and, potentially, a shorter total duration of anticoagulation.

The validity of TEE-guided cardioversion was shown in a randomized clinical trial involving 1222 patients.[17] Patients who had AF requiring cardioversion were randomized to 24 hours of unfractionated heparin and TEE-guided cardioversion versus empiric anticoagulation for 3 weeks

before cardioversion. In both strategies, patients were anticoagulated for 4 weeks postcardioversion. After 8 weeks, no significant difference was seen in the rate of embolic events (0.8% versus 0.5%; $P = .50$) between the TEE-guided versus warfarin-only groups. However, a significantly decreased rate of hemorrhagic events (2.9% versus 5.5%; $P = .03$) and a shorter time to cardioversion (3.0 versus 30.6 days; $P<.001$) were seen in the TEE-guided versus warfarin-only groups.

A smaller, randomized, controlled trial compared low molecular weight heparin with unfractionated heparin plus oral anticoagulation.[15] Of the 496 patients in the trial, 431 underwent TEE-guided cardioversion, whereas the remaining 65 were anticoagulated empirically and cardioverted after 3 weeks. In all strategies, patients underwent 4 weeks of anticoagulation postcardioversion. The use of low molecular weight heparin was found to be noninferior in the empiric-anticoagulation and TEE-guided treatment arms, compared with the use of unfractionated heparin plus oral anticoagulation, for the primary end point of preventing ischemic and embolic events, bleeding complications, and death.

Again, given the delay of up to 4 weeks for recovery of atrial mechanical function postcardioversion, patients should undergo at least 4 weeks of therapeutic anticoagulation postcardioversion.[1,12] Especially in the early postcardioversion period, meticulous attention should be given to anticoagulation status, because most thromboembolic events occur within the first few days postcardioversion (**Fig. 2**).[18] In particular, overlapping therapy with heparin (unfractionated or low molecular weight) should be administered if the INR is less than 2.0.

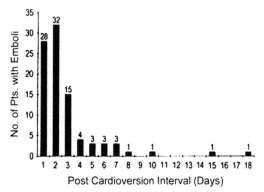

Fig. 2. Interval between cardioversion and thromboembolic events in 92 patients. (*From* Berger M, Schweitzer P. Timing of thromboembolic events after electrical cardioversion of atrial fibrillation or flutter: a retrospective analysis. Am J Cardiol 1998;82:1545–7, © Elsevier 1998; with permission.)

One analysis that pooled data from 32 studies and included 4621 patients examined the timing of embolic events,[18] finding that 92 (2%) patients experienced embolic events. Only 11 of the patients were anticoagulated before cardioversion. Of the 92 episodes, 75 (82%) occurred within the first 72 hours postcardioversion (see **Fig. 2**). Notably, 98% of the embolic events occurred within the first 10 days postcardioversion.

For AF episodes lasting less than 48 hours, the likelihood of thrombus formation and subsequent embolization after cardioversion is low. Therefore, anticoagulation is not recommended routinely for patients who have episodes lasting less than 48 hours.[1] Neither pre- nor postcardioversion anticoagulation is recommended for these short-duration episodes.

One prospective observational study followed 375 patients admitted to the hospital for AF who were found to have an episode lasting less than 48 hours.[19] Patients treated with anticoagulation using warfarin (INR >1.6) or heparin at presentation were excluded. Spontaneous conversion occurred in 250 patients, whereas 107 underwent pharmacologic or electrical conversion. Three patients (0.8%; 95% CI, 0.2%–2.4%) had a clinical thromboembolic event. Thus, overall, the thromboembolic risk for patients who have short-duration AF seems low.

Determining the true onset of an AF episode can be difficult in the absence of electrocardiographic documentation (eg, telemetry or 12-lead ECG). Symptoms generally are unreliable as a marker of the presence of absence of AF. One study in patients who had pacemakers showed that more than 90% of atrial tachyarrhythmia events documented by the pacemaker were not perceived by the patients, even in those who were believed to have symptomatic arrhythmias.[20] Therefore, in the absence of electrocardiographic evidence of the true onset of an episode of AF, it is most prudent to assume that the episode has been ongoing for more than 48 hours.

CARDIOVERSION

Most patients who require cardioversion undergo transthoracic electrical cardioversion rather than an attempt at pharmacologic conversion because of its shorter overall procedure duration and high rate of success (as high as >90%).[21] Although at least deep sedation is required for transthoracic electrical cardioversion, if short-acting agents are used, patients may be discharged within hours after recovery from anesthesia. Antiarrhythmic medications play two primary roles in cardioversion for AF. Used alone, they are effective in timely termination of symptomatic AF of short duration. Used together with electrical cardioversion, they help facilitate persistent sinus rhythm in two distinct populations of patients: those who have IRAF (successful conversion to sinus rhythm, even just one beat, followed by recurrence of AF within minutes) and those for whom cardioversion truly fails with no achievement of sinus rhythm.

Electrical Cardioversion

Biphasic waveforms superior to monophasic waveforms

The success of cardioversion and defibrillation depends on the delivery of adequate current flow through the heart.[22] However, excessive current delivery can lead to myocardial damage, leading to ST-segments changes, enzyme release, depression of myocardial function, and reduced mean arterial pressures.[23,24]

The two major determinants of current delivery through an external defibrillator are energy selection and the shock waveform used. When Bernard Lown[25] reported the first series of AF cardioversions using an external defibrillator in 1963, he was using what is termed *monophasic damped sinusoidal (MDS) waveform*, or the *Lown waveform*, for energy delivery (**Fig. 3**).[26] This waveform, displayed as current amplitude over time, is characterized by an initial high peak followed by an exponential decay of the current to zero. The MDS waveform remained the dominant waveform in external defibrillators until biphasic waveforms emerged. Under pressure to reduce the size of implantable defibrillator generators, device manufactures developed biphasic waveforms, which showed a significant decrease in defibrillation energy requirements for ventricular fibrillation.[27,28] Given their superiority in implantable defibrillators, biphasic waveforms then were tried in external defibrillators. Currently, two types of biphasic waveforms are used in most commercially available external defibrillators: biphasic truncated exponential (BTE) waveforms and rectilinear biphasic waveforms (RBW) (see **Fig. 3**). Both biphasic waveforms are characterized by lower peak current amplitudes (compared with monophasic waveform energies of similar clinical efficacy) and a second phase with a negative or inverted polarity. The lower peak current amplitudes may be associated with less myocardial injury than higher peak current shocks.[29]

Biphasic waveforms have proven to convert AF at much lower energies and higher rates than the MDS waveform. In one study comparing the RBW and MDS waveforms,[21] 165 patients who had AF were randomized to monophasic shocks

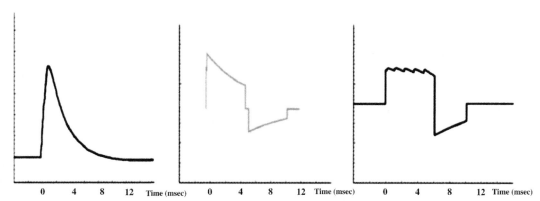

Fig. 3. Shock waveforms: (*left*) MDS waveform; (*middle*) BTE waveform; (*right*) RBW. The vertical axis represents current amplitude. (*From* Mittal S, Stein KM, Markowitz SM, et al. An update on electrical cardioversion of atrial fibrillation. Card Electrophysiol Rev 2003;7:285–9, © 2003 Springer; with permission from Springer Science and Business Media.)

using a dose escalation of 100, 200, 300, and 360 J or biphasic shocks using 70, 120, 150, and 170 J. With the first shock, the RBW was significantly more successful than the MDS shock, with a 60/88 (68%) versus 16/77 (21%) (P<.0001) conversion rate. A significantly higher success rate was still seen in the biphasic shock group after the highest energy shock (83/88 [94%] versus 61/77 [79%]; P = .005). At all comparable energy levels and across all impedances, peak currents in the biphasic shocks measured at approximately 50% of the peak current amplitude seen with monophasic shocks.

Two randomized studies compared the BTE waveform with the MDS waveform for AF cardioversion. In the first study, 57 patients were randomized to either cardioversion with 150 J and then 360 J with a MDS defibrillator or 150 J followed by another 150 J with a BTE defibrillator. With the first shock (each at 150 J), the cardioversion success rate was 16/27 (59%) in the MDS group versus 26/30 (86%) in the BTE group.[30] Cumulative success rates after the second shock and after crossover were not significantly different between the groups (88% versus 93% and 92% versus 96%, respectively).

In the second study, 203 patients were randomized to an MDS versus a BTE waveform with delivery of 100, 150, or 200 J, then maximum-output (360 and 200 J, respectively) shocks.[31] At each of the first three energy levels, the cumulative cardioversion success rate was significantly higher in the BTE group versus the MDS group: for example, at 200 J, the success rate was 86/96 (90%) versus 57/107 (53%), respectively (P<.0001). At the highest energies, no statistically significant difference in outcome was seen between the groups: 87/96 (91%) versus 91/107 (85%), respectively

(P = .29). Also, at equal energy levels, the BTE waveform was associated with significantly less dermal injury than the MDS waveform.

Finally, biphasic external defibrillators are more efficacious in patients who have AF resistant to monophasic cardioversion.[32] Fifty-six patients who had AF for whom at least one 360-J monophasic shock had failed were randomized to progressive 150-J, 200-J, and 360-J BTE shocks or one 360-J monophasic shock. Sinus rhythm was restored in 17 of 28 (61%) patients who had biphasic versus 5 of 28 (18%) who had monophasic shocks (P = .001). With crossover allowed after failed shocks, 78% of patients who had a failed monophasic shock were cardioverted successfully with a biphasic shock, whereas only 27% of those patients who had failed biphasic shocks converted with the high-energy monophasic shock.

Currently, most evidence favors the use of biphasic external defibrillators for AF cardioversion because of their categorically lower energy requirements and greater efficacy compared with monophasic defibrillators.

Practical considerations

Anesthesia Patients undergoing elective cardioversion should receive at least deep sedation, because high-energy shock can cause significant discomfort. Short-acting agents, such as midazolam, fentanyl, and propofol, are desirable given their rapid onset and short half-life. In some cases, general anesthesia may be indicated. Anesthesia and cardioversion should be performed in the postabsorptive state. Even when urgent cardioversion is required, as in cases of hypotension, severe decompensated heart failure, angina, or ischemia, attempts should be made to sedate patients when circumstances allow.

Pad or paddle positioning and size A handful of studies have examined the effect of anterior-posterior (AP) versus anterior-lateral (AL) electrode (pad or paddle) positioning on cardioversion success. One study randomized 301 patients who had AF to AP or AL pad positioning. The AP position was associated with a significantly higher rate of successful cardioversion and lower cumulative energy requirement (**Fig. 4**).[33] Two subsequent studies show no effect of pad placement on cardioversion success in AF.[34,35] The second study also showed that an increased pad size (13 cm versus the standard 8.5 cm) did not improve the likelihood of cardioversion.[35]

Shock delivery To avoid shock delivery during the vulnerable phase of the cardiac cycle ("shock on T") and subsequent ventricular fibrillation, shocks should be delivered in a synchronized fashion. In the synchronized mode, intrinsic R waves are sensed and shock delivery is timed to minimize the risk associated with delivery during the vulnerable period. This technique is different from the defibrillation mode, which delivers shocks in an asynchronous or random fashion without regard to the cardiac cycle. This mode is appropriate for ventricular fibrillation or very rapid ventricular tachycardia, for which synchronized delivery is not possible and immediate shock is desired.

Energy selection Energy level is related directly to current amplitude, and adequate current delivery

determines successful cardioversion. Therefore, one choice may be to start with the highest energy for every cardioversion (360 J with monophasic defibrillators and 200 J or even 360 J in some biphasic defibrillators). The advantage is a high probability of successful cardioversion and, thus, a shorter duration of sedation. The greatest disadvantage of higher energy shocks, especially with monophasic defibrillators, is thermal injury to the skin.[31,36] Any potential myocardial damage, from even high-energy cardioversion, rarely is of clinical consequence.

Because current is related inversely to impedance, increased transthoracic impedance can diminish current delivery to myocardium. One study found increased transthoracic impedance to be significantly and independently associated with lower rates of successful cardioversion.[21] Incomplete pad or paddle contact also may increase transthoracic impedance. Adequate contact medium (usually gel or paste) and firm pad or paddle contact should be assured. Other factors that increase transthoracic impedance include obesity, emphysema, and asthma. In patients who have these conditions, selecting a high level of energy is appropriate. Delivering shocks during the expiratory phase of the respiratory cycle also may decrease transthoracic impedance.

Patients who have AF of longer duration have lower rates of successful cardioversion.[21,33] They also may have more success with higher energy shocks.

Lower-energy shocks are appropriate when patients are smaller in size or have AF of shorter

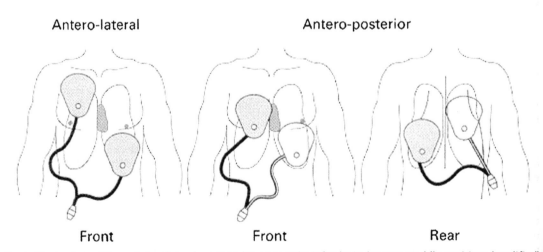

Antero-lateral   Antero-posterior

Front   Front   Rear

Fig. 4. Electrode positions. Anterolateral, ventricular apex-right infraclavicular area paddle position; (modified) anteroposterior, right sternal body at the third intercostal space-angle of the left scapula paddle position; front, front view; rear, rear view. (*From* Botto GL, Politi A, Bonini W, et al. External cardioversion of atrial fibrillation: role of paddle position on technical efficacy and energy requirements. Heart 1999;82:726–30; with permission from the BMJ Publishing Group.)

duration. Furthermore, patients who have atrial flutter may successfully convert with low energies (as low as 100 J monophasic or 50 J biphasic) for successful cardioversion. Even with lower energy shocks, patients can experience significant discomfort and still should undergo at least deep sedation.

Patients who have implanted devices Under the proper circumstances, patients who have implanted devices (permanent pacemakers or implantable cardioverter-defibrillators [ICDs]) can undergo external cardioversion with minimal risk to their devices and themselves. Potential risks at shocking include alteration of programmed data or, if electricity is conducted down an implanted lead, endocardial injury with transient or permanent exit block. These risks are maximized when pads or paddles are placed with one over the pulse generator and one at the apex of the heart. AP positioning seems to lower these risks.[1] Pre- and postcardioversion, devices should be interrogated with complete lead testing and device reprogramming as needed.

In patients who have ICDs, cardioversion may be achieved with a commanded internal shock delivered through the device. Device-mediated cardioversion has the advantage of avoiding potential damage to the implanted system. A disadvantage is that each shock contributes to significant decrease in battery life of up to approximately 1 month for each maximum-energy shock. Internal shocks can cause significant discomfort, and therefore patients still should receive at least deep sedation. For patients who have atrial flutter, device-delivered antitachycardia pacing should be attempted because it is painless and sedation is unnecessary.

Internal by way of intracardiac catheters This article has primarily discussed external transthoracic cardioversion. Before the development of biphasic defibrillators, AF cardioversion failure rates were significantly higher. In that setting, internal cardioversion was established as next-line therapy for patients for whom external cardioversion failed. The technique eventually evolved to placement of intracardiac catheters in the right atrium, coronary sinus, and left pulmonary artery, through which low-energy shocks were delivered.[37] This treatment option may be useful in patients for whom all other cardioversion techniques have failed.

Outcomes The three potential outcomes after electrical cardioversion are (1) persistent restoration of sinus rhythm, (2) restoration of sinus rhythm (at

least one sinus beat) followed by IRAF, or (3) failed cardioversion with no evidence of sinus rhythm. Results from many studies show that patients who have IRAF can experience rates of long-term freedom from AF[38,39] comparable to patients who have persistent sinus rhythm postcardioversion. The rates of long-term freedom from AF are significantly worse, however, in patients who have true failed cardioversion who ultimately achieve sinus rhythm. Thus, it is critical to distinguish between patients who have IRAF (those who have even just one sinus beat after cardioversion) and those who have true failed cardioversion. Because patients who have IRAF can have favorable long-term outcomes, aggressive measures should be taken to facilitate persistent postcardioversion sinus rhythm.

Immediate recurrence of atrial fibrillation IRAF is defined as AF recurring within the first few minutes after cardioversion. One study suggests that if AF recurs within the first 24 hours postcardioversion, it will occur within the first few minutes after cardioversion.[40] Even when only one beat of sinus rhythm is seen, the subsequent AF is considered IRAF as opposed to true failed cardioversion. The incidence of IRAF ranges from 5% to 25%.[41]

The distinction between IRAF and true failed cardioversion is important because the two populations have different long-term outcomes:[39] patients who have IRAF who ultimately achieve persistent sinus rhythm postcardioversion (usually pharmacologically facilitated) have better rates of long-term freedom from AF than those who have true failed cardioversion who subsequently achieve sinus rhythm.

IRAF seems to be triggered by very early coupled premature atrial beats (PABs). In one study of patients undergoing internal cardioversion for AF, IRAF was noted in 13% (5/38). IRAF in these patients always was seen to reinitiate with non-catheter-induced PABs. PAB-coupling intervals that led to IRAF were significantly shorter than those that did not.[38] Pretreatment with atropine or flecainide facilitated cardioversion without IRAF in three patients, whereas repeat shock alone was successful for two.

In another study in patients undergoing catheter ablation for AF, PABs triggering IRAF also were significantly shorter than PABs not triggering AF.[42] This study documented that 20% of IRAF episodes were initiated by pulmonary vein activity. In every case, the pulmonary vein activity took the form of a rapid pulmonary vein tachycardia.

In a third study, also in patients undergoing catheter ablation for AF, coupling intervals for IRAF-initiating PABs were again significantly shorter than those not initiating IRAF. IRAF was seen more frequently in patients who had AF lasting less than 1 month than in those who had longer episodes. Long-term, patients who had IRAF experienced similar freedom from AF to those who did not have IRAF.[43]

Another study also showed the increased incidence of IRAF in patients who have shorter-duration episodes of AF.[41] This study involved patients who had implantable atrial defibrillators and those undergoing external transthoracic cardioversion. In patients who underwent cardioversion within 1 hour of the onset of AF, IRAF occurred at a rate of 56%, compared with those whose AF lasted more than 24 hours who had a rate of 12%. This finding suggests a possible lower limit of AF duration below which cardioversion may be less likely to lead to persistent sinus rhythm.

Patients who have IRAF have experienced successful persistent postcardioversion sinus rhythm or suppression of IRAF in many studies using various antiarrhythmic medications. An early demonstration of successful pharmacologic suppression of IRAF was published in 1967 with the use of quinidine.[44] Fifty patients received oral quinidine (1200 mg) 1 day before cardioversion. Successful cardioversion was achieved in 92% patients receiving quinidine versus 64% in control patients (P<.01), predominantly because of the prevention of IRAF. Another Vaughan-Williams class IA agent, procainamide, has no effect on the rate of successful cardioversion compared with placebo.[45]

In another study, 50 patients were randomized to propafenone (750 mg/d) or placebo for 2 days before cardioversion. Patients treated with propafenone had a significantly lower likelihood of IRAF and, thus, a higher overall likelihood of persistent sinus rhythm postcardioversion compared with patients receiving placebo (0% versus 17% IRAF, respectively, and 84% versus 65% sinus rhythm, respectively, at 48 hours).[46] A subsequent study showed that adding verapamil to propafenone was superior to propafenone alone in suppressing IRAF.[47]

Sotalol and amiodarone suppress IRAF effectively. Sotalol suppressed IRAF effectively in patients undergoing internal cardioversion.[48] Amiodarone was studied in 27 patients who had either IRAF (group A) or a failed cardioversion (group B).[39] All patients received oral amiodarone loading (600 mg/d for 4 weeks) followed by 200 mg/d for 4 weeks if sinus rhythm was ultimately achieved. Among patients in group A, 5 of 11 (46%) converted during loading compared with only 1 of 16 (6%) patients in group B. After electrical cardioversion, the number of patients in group A

in sinus rhythm was 10 of 11 (91%), versus 7 of 16 (44%) in group B. At 1-month follow-up, all 10 of 11 (91%) patients in group A versus only 5 of 16 (33%) patients in group B remained in sinus rhythm. This study, although small, showed a significant outcome difference between patients who had IRAF postcardioversion versus those who underwent failed cardioversion. These findings suggest that restoration of persistent sinus rhythm should be pursued aggressively in patients who have IRAF.

Another study showed favorable outcomes in pharmacologically facilitated cardioversion in patients who had IRAF, this time using intravenous verapamil or ibutilide. These medications have been shown to attenuate the shortening of the atrial refractory period seen in patients post-AF; that is, they prolong the atrial refractory period.[49] Subsequently, both medications were studied in patients who had IRAF.[50] Verapamil (0.15 mg/kg at 2 mg/min) was assigned randomly to 11 patients versus ibutilide (1 mg) over 10 minutes in 9 patients. IRAF occurred in 73% of patients treated with verapamil and in only 22% of patients treated with ibutilide (P<.05). After crossover, ibutilide continued to have a higher rate of IRAF suppression than verapamil. These findings correlated with ibutilide's much greater effect on the atrial refractory period compared with verapamil's in the earlier study.[49]

Verapamil was used alone in one uncontrolled study of 19 patients who had IRAF after each of three cardioversions.[51] Each patient received 10 mg intravenously followed by a fourth cardioversion attempt. IRAF was suppressed in 9 of 19 (47%) patients, and sinus rhythm duration before IRAF was increased in patients who experienced IRAF.

For patients undergoing transthoracic cardioversion, same-day options for pharmacologic suppression of IRAF include intravenous verapamil and ibutilide, with higher success rates seen with ibutilide. Because ibutilide is contraindicated in patients who have depressed left ventricular systolic function, intravenous verapamil (in the absence of decompensated heart failure) or outpatient loading with amiodarone should be used.

Failed cardioversion Even in the era of biphasic defibrillation, up to 10% or more of patients may have true failed cardioversion; that is, no evidence of any sinus activity after cardioversion. Certainly the use of monophasic rather than biphasic waveforms is associated with higher failure rates.[21,30,31] Longer duration of episodes and increased transthoracic impedance also are associated with higher cardioversion failure rates.[21,33] In contrast, younger age and smaller left atrial size are found to be independently associated with successful cardioversion.[5,52]

When conventional external cardioversion fails, several tactics may be effective. First, shocks should be repeated at highest energy. Because success of cardioversion is probabilistic, a failed attempt at maximum output does not imply that it never will work. Although most biphasic defibrillators deliver a maximum of 200 J, some biphasic defibrillators can deliver up to 360 J. The pads or paddles should be repositioned. If the electrodes are in the AL position, they should be moved to the AP position (right sternal body at the third intercostal space and angle of the left scapula [see **Fig. 4**]).[33] The goal is to direct the energy vector optimally through the atria. Manual pressure should be applied on the anterior pad at shock delivery. With the pads in the AP position, while ensuring electrical insulation, mechanical pressure should be applied to the anterior pad to decrease the distance (thus, the impedance) between the two pads. The shock should be delivered during the expiration. In theory, this may decrease transthoracic impedance. Pharmacologic facilitation of cardioversion should be considered (discussed later). The "double-paddle" technique should be attempted. In one study, patients who had AF and had failed 360-J monophasic cardioversion were loaded with amiodarone orally. If repeat 360-J monophasic cardioversion failed again, the patients underwent the double-paddle technique: two monophasic defibrillators were used with two sets of paddles for each patient; each defibrillator was set for a synchronous shock at the maximum output of 360 J; they then were discharged simultaneously, resulting in successful conversion of 13 of 15 patients.[53] Finally, internal cardioversion should be considered.

In addition to facilitating persistent sinus rhythm for patients who have IRAF, antiarrhythmic medications are effective in facilitating successful cardioversion for patients who have true failed cardioversion (ie, no evidence of any sinus activity).

Amiodarone and ibutilide show the strongest success in pharmacologic facilitation of cardioversion after true failed cardioversion. Although some data show decreased IRAF when using propafenone, verapamil, and quinidine, it is less clear whether they increase the likelihood of cardioversion in patients who have had true cardioversion failure.

Amiodarone, used pre- and postcardioversion, increases the rate of successful cardioversion in patients undergoing initial cardioversion[54] and in those for whom past cardioversion failed.[39,55] In patients for whom past cardioversion failed, success rates were 7 of 16 (44%) with 4 weeks of amiodarone (600 mg/d by mouth) and 32 of 49 (65%) with amiodarone (6.0-g load by mouth) given before cardioversion.

Ibutilide clearly is shown to facilitate successful cardioversion in patients for whom direct current cardioversion failed.[56] In one study, 100 patients who had long-duration AF (mean 117 ± 201 days) and a high prevalence of structural heart disease (89%) were randomized to undergo transthoracic electrical cardioversion with or without pretreatment with ibutilide (1 mg). Remarkably, conversion to sinus rhythm occurred in 50 of 50 (100%) of patients pretreated with ibutilide compared with 36 of 50 (72%) of those who did not have pretreatment. Additionally, all 14 patients in the untreated group were cardioverted successfully after ibutilide pretreatment. Sustained polymorphic ventricular tachycardia occurred in 2 of 64 patients treated with ibutilide; both patients had ejection fractions less than or equal to 20%.

Thus, amiodarone and ibutilide facilitate cardioversion effectively in patients who have true failed cardioversion. Conveniently, ibutilide can be administered over a short time frame for same-day treatment. Ibutilide, however, should not be used in patients who have low ejection fractions. In patients who have ejection fractions less than or equal to 30%, oral loading with amiodarone is the preferred option.

Complications The risks and complications of cardioversion fall largely into three categories: (1) risks associated with sedation, (2) thromboembolic events (<1% with appropriate anticoagulation),[15,17] and (3) postcardioversion arrhythmias. Overall, the risk for electrical cardioversion is low in patients who are selected properly.[1,57]

Pharmacologic Cardioversion

General considerations

Because of the relative simplicity and high efficacy, most cardioversions are performed electrically. Pharmacologic cardioversion is used primarily in two settings: (1) for short-duration AF in highly symptomatic patients who have little or no structural heart disease, and (2) as adjunct therapy to facilitate electrical cardioversion in patients who have undergone failed cardioversion or have IRAF. In rare instances, such as to avoid anesthesia, pharmacologic cardioversion also may be indicated.

The principles of pericardioversion anticoagulation apply whether cardioversion is performed electrically or pharmacologically. That is, if patients' AF episodes have persisted for more than 48 hours or for unknown duration, those patients should undergo therapeutic anticoagulation for 3 weeks or TEE with heparin administration before initiation of any antiarrhythmic medication, even those with low efficacy. In particular, amiodarone frequently is used in patients who have AF. Because amiodarone has the potential to convert the AF to sinus rhythm, pericardioversion anticoagulation principles should be applied.

Short-duration atrial fibrillation

In patients who have little comorbid disease and short-duration AF, antiarrhythmic agents show no significant difference in long-term cardioversion outcomes compared with placebo. Class IC agents, however, show a faster time to cardioversion and therefore may be useful in terminating short-duration episodes of AF more rapidly for patients who are highly symptomatic.[58,59]

This finding underlies the "pill-in-the-pocket" approach to management of symptomatic, short-duration AF in patients who have little to no structural heart disease. One study examined 268 patients who had little structural heart disease and presented to an emergency department for symptomatic AF.[60] On discharge from the hospital, patients were instructed in out-of-hospital self-administration of flecainide or propafenone after the onset of symptoms. Patients weighing more than 70 kg received flecainide (300 mg) or propafenone (600 mg); those weighing less than 70 kg in weight received flecainide (200 mg) or propafenone (450 mg). This approach was successful in 94% of episodes (534/569), with time to resolution of symptoms at 113 ± 93 minutes. In 139 of 165 patients, the medication was effective for all arrhythmic episodes. Also, the number of monthly emergency room visits and hospitalizations decreased significantly after the initiation of this management strategy. Overall, 12 of 268 patients (7%) experienced adverse effects, including nausea, asthenia, and vertigo. One episode of atrial flutter with 1:1 AV conduction occurred. Given its overall safety and efficacy, the pill-in-the-pocket strategy can be useful in a select population of patients who have AF.

Longer-duration atrial fibrillation

In patients who have structural heart disease and longer-duration AF, pharmacologic cardioversion shows only modest success (20%–30%).[56,61] Therefore, electrical cardioversion is used more commonly. Antiarrhythmic medications provide useful adjunct therapy for patients experiencing IRAF postcardioversion or those who have true cardioversion failure.

ATRIAL FLUTTER

Generally, the principles discussed previously are valid for atrial flutter, except as specifically noted. In particular, anticoagulation for patients who have atrial flutter should be handled just as it would for patients who have AF.

SUMMARY

In summary, cardioversion is a useful option in managing patients who have AF. It is useful especially for patients who are symptomatic or newly diagnosed or for some patients who have postoperative AF. To minimize the presence of thrombus at cardioversion, patients who have AF of more than 48 hours' duration should undergo therapeutic anticoagulation for 3 weeks prior (full-dose low molecular weight heparin or warfarin; INR target, 2.5; range, 2.0–3.0) or TEE accompanied by heparin before cardioversion. To minimize the formation of thrombus post-cardioversion in patients who experience AF for more than 48 hours, therapeutic anticoagulation should be continued for 4 weeks, keeping in mind that the greatest risk for systemic embolization occurs during the first few days postcardioversion. Electrical, pharmacologic, or a combined approach to cardioversion can be taken. In most cases, transthoracic electrical cardioversion is indicated, given its simplicity and high efficacy, especially in the era of biphasic-waveform defibrillators, even in patients who have multiple comorbid conditions and significant structural heart disease.

Pharmacologic cardioversion with class IC agents may be useful for early conversion to sinus rhythm in patients who have minimal structural heart disease and short-duration, symptomatic AF. Antiarrhythmic agents also are useful in the setting of two distinct postcardioversion outcomes: (1) IRAF, which is recurrence within minutes post cardioversion after even just one sinus beat, and (2) true failed cardioversion (no sinus beats seen). Patients who have IRAF and who experience persistent sinus rhythm may have good rates of long-term freedom from AF and should be treated aggressively with pharmacologically facilitated cardioversion. Ibutilide, amiodarone, and verapamil along with propafenone and quinidine are effective. For patients who have true failed cardioversion, ibutilide and amiodarone are effective. Given its short administration period and strong clinical efficacy, ibutilide is an excellent agent for facilitated cardioversion, except in patients who have ejection fractions less than or equal to 30%. Because of the potential for cardioversion, regardless of indication or level of efficacy, antiarrhythmic medications should be given only with proper application of the principles of pericardio-version anticoagulation.

REFERENCES

1. Fuster V, Ryden LE, Cannom DS, et al. ACC/AHA/ESC 2006 guidelines for the management of patients with atrial fibrillation: a report of the American College of Cardiology/American Heart Association Task Force on practice guidelines and the European Society of Cardiology Committee for Practice Guidelines (Writing Committee to Revise the 2001 guidelines for the management of patients with atrial fibrillation): developed in collaboration with the European Heart Rhythm Association and the Heart Rhythm Society. Circulation 2006;114(7):E257–354.

2. Wijffels MCEF, Kirchhof CJHJ, Dorland R, et al. Atrial fibrillation begets atrial fibrillation. Circulation 1995; 92:1954–68.

3. Kopecky SL, Gersh BJ, McGoon MD, et al. The natural history of lone atrial fibrillation: a population based study over three decades. N Engl J Med 1987;317:669–74.

4. Godtfredsen J. Atrial fibrillation: etiology, course and prognosis: a follow-up study of 1212 cases. Copenhagen (Denmark): Munksgaard; 1975.

5. Van Gelder IC, Crijns HJ, Van Gilst WH, et al. Prediction of uneventful cardioversion and maintenance of sinus rhythm from direct-current electrical cardioversion of chronic atrial fibrillation and flutter. Am J Cardiol 1991;68(1):41–6.

6. The Atrial Fibrillation Follow-up Investigation of Rhythm Management (AFFIRM) Investigators. A comparison of rate control and rhythm control in patients with atrial fibrillation. N Engl J Med 2002;347: 1825–33.

7. Van Gelder IC, Hagens VE, Bosker HA, et al. Rate Control versus Electrical Cardioversion for Persistent Atrial Fibrillation Study Group. A comparison of rate control and rhythm control in patients with recurrent persistent atrial fibrillation. N Engl J Med 2002; 347(23):1834–40.

8. Alegret JM, Viñolas X, Sagristá J, et al. REVERSE Study Investigators. Predictors of success and effect of biphasic energy on electrical cardioversion in patients with persistent atrial fibrillation. Europace 2007;9(10):942–6.

9. Boriani G, Diemberger I, Biffi M, et al. Electrical cardioversion for persistent atrial fibrillation or atrial flutter in clinical practice: predictors of long-term outcome. Int J Clin Pract 2007;61(5):748–56.

10. Dudley SC Jr, Hoch NE, McCann LA, et al. Atrial fibrillation increases production of superoxide by the left atrium and left atrial appendage: role of the NADPH and xanthine oxidases. Circulation 2005; 112(9):1266–73.

11. O'Neill PG, Puleo PR, Bolli R, et al. Return of atrial mechanical function following electrical conversion of atrial dysrhythmias. Am Heart J 1990;120(2):353–9.

12. Laupacis A, Albers G, Dalen J, et al. Antithrombotic therapy in atrial fibrillation. Chest 1998;114(5 Suppl): 579S–89S.

13. Manning WJ, Leeman DE, Gotch PJ, et al. Pulsed Doppler evaluation of atrial mechanical function after electrical cardioversion of atrial fibrillation. J Am Coll Cardiol 1989;13(3):617–23.

14. Bjerkelund C, Orning O. The efficacy of anticoagulant therapy in preventing embolism related to DC electrical conversion of atrial fibrillation. Am J Cardiol 1969; 23:208–16.

15. Stellbrink C, Nixdorff U, Hofmann T, et al. ACE (Anticoagulation in Cardioversion using Enoxaparin) Study Group. Safety and efficacy of enoxaparin compared with unfractionated heparin and oral anticoagulants for prevention of thromboembolic complications in cardioversion of nonvalvular atrial fibrillation: the Anticoagulation in Cardioversion using Enoxaparin (ACE) trial. Circulation 2004;109(8): 997–1003.

16. Gallagher MM, Hennessy BJ, Edvardsson N, et al. Embolic complications of direct current cardioversion of atrial arrhythmias: association with low intensity of anticoagulation at the time of cardioversion. J Am Coll Cardiol 2002;40(5):926–33.

17. Klein AL, Grimm RA, Murray RD, et al. Assessment of Cardioversion Using Transesophageal Echocardiography Investigators. Use of transesophageal echocardiography to guide cardioversion in patients with atrial fibrillation. N Engl J Med 2001;344(19): 1411–20.

18. Berger M, Schweitzer P. Timing of thromboembolic events after electrical cardioversion of atrial fibrillation or flutter: a retrospective analysis. Am J Cardiol 1998;82(12):1545–7 A8. Full-Text PDF (62 KB).

19. Weigner MJ, Caulfield TA, Danias PG, et al. Risk for clinical thromboembolism associated with conversion to sinus rhythm in patients with atrial fibrillation lasting less than 48 hours. Ann Intern Med 1997; 126(8):615–20.

20. Strickberger SA, Ip J, Saksena S, et al. Relationship between atrial tachyarrhythmias and symptoms. Heart Rhythm 2005;2(2):125–31.

21. Mittal S, Ayati S, Stein KM, et al. Transthoracic cardioversion of atrial fibrillation: comparison of rectilinear biphasic versus damped sine wave monophasic shocks. Circulation 2000;101(11): 1282–7.

22. Zhou X, Daubert JP, Wolf PD, et al. Epicardial mapping of ventricular defibrillation with monophasic and biphasic shocks in dogs. Circ Res 1993;72(1): 145–60.

23. Dahl CF, Ewy GA, Warner ED, et al. Myocardial necrosis from direct current countershock: effect of

paddle electrode size and time interval between discharges. Circulation 1974;50:956–61.

24. Joglar JA, Kessler DJ, Welch PJ, et al. Effects of repeated electrical defibrillations on cardiac troponin I levels. Am J Cardiol 1999;83:270–2.

25. Lown B, Perlroth MG, Kaidbey S, et al. "Cardioversion" of atrial fibrillation. A report on the treatment of 65 episodes in 50 patients. N Engl J Med 1963;269:325–31.

26. Mittal S, Stein KM, Markowitz SM, et al. An update on electrical cardioversion of atrial fibrillation. Card Electrophysiol Rev 2003;7(3):285–9.

27. Winkle RA, Mead H, Ruder MA, et al. Improved low energy defibrillation efficacy in man with the use of a biphasic truncated exponential waveform. Am Heart J 1989;117:122–7.

28. Kroll M, Anderson K, Supino C, et al. Decline in defibrillation thresholds. Pacing Clin Electrophysiol 1993;16(1 pt 2):213–7.

29. Bardy GH, Marchlinski FE, Sharma AD, et al. Multicenter comparison of truncated biphasic shocks and standard damped sine wave monophasic shocks for transthoracic ventricular defibrillation. Transthoracic investigators. Circulation 1996; 94(10):2507–14.

30. Ricard P, Levy S, Boccara G, et al. External cardioversion of atrial fibrillation: comparison of biphasic vs. monophasic waveform shocks. Europace 2001; 3(2):96–9.

31. Page RL, Kerber RE, Russell JK, et al. BiCard Investigators. Biphasic versus monophasic shock waveform for conversion of atrial fibrillation: the results of an international randomized, double-blind multicenter trial. J Am Coll Cardiol 2002;39(12):1956–63.

32. Khaykin Y, Newman D, Kowalewski M, et al. Biphasic versus monophasic cardioversion in shock-resistant atrial fibrillation. J Cardiovasc Electrophysiol 2003;14(8):868–72.

33. Botto GL, Politi A, Bonini W, et al. External cardioversion of atrial fibrillation: role of paddle position on technical efficacy and energy requirements. Heart 1999;82:726–30.

34. Brazdzionyte J, Babarskiene RM, Stanaitiene G. Anterior-posterior versus anterior-lateral electrode position for biphasic cardioversion of atrial fibrillation. Medicina (Kaunas) 2006;42(12):994–8.

35. Kerber RE, Jensen SR, Grayzel J, et al. Elective cardioversion: influence of paddle-electrode location and size on success rates and energy requirements. N Engl J Med 1981;305:658–62.

36. Ambler JJ, Deakin CD. A randomised controlled trial of the effect of biphasic or monophasic waveform on the incidence and severity of cutaneous burns following external direct current cardioversion. Resuscitation 2006;71(3):293–300.

37. Levy S. Internal defibrillation: where we have been and where we should be going? J Interv Card Electrophysiol 2005;13(Suppl 1):61–6.

38. Timmermans C, Rodriguez LM, Smeets JL, et al. Immediate reinitiation of atrial fibrillation following internal atrial defibrillation. J Cardiovasc Electrophysiol 1998;9(2):122–8.

39. Van Noord T, Van Gelder IC, Schoonderwoerd BA, et al. Immediate reinitiation of atrial fibrillation after electrical cardioversion predicts subsequent pharmacologic and electrical conversion to sinus rhythm and amiodarone. Am J Cardiol 2000;86(12):1384–5, A5.

40. Tieleman RG, Van Gelder IC, Crijns HJ, et al. Early recurrences of atrial fibrillation after electrical cardioversion: a result of fibrillation-induced electrical remodeling of the atria? J Am Coll Cardiol 1998;31(1): 167–73.

41. Oral H, Ozaydin M, Sticherling C, et al. Effect of atrial fibrillation duration on probability of immediate recurrence after transthoracic cardioversion. J Cardiovasc Electrophysiol 2003;14(2):182–5.

42. Chugh A, Ozaydin M, Scharf C, et al. Mechanism of immediate recurrences of atrial fibrillation after restoration of sinus rhythm. Pacing Clin Electrophysiol 2004;27(1):77–82.

43. Husser D, Bollmann A, Kang S, et al. Determinants and prognostic significance of immediate atrial fibrillation recurrence following cardioversion in patients undergoing pulmonary vein isolation. Pacing Clin Electrophysiol 2005;28(2):119–25.

44. Rossi M, Lown B. The use of quinidine in cardioversion. Am J Cardiol 1967;19(2):234–8.

45. Jacobs LO, Andrews TC, Pederson DN, et al. Effect of intravenous procainamide on direct-current cardioversion of atrial fibrillation. Am J Cardiol 1998;82(2):241–2.

46. Bianconi L, Mennuni M, Lukic V, et al. Effects of oral propafenone administration before electrical cardioversion of chronic atrial fibrillation: a placebo-controlled study. J Am Coll Cardiol 1996;28(3):700–6.

47. De Simone A, Stabile G, Vitale DF, et al. Pretreatment with verapamil in patients with persistent or chronic atrial fibrillation who underwent electrical cardioversion. J Am Coll Cardiol 1999;34(3):810–4.

48. Tse HF, Lau CP, Ayers GM. Incidence and modes of onset of early reinitiation of atrial fibrillation after successful internal cardioversion, and its prevention by intravenous sotalol. Heart 1999;82(3):319–24.

49. Sticherling C, Hsu W, Tada H, et al. Effects of verapamil and ibutilide on atrial fibrillation and postfibrillation atrial refractoriness. J Cardiovasc Electrophysiol 2002;13(2):151–7.

50. Sticherling C, Ozaydin M, Tada H, et al. Comparison of verapamil and ibutilide for the suppression of immediate recurrences of atrial fibrillation after transthoracic cardioversion. J Cardiovasc Pharmacol Ther 2002;7(3):155–60.

51. Daoud EG, Hummel JD, Augostini R, et al. Effect of verapamil on immediate recurrence of atrial fibrillation. J Cardiovasc Electrophysiol 2000;11(11): 1231–7.

52. Frick M, Frykman V, Jensen-Urstad M, et al. Factors predicting success rate and recurrence of atrial fibrillation after first electrical cardioversion in patients with persistent atrial fibrillation. Clin Cardiol 2001;24(3):238–44.

53. Kabukcu M, Demircioglu F, Yanik E, et al. Simultaneous double external DC shock technique for refractory atrial fibrillation in concomitant heart disease. Jpn Heart J 2004;45(6):929–36.

54. Manios EG, Mavrakis HE, Kanoupakis EM, et al. Effects of amiodarone and diltiazem on persistent atrial fibrillation conversion and recurrence rates: a randomized controlled study. Cardiovasc Drugs Ther 2003;17(1):31–9.

55. Opolski G, Stanislawska J, Gorecki A, et al. Amiodarone in restoration and maintenance of sinus rhythm in patients with chronic atrial fibrillation after unsuccessful direct-current cardioversion. Clin Cardiol 1997;20(4):337–40.

56. Oral H, Souza JJ, Michaud GF, et al. Facilitating transthoracic cardioversion of atrial fibrillation with ibutilide pretreatment. N Engl J Med 1999;340(24):1849–54.

57. Ditchey RV, Karliner JS. Safety of electrical cardioversion in patients without digitalis toxicity. Ann Intern Med 1981;95(6):676–9.

58. Capucci A, Lenzi T, Boriani G, et al. Effectiveness of loading oral flecainide for converting recent-onset atrial fibrillation to sinus rhythm in patients without organic heart disease or with only systemic hypertension. Am J Cardiol 1992;70:69–72.

59. Crijns HJ, van Wijk LM, van Gilst WH, et al. Acute conversion of atrial fibrillation to sinus rhythm: clinical efficacy of flecainide acetate. Comparison of two regimens. Eur Heart J 1988;9(6):634–8.

60. Alboni P, Botto GL, Baldi N, et al. Outpatient treatment of recent-onset atrial fibrillation with the "pill-in-the-pocket" approach. N Engl J Med 2004; 351(23):2384–91.

61. Singh S, Zoble RG, Yellen L, et al. Efficacy and safety of oral dofetilide in converting to and maintaining sinus rhythm in patients with chronic atrial fibrillation or atrial flutter the symptomatic atrial fibrillation investigative research on dofetilide (SAFIRE-D) study. Circulation 2000;102:2385–90.

Drug Therapy for Atrial Fibrillation

Emily L. Conway, MD[a], Simone Musco, MD[a],
Peter R. Kowey, MD[a,b],*

KEYWORDS

- Atrial fibrillation • Pharmacologic therapy
- Rhythm control • Prevention

Atrial fibrillation (AF) is the most frequently diagnosed arrhythmia, affecting an estimated 2.3 million people in the United States. Prevalence increases with age, occurring in 3.8% of people age 60 and older and in up to 9% of people over age 80.[1]

One of the fundamental considerations in the management of AF is whether or not to attempt to restore sinus rhythm or to allow AF to continue while controlling the ventricular rates. The decision depends on the severity of symptoms, associated heart disease, age, and other comorbidities that may limit therapeutic options.

AF can be classified as paroxysmal, persistent, or permanent. Paroxysmal AF terminates spontaneously, with episodes typically lasting less than 24 hours but possibly lasting up to 7 days. Persistent AF requires cardioversion (pharmacologic or electrical) to terminate, and episodes last greater than 7 days. Permanent AF describes continuous AF that has failed cardioversion or where cardioversion never has been attempted. Recurrent AF describes two or more episodes of paroxysmal or persistent AF.

Determining how symptomatic patients are from AF can be difficult. Symptoms of palpitations, dyspnea, lightheadedness, or syncope generally are related to rapid, irregular ventricular rates. By slowing the heart rate with atrioventricular (AV) nodal blocking agents, these symptoms may abate. Some patients may notice a subtle decline in exercise tolerance or complain of generalized fatigue despite adequate rate control resulting from loss of atrial mechanical function. Patients who have hypertension, left ventricular hypertrophy, impaired diastolic relaxation, and restrictive cardiomyopathy are particularly sensitive to the loss of AV synchrony and the resultant decrease in diastolic filling. Patients who clearly are symptomatic from AF may benefit from an attempt to control rhythm. In asymptomatic patients who have no appreciable decline in functional status in AF, rate control may be sufficient.

RHYTHM VERSUS RATE CONTROL

Multiple prospective randomized studies have examined the issue of rhythm versus rate control. The two largest trials, Atrial Fibrillation Follow-up Investigation of Rhythm Management (AFFIRM) and Rate Control Versus Electrical Cardioversion for Persistent Atrial Fibrillation (RACE), failed to show any benefit in the rhythm-control arm.[2,3] The AFFIRM trial enrolled more than 4000 patients who had paroxysmal and persistent AF. Patients were randomized to receive rate control or antiarrhythmic drug therapy. All patients initially were anticoagulated, but patients in the rhythm-control group who had remained in sinus rhythm for at least 3 months could stop warfarin. There was no significant difference in the primary end point of overall mortality, with a trend toward increased risk in the rhythm-control group (5-year mortality,

A version of this article originally appeared in *Medical Clinics of North America*, volume 92, issue 1. Support for research provided by the WW Smith Charitable Trust and the Albert Greenfield Foundation.
[a] Lankenau Hospital, Division of Cardiovascular Diseases, Main Line Heart Center, Suite 556, Medical Office Building East, 100 Lancaster Avenue, Wynnewood, PA 19096, USA
[b] Thomas Jefferson University, 1020 Walnut Street, Philadelphia, PA 19107, USA
* Corresponding author. Lankenau Hospital and Institute for Medical Research, Division of Cardiovascular Diseases, Main Line Heart Center, Suite 556, Medical Office Building East, 100 Lancaster Avenue, Wynnewood, PA 19096, USA.
E-mail address: Koweypr@mlhheart.org (P.R. Kowey).

Cardiol Clin 27 (2009) 109–123
doi:10.1016/j.ccl.2008.10.003
0733-8651/08/$ – see front matter © 2009 Elsevier Inc. All rights reserved.

24% versus 21%). A trend toward higher risk for ischemic stroke was seen in the rhythm-control group, however, mainly in patients who were not receiving adequate anticoagulation. This emphasizes the need for indefinite anticoagulation for rate- and rhythm-control methods in high-risk patients, because asymptomatic recurrences of AF predispose to thromboembolic events.

The RACE trial randomized 522 patients who had persistent AF, despite previous electrical cardioversion, into rate- or rhythm-control groups. All patients were anticoagulated. The study protocol allowed patients in the rhythm-control group who had maintained sinus rhythm for 1 month the option of discontinuing warfarin therapy. The primary end point was a composite of death from cardiovascular causes, heart failure, thromboembolic complications, bleeding, implantation of a pacemaker, or severe adverse reactions to drugs. After a mean of 2.3 years of follow-up, the trial found rate control was not inferior to rhythm control for the prevention of death or morbidity. Only 39% of the rhythm-control group was in sinus rhythm compared with 10% of the rate-control group. Within the rhythm-control group, hypertension and female gender were associated with a higher risk for an event. Higher rates of thromboembolic events occurred in the rhythm-control group, with most of the events associated with subtherapeutic anticoagulation. Cessation of anticoagulation also was associated with a higher risk for thromboembolic events.

To address the issue of whether or not patients had any difference in exercise tolerance with rate versus rhythm control, a substudy of the AFFIRM trial performed serial 6-minute walk tests on 245 study patients.[4] Walk distances improved in both groups over time, with slightly longer distances observed in the rhythm-control group. It was unclear whether or not the difference in walk distances was clinically significant.

Focusing on the heart failure population, a recent multicenter, randomized study from the Atrial Fibrillation and Congestive Heart Failure investigators compared rhythm versus rate control in 1376 patients with a left ventricular ejection fraction of 35% or less. There was no difference between the two groups in cardiovascular mortality, all-cause mortality, stroke, or worsening heart failure.[5]

The results from the AFFIRM and RACE trials are most applicable to elderly patients (mean ages of study patients were 70 and 68, respectively) who have few or no symptoms from AF, for whom anticoagulation and a strategy of rate control may be most appropriate. For younger, symptomatic patients who do not have underlying heart disease, restoration of sinus rhythm must still be considered a valid approach.

RATE CONTROL AGENTS

The goal of rate control is to control the resting heart rate and the heart rate during exercise while avoiding excessive bradycardia. Persistent tachycardia may lead to development of cardiomyopathy, which usually is reversible with adequate rate control. Although criteria for adequate rate control vary among trials, typical goals for ventricular rates range from 60 to 80 beats per minute at rest and between 90 and 115 beats per minute during exercise.[6] Given that rates may be well controlled at rest but may increase significantly during exercise, it is useful to record heart rates during exercise stress testing or by 24-hour ambulatory EKG monitoring.

Ventricular rate during AF is a function of the refractoriness of the AV node, sympathetic and parasympathetic tone, and intrinsic conduction. Agents that prolong the refractory period of the AV node effectively control ventricular rate. β-Blockers, calcium channel blockers, and digoxin all slow conduction through the AV node and may be used alone or in combination for rate control.

β-Blockers are the most effective monotherapy for rate control, especially in high adrenergic states. In the AFFIRM trial, 70% of patients on β-blockers achieved adequate rate control (as defined previously) compared with 54% of patients on calcium channel blockers.[2] In the acute setting, intravenous β-blockade with esmolol, metoprolol, propanolol, or atenolol has a rapid onset. Esmolol may be given as a continuous intravenous infusion. Caution is advised when starting β-blockers in patients who have heart failure or hypotension. In hemodynamically stable patients, oral β-blockade is safe and effective for controlling ventricular rates. Sotalol, a β-blocker with Vaughan-Williams class III antiarrhythmic properties that suppresses AF, is associated with slower ventricular rates with AF recurrences.

Calcium channel blockers (nondihydropyridines) may be preferred in patients who have preserved left ventricular systolic function and severe chronic obstructive pulmonary disease. Verapamil and diltiazem are equally effective in controlling ventricular rates. Given intravenously, calcium channel blockers have a rapid onset of action (2–7 minutes). To maintain effectiveness, a continuous drip usually is given because of the drugs' short half-lives.

Digoxin, once considered first-line treatment for rate control in the acute management of AF, is less effective than β-blockers or calcium channel blockers. Intravenous digoxin requires 60 minutes to take effect, whereas its peak effect may not be seen for 6 hours. Digoxin is not shown more effective than placebo in converting AF to sinus rhythm. Digoxin may be used in patients who cannot tolerate β-blockers or calcium channel blockers because of heart failure or hypotension. Digoxin is less effective in settings of high sympathetic tone and does not slow heart rates during exercise. In sedentary patients who do not exercise, digoxin alone may be sufficient to control rates at rest.[6] Often, patients require combination therapy to achieve sufficient rate control.

RHYTHM CONTROL: PHARMACOLOGIC CARDIOVERSION

Once the decision is made to proceed with restoration of sinus rhythm, it can be pursued pharmacologically or electrically. The duration of AF is an important factor. Patients who have recent-onset AF (<48 hours) have a high rate of spontaneous conversion, up to 60% at 24 hours.[7] Pharmacologic or electrical cardioversion in this setting allows faster restoration of sinus rhythm, with resolution of symptoms and shorter lengths of stay. Success rates for direct current electrical cardioversion range from 75% to 93%. Administration of antiarrhythmic drugs before electrical cardioversion increases long-term success rates. Achievement of sinus rhythm with pharmacologic cardioversion alone varies by agent, averaging approximately 50% after 1 to 5 hours.[8] Biphasic electrical cardioversion may be more effective than pharmacologic cardioversion but requires pain control (general anesthesia or conscious sedation) and a 6- to 8-hour fasting period.

Once an episode of AF is present for more than 7 days, electrical cardioversion is preferred. Spontaneous conversion rates are much lower after 1 week, and pharmacologic therapy also is less effective. With either method, adequate anticoagulation must be achieved before cardioversion and for a period of 4 weeks after, as the risks for thromboembolic events are similar.

MAINTENANCE OF SINUS RHYTHM

For patients who have recurrent paroxysmal or persistent AF, the choice of agent for long-term antiarrhythmic therapy must be individualized. The benefit of maintaining sinus rhythm must be balanced against the side-effect profile of the antiarrhythmic drug. Even after successful cardioversion, recurrence of AF is high in untreated patients, with relapse rates of 71% to 84% at 1 year.[9] Using a rhythm control strategy, recurrence is reduced by 30% to 50%.[9]

Amiodarone is the most effective drug for preventing recurrence of AF.[9–11] In the Sotalol Amiodarone Atrial Fibrillation Efficacy Trial, 665 patients who had persistent AF were randomized to receive amiodarone, sotalol, or placebo and followed for 1 to 4.5 years. Recurrence rates at 1 year were 48% with amiodarone, 68% with sotalol, and 87% in the placebo group. A higher incidence of minor bleeding episodes was seen in the amiodarone group, likely because of interaction with warfarin levels.[12] The Canadian Trial of Atrial Fibrillation found similar results among 403 patients assigned to amiodarone, sotalol, or propafenone. After a mean follow-up period of 16 months, the recurrence rate for the amiodarone group was 35%, compared with 63% in the sotalol or propafenone group. A total of 18% of patients in the amiodarone group withdrew because of adverse events, however, compared with 11% in the sotalol or propafenone group.[10] In a post hoc analysis of the Veterans Affairs Congestive Heart Failure: Survival Trial of Antiarrhythmic Therapy, amiodarone facilitated conversion to and maintenance of sinus rhythm in patients who had left ventricular systolic dysfunction. Furthermore, the subset of patients who were maintained in sinus rhythm had lower overall mortality. Amiodarone was not linked to worsening of heart failure.[13] Despite its effectiveness over other agents, the lengthy list of potential adverse effects associated with amiodarone use makes it a second-line agent in patients who do not have contraindications to other antiarrhythmic drugs. Major side effects of amiodarone include potentially fatal pulmonary toxicity, thyroid dysfunction, hepatic toxicity, optic neuropathy, peripheral neuropathy, gastrointestinal upset, skin discoloration, and rarely torsades de pointes.

In patients who have no evidence of structural heart disease, class IC agents are first-line therapy for maintaining sinus rhythm, based on the guidelines recently issued by the American College of Cardiology, American Heart Association, and European Society of Cardiology.[6] Propafenone and flecainide generally are well tolerated, show similar effectiveness, and have a low risk for toxicity.[14] The Rythmol Atrial Fibrillation Trial, a randomized control trial of 523 patients, tested sustained-release propafenone in three doses (225 mg, 325 mg, and 425 mg). At the end of the 39-week follow-up period, recurrence rate of AF was 69% in the placebo group compared with 52%, 42%, and 30% in the propafenone groups (225 mg, 325 mg, and 425 mg, respectively). Similar results were found in the European Rythmol/Rytmonorm Atrial Fibrillation Trial of similar design.[15] There were significantly higher withdrawals because of adverse events in the 425-mg group than any other group.[16] Propafenone may cause gastrointestinal symptoms, such as nausea, and should be avoided in patients who have severe obstructive lung disease. Flecainide may cause mild neurologic side effects. Side effects of both agents may include hypotension and bradycardia after conversion to sinus rhythm. Class IC agents also may convert AF into a slow atrial flutter. The slow flutter rate may conduct 1:1, causing rapid ventricular conduction with a wide complex QRS, which may be mistaken for ventricular tachycardia. To prevent rapid ventricular rates, an agent to slow AV nodal conduction, such as a β-blocker or calcium channel blocker, may be coadministered with propafenone or flecainide. Because of the negative inotropic effect and proarrhythmic potential of class IC drugs, they should be avoided in patients who have heart failure or ischemic heart disease.

Sotalol, although not a useful agent for cardioverting AF to sinus rhythm, can be used to maintain sinus rhythm. Sotalol is a nonselective β-blocker, in addition to its class III potassium channel-blocking effects. Sotalol has the added benefit of slowing AV nodal conduction should AF recur, which may decrease symptoms during AF episodes. In the Sotalol Amiodarone Atrial Fibrillation Efficacy Trial and Canadian Trial of Atrial Fibrillation studies, recurrence rates of AF with sotalol were significantly lower compared with placebo, although higher than with amiodarone.[10,12] Sotalol prolongs the QT interval and has a risk for torsades de pointes. Sotalol should not be used in patients who have significant left ventricular hypertrophy or heart failure.

Dofetilide is a class III antiarrhythmic drug that selectively inhibits the delayed rectifier potassium current and increases the atrial and ventricular effective refractory period, prolonging repolarization. Plasma concentrations peak 2 to 3 hours after oral dosing. The corrected QT interval (QTc) lengthens in a linear, dose-dependent fashion. Unlike class IC agents, dofetilide has no negative inotropic effects. The safety of dofetilide in heart failure has been studied by the Danish Investigations of Arrhythmia and Mortality ON Dofetilide (DIAMOND) study group in two large randomized control trials, DIAMOND-CHF and DIAMOND-AF.[17,18] DIAMOND-CHF enrolled 1518 patients who had severe symptomatic left ventricular dysfunction randomized to dofetilide or placebo. The primary end point was all-cause mortality. After a median of 18 months' follow-up, there was no difference in survival in the two groups (41% versus 42%). DIAMOND-AF was a substudy of 506 heart failure patients who had baseline AF or flutter. Over the course of the study, 44% in the dofetilide group converted to sinus rhythm by 1 year

compared with 14% in the placebo group. At 1 year, patients receiving dofetilide had a 79% probability of maintaining sinus rhythm versus 42% in the placebo arm.

Because of its QTc prolonging effect, dofetilide use carries a risk for torsades de pointes. In the DIAMOND-CHF study, the incidence of torsades de pointes was 3.3%, with 76% of cases occurring within 3 days of initiation of dofetilide. During the study, dose reduction based on creatinine clearance decreased the incidence of torsades de pointes.[17] The risk for torsades de pointes can be minimized by adjusting the dose for renal function, along with instituting a 72-hour in-hospital monitoring period on initiation of dofetilide.

The Symptomatic Atrial Fibrillation Investigative Research on Dofetilide tested the safety and efficacy of dofetilide in a group of 325 patients who had persistent AF. The trial reported a 58% efficacy for maintaining sinus rhythm at 1 year (versus 25% with placebo) along with a much lower incidence of torsades de pointes (0.8%) compared with DIAMOND-AF. Dofetilide dosing in this study was reduced for impaired renal function and for prolongation of the QTc over 15% of baseline.[19] Similar results were reported in the European and Australian Multicenter Evaluative Research on Atrial Fibrillation and Dofetilide study.[20] Because of the complexity of dosing regimens, the US Food and Drug Administration has restricted prescription of dofetilide to registered hospitals, physicians, pharmacists, and nurses who have completed specific training in the use of the drug.

Selection of a specific antiarrhythmic agent usually is determined by the presence or absence of underlying cardiac disease (Fig. 1). Class IC antiarrhythmic drugs are contraindicated in patients who have marked left ventricular hypertrophy, coronary artery disease, or congestive heart failure because of the risk for ventricular arrhythmias. In patients who do not have structural heart disease, flecainide, propafenone, or sotalol is preferred because of their effectiveness and low risk for toxicity. Among class III drugs, dofetilide and sotalol are associated with QT prolongation and torsades de pointes and should be avoided in the presence of marked left ventricular hypertrophy. In patients who have congestive heart failure, only amiodarone and dofetilide are safe for use.

OUTPATIENT VERSUS INPATIENT INITIATION OF THERAPY

For paroxysmal AF, inpatient versus outpatient initiation of antiarrhythmic drug therapy is an important consideration. For symptomatic

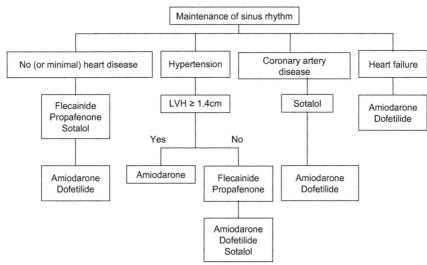

Fig. 1. Algorithm for antiarrhythmic drug selection for maintenance of sinus rhythm.

patients, the "pill-in-the-pocket" approach uses self-administration of a single dose of a drug shortly after the start of palpitations. The goal of this method is to terminate an episode and prevent recurrence while decreasing the need for emergency room visits, hospitalizations, and direct current cardioversions. This approach has been studied in patients who do not have structural heart disease, primarily with flecainide and propafenone.[21] After oral administration, an effect usually is seen in 3 to 4 hours.[22]

Certain class III agents may be started as outpatient treatment in certain patient populations under careful observation. Sotalol may be initiated as outpatient treatment in patients who have little or no heart disease, if the baseline QT interval is less than 450 milliseconds, the electrolytes are normal, and there are no predisposing factors to development of torsades de pointes.[6] Amiodarone has low proarrhythmic potential and may be prescribed without an inpatient evaluation in patients who do not have severe conduction disease. Dofetilide, by Food and Drug Administration mandate, requires inpatient monitoring for initiation.

Patients maintained on antiarrhythmic drugs need close follow-up.[23] Those on class III agents should have renal function, potassium, and magnesium levels checked periodically. An EKG should be performed every 6 months to measure the QT interval. Echocardiograms and stress testing should be checked at appropriate intervals for ischemic disease in patients on class IC antiarrhythmics. Amiodarone use mandates semiannual monitoring of thyroid, liver, and pulmonary function and yearly ocular examinations.

FUTURE PHARMACOLOGIC THERAPY

The marginal efficacy and safety of commercially available drugs has stimulated the development of new compounds in two major directions: modification of existing drugs and designing drugs with new targets. **Table 1** is a list of investigational compounds and their putative mechanism of action.[24,25] Although much interest has been generated by the modification of current class III agents, the discovery and characterization of novel ion channels believed to participate in onset and perpetuation of AF has provided a new way forward in drug development. Much of the research has focused on blocking potassium channels but several new ideas are being explored. The next paragraphs review the current evidence that supports the potential usefulness of these novel compounds.

AMIODARONE ANALOGUES
Dronedarone

Dronedarone is an amiodarone-like compound that lacks the iodine moiety that may be responsible for the pulmonary, thyroid, hepatic, and ocular toxicity of amiodarone. Like amiodarone, dronedarone has complex antiarrhythmic properties that span all classes of the Vaughan-Williams classification. Dronedarone inhibits potassium currents INa, IKr, and IKAch and L-type calcium current; has α- and β-adrenergic blocking properties; and prolongs the action potential duration in atria and ventricles with no significant reverse-use dependence. Dronedarone and amiodarone have similar

Table 1 Investigational antiarrhythmic drugs in development[a]	
Modification of Existing Compound	**Novel Mechanism of Action**
Amiodarone analogues	Serotonin type 4 antagonists
Dronedarone (I_{Kr} I_{Ks} $\beta1$ I_{Ca} I_{to} I_{Na})	Piboserod
Celivarone (I_{Kr} I_{Ks} $\beta1$ I_{Ca} I_{to} I_{Na})	RS100302
ATI-2042 (I_{Kr} I_{Ks} $\beta1$ I_{Ca} I_{to} I_{Na})	SB203186
ATI-2001 (I_{Kr} I_{Ks} $\beta1$ I_{Ca} I_{to} I_{Na})	Atrial selective repolarization delaying agents
GYKI-16638 (I_{Kr} I_{KI} I_{Na})	AZD 7009 (I_{Kr} I_{Na} I_{Kur})
KB 130015 (I_{KAch} I_{Ca} I_{KATP} I_{Na})	AVE 0118 (I_{Kr} I_{to})
Conventional class III agents	AVE 1231 (I_{Kr} I_{to})
Azimilide (I_{Kr} I_{Ks})	Vernakalant (I_{Kr} I_{to} I_{Na} I_{Ach})
Tedisamil (I_{Kr} I_{to} I_{KTAP} I_{Kur} I_{Na})	Almokalant (I_{Kr} I_{to} I_{Na} I_{Ach})
Bertosamil (I_{Kr} I_{to} I_{KTAP} I_{Kur} I_{Na})	Terikalant (I_{Kr} I_{to} I_{Na} I_{Ach})
SB-237376 (I_{Kr})	Nifekalant (I_{Kr} I_{to} I_{Na} I_{Ach})
NIP-142 (I_{Kur} I_{KAch})	S-9947 (I_{Kur})
L-768673 (I_{Ks})	S-20951 (I_{Kur})
HMR-1556 (I_{Ks})	Miscellaneous compounds
HMR-1402 (I_{Ks} I_{ATP})	ZP-123 (GAP 486)
Miscellaneous compounds	AAP 10 (connexin modulator)
Ersentilide (I_{Kr} β)	GsMtx (stretch receptor)
Trecetilide (I_{Kr} β)	
CP060S (I_{Na} I_{Ca})	
KB-R7943 (I_{Na} I_{Ca})	
Cariporide (I_{Na} I_H)	
JTV-519 (I_{Na} I_{Kr} I_{CA})	

Abbreviations: β, β-adrenergic antagonist; ICa, inward calcium current; IKach, Ach-sensitive inward potassium current; IKATP, ATP-sensitive inward potassium current; IKI, inward potassium rectifier; IKr, rapid component of the delayed rectifier potassium inward current; IKs, slow component of the delayed rectifier potassium inward current; IKur, ultra rapid component of the delayed rectifier potassium inward current; INa, inward sodium current; Ito, transient outward potassium current.

[a] The drugs are classified by mechanism of action.

Data from Goldstein RN, Stambler BS. New antiarrhythmic drugs for prevention of atrial fibrillation. Prog Cardiovasc Dis 2005;48:193–208; and Pecini R, Elming H, Pedersen OD, et al. New antiarrhythmic agents for atrial fibrillation and atrial flutter. Expert Opin Emerg Drugs 2005;10:311–22.

electrophysiologic properties in animal models, but their pharmacokinetic profiles differ significantly. Dronedarone has a 24-hour half-life and far less tissue accumulation.[26,27]

The Dronedarone Atrial Fibrillation Study After Electrical Cardioversion trial was designed to determine the most appropriate dose of dronedarone for prevention of AF after cardioversion. After 6-months' follow-up, 800 mg daily was deemed the optimal dose.[28] Thyroid, pulmonary, ocular, hepatic toxicity, or proarrhythmic effects were not seen at any of the study doses.

In the European Trial in Atrial Fibrillation or Flutter Patients Receiving Dronedarone for the Maintenance of Sinus Rhythm and its sister trial, the American-Australian-African Trial with Dronedarone in Atrial Fibrillation or Flutter Patients for the Maintenance of Sinus Rhythm, dronedarone administered at a dose of 400 mg twice daily was effective in preventing symptomatic and asymptomatic recurrences of AF or atrial flutter, the primary end point of the trials. A secondary end point of both trials, mean ventricular rate during AF atrial flutter at first recorded recurrence, also was reduced significantly. The incidence of adverse events in both trials was similar in the dronedarone and placebo groups.[29]

In the phase III study, Efficacy and Safety of Dronedarone for the Control of Ventricular Rate, dronedarone was tested in patients who had symptomatic permanent AF for its effect on heart rate. Dronedarone significantly reduced average resting and maximal exercise heart rates compared with placebo.[30]

The Antiarrhythmic Trial with Dronedarone in Moderate to Severe Congestive Heart Failure Evaluating Morbidity Decrease (ANDROMEDA) was a double-blind, placebo-controlled study evaluating the tolerability of dronedarone in high-risk patients who had congestive heart failure and ventricular dysfunction. The primary end point of the trial was death or hospitalization for heart failure. The study was ended prematurely after an interim safety analysis showed an excess risk for death in patients on active treatment.[31]

Because ANDROMEDA raised concerns over the safety of dronedarone in the heart failure population, further studies are needed. The ongoing trial, A Trial With Dronedarone to Prevent Hospitalization or Death in Patients With Atrial Fibrillation, was designed to examine further the safety and efficacy of dronedarone compared with placebo in a larger study group of 4628 patients.[32] Twenty-nine percent of the study population had a history of heart failure, although only 12% had evidence of systolic dysfunction. Preliminary results after 21 months of follow-up demonstrated a significant decrease in the combined end point of cardiovascular hospitalization or death in the dronedarone arm. This difference was mainly caused by a decrease in cardiovascular hospitalization and deaths from arrhythmia.[33]

Celivarone

Celivarone (SSR149744C) is a new noniodinated benzofuran derivative structurally related to amiodarone and dronedarone. Like its parent compounds, celivarone inhibits several potassium currents: IKr, IKs, IKAch, IKv1.5, and the L-type calcium current. Studies in canine models show relative atrial selectivity.[34] Two clinical trials currently are evaluating the role of celivarone in conversion and maintenance of AF.

The Maintenance of Sinus Rhythm in Patients with Recent Atrial Fibrillation/Flutter trial, a placebo-controlled, double-blind study of 673 patients, compared celivarone in a range of dosages (50, 100, 200, or 300 mg daily) with placebo for maintenance of sinus rhythm after electrical, pharmacologic, or spontaneous conversion of AF or atrial flutter.[35] The primary end point was recurrence of arrhythmia by ECG or transtelephonic ECG monitoring. Incidence of recurrence at 90 days was 52% in the celivarone, 50-mg arm, compared with 67% in the placebo arm. No thyroid dysfunction or proarrhythmia was seen.

The Double Blind Placebo Controlled Dose Ranging Study of the Efficacy and Safety of ssr149744c 300 or 600 mg for the Conversion of Atrial Fibrillation/Flutter trial has recently been completed and assesses the efficacy of celivarone in converting AF or flutter to sinus rhythm at the time of planned electrical cardioversion.[36]

ATI-2001 and Related Compounds

ATI-2001 is a synthetic amiodarone analogue shown to retain the electrophysiologic properties of amiodarone in regards to ventricular tachyarrhythmia initiation, perpetuation, and termination in guinea pigs isolated hearts.[37] In the same animal model, ATI-2001 was significantly more potent than amiodarone in its atrial and AV nodal electrophysiologic properties.[38] A recent study, however, showed that the half-life of ATI-2001 in human plasma is only 12 minutes, making the drug more suitable for acute termination of arrhythmias than for long-term management.[39] Of the ATI-2001 congeners, ATI-2042 may have more favorable pharmacokinetic properties and currently is in phase 2 development.[40]

TRADITIONAL CLASS III AGENTS
Azimilide

Azimilide is a selective once-daily class III antiarrhythmic agent that prolongs action, potential duration, and refractory periods in both atria and lacks reverse-use dependence.[41] The optimal dose, as determined in the Azimilide Supraventricular Arrhythmia Program, was 125 mg daily.[42] Unfortunately, after 180 days' follow-up, only 50% of patients enrolled maintained sinus rhythm.

The Azimilide Postinfarct Survival Evaluation, a large randomized trial of high-risk patients, as defined by low ejection fraction and recent myocardial infarction, showed no difference in all-cause mortality. The azimilide group, however, had fewer occurrences of AF and higher maintenance of sinus rhythm at 1 year.[43]

Three other studies have evaluated the role of azimilide in the treatment of symptomatic supraventricular arrhythmias.[44] The North American Azimilide Cardioversion Maintenance Trial-I investigated the role of azimilide compared with placebo for maintenance of sinus rhythm after electrical cardioversion of patients who had symptomatic AF. There was no significant difference between placebo and azimilide.[45]

The North American Azimilide Cardioversion Maintenance Trial-II, conducted in Europe, compared azimilide (125 mg daily) with sotalol (160 mg twice daily) or placebo in patients undergoing electrical cardioversion. Although azimilide was superior to placebo, it was inferior to sotalol with regard to efficacy and safety.[46] The Azimilide

Supraventricular Tachyarrhythmia Reduction trial also tested 125 mg of azimilide daily compared with placebo in patients who had symptomatic paroxysmal AF and structural heart disease. The primary end point was the time to the first symptomatic recurrence. No statistically significant difference was seen in the study groups.[47]

Although in these trials azimilide generally was well tolerated, early onset, reversible neutropenia has been reported in 0.2% and torsades de pointes in 0.9% of patients.[48] Based on its modest efficacy and these safety issues, it is unlikely that azimilide will be available for the treatment of AF.

Tedisamil

Tedisamil is a class III antiarrhythmic agent that blocks multiple potassium channels and slows sinus rate. Tedisamil prolongs action potential duration more strongly in the atria than in the ventricles.[49] Tedisamil also possesses significant antianginal and anti-ischemic properties.

In a study of 175 patients, tedisamil was shown to be superior to placebo in acutely terminating AF or atrial flutter.[50] The study, however, showed significant lengthening of the QTc. Two of the patients receiving the higher dose of the drug developed ventricular tachycardia during administration. Larger-scale studies are in progress to assess the safety and efficacy of tedisamil, although the initial report of torsades de pointes may make it a less desirable compound for widespread clinical use. Bertosamil, a structural analog of tedisamil, has similar pharmacologic properties. It has been studied in vitro but no clinical trials to date have been performed to validate its safety and efficacy.

ATRIAL REPOLARIZATION DELAYING AGENTS
Vernakalant

Vernakalant (RSD1235) is a sodium and potassium channel blocker with atrial selectivity and a short half-life (2–3 hours).[51,52] These attributes suggest vernakalant may be an appealing agent for pharmacologic cardioversion. Vernakalant has been demonstrated to be safe in a variety of doses in healthy volunteers.[53] Initial studies showed vernakalant superior to placebo in the acute termination of recent-onset AF, with a 61% conversion rate.[54]

Intravenous vernakalant has been studied in four trials for pharmacologic cardioversion. Atrial Arrhythmia Conversion Trial I and III (ACT I, N = 396; ACT III, N = 285) were phase 3, randomized, placebo-controlled trials of patients with AF or flutter of either short duration (3 hours–7 days) or long duration (8–45 days).[55,56] Vernakalant, 3 mg/kg, or placebo was administered over 10 minutes. If the patient failed to convert to sinus rhythm after 15 minutes, a second infusion of vernakalant, 2 mg/kg, was given. The primary end point was conversion to sinus rhythm within 90 minutes of drug dosage. In both trials, 51% of patients who received vernakalant converted to sinus rhythm, compared with 4% in the placebo group. Median time to conversion was 11 minutes in ACT I and 8 minutes in ACT III. Patients with short duration AF had the highest success rates, with 78% and 71%, respectively. Conversion rates fell to 8% to 9% in the long-duration AF group. The results of ACT IV, an open-label study of 167 patients, were presented at the Boston Atrial Fibrillation Symposium in January 2008, and also demonstrated a 51% conversion rate, with a median time to conversion of 14 minutes.

ACT II assessed the efficacy of intravenous vernakalant for cardioversion in 150 patients who developed AF within 7 days after coronary artery bypass grafting or valve replacement surgery.[57] All patients had AF of short duration (3–72 hours). Forty-seven percent of the vernakalant group converted to sinus rhythm, compared with 14% in the placebo group. Median time to conversion was 12 minutes.

The most commonly reported side effects of verkalant were dysguesia, sneezing, and nausea, occurring in 5% of patients. In ACT I, the QTc was greater than 500 milliseconds in 24% of the vernakalant group compared with 15% in the placebo group. No episodes of torsades de pointes were seen up to 24 hours postinfusion. Analysis of data from two phase II trials showed 5% of patients who received vernakalant developed ventricular arrhythmias in the first 2 hours, and 9% in the 2 to 24 hours after dosing.[58]

A phase 3 superiority study comparing intravenous vernakalant with intravenous amiodarone for pharmacologic cardioversion of recent-onset AF is currently underway.[59]

AVE0118

AVE0118 selectively blocks IKur, Ito, and IKACh in atrial tissue in several preclinical models.[60,61] In animal models, AVE0118 successfully converted 63% of persistent AF and increased the fibrillation wavelength significantly. Unlike dofetilide and ibutilide, AVE0118 did not have any appreciable effect on QT duration. Although preliminary studies of AVE0118 in animal models show promise, safety and efficacy in humans are not yet established.

AZD7009

AZD7009 is a mixed ion channel blocker (IKr, INa, and IKur) that prolongs atrial repolarization.[62] Animal models showed that AZD7009 effectively terminated all sustained episodes of induced AF and atrial flutter and prevented 95% of recurrences. Although QTc interval prolongation was noted, torsades de pointes were not induced.[63] A phase II clinical trial designed to assess the efficacy and safety of intravenous AZD7009 in conversion of AF currently is in progress.[64]

SEROTONIN ANTAGONISTS

The serotonin type 4 receptors are found in the atria but not in the ventricles. Stimulation of serotonin type 4 receptors of atrial human cells in vitro produces positive chronotropic effects and induces arrhythmias.[65,66] Efficacy of RS-100302, a selective serotonin type 4 antagonist, was tested in a pig model of AF and atrial flutter.[67] In experimental conditions, the agent terminated atrial flutter in 75% of the animals and AF in 88% of the animals and prevented reinduction of sustained tachycardia in all animals. At this time, there are not any positive clinical trial data with serotonin type 4 antagonists.

ADJUVANT THERAPY FOR PREVENTION OF ATRIAL FIBRILLATION
Angiotensin-Converting Enzyme Inhibitors

Remodeling of atrial tissue may contribute to the initiation and perpetuation of AF, especially in the heart failure population (**Table 2**). Recent studies show that blockade of the renin-angiotensin-aldosterone system prevents left atrial dilatation and atrial fibrosis, slows atrial conduction velocity, and reduces inflammation.[68,69] Several human and animal models show that the inhibition of the renin-angiotensin-aldosterone system may help prevent AF.[70] A substudy of the Trandolapril Cardiac Evaluation trial analyzed patients who had sinus rhythm at the time of randomization. After 2 to 4 years of follow-up, significantly more patients in the placebo group developed AF compared with the trandolapril group.[71] Similarly, a retrospective analysis conducted by a single center participating in the Studies of Left Ventricular Dysfunction revealed that treatment with enalapril markedly reduced the risk for developing AF in patients who had heart failure.[72] In a longitudinal cohort study that included hypertensive patients treated with angiotensin-converting enzyme inhibitors or calcium channel blockers, angiotensin-converting enzyme inhibitors were associated with a lower incidence of developing AF.[73] This favorable effect of angiotensin-converting enzyme inhibitors is supported further by meta-analyses of published data.[74,75]

In the Heart Outcomes Prevention Evaluation Study, however, which randomized 8335 patients without heart failure or left ventricular dysfunction to receive either ramipril or placebo, there was no difference in the incidence of new AF after median follow-up of 4.5 years. The overall incidence of new AF in the study was low (2.1%).[76]

The addition of enalapril to amiodarone increases the chances of maintaining sinus rhythm after cardioversion compared with amiodarone alone.[77] A study currently in progress is testing the hypothesis that angiotensin-converting enzyme inhibition with ramipril or aldosterone receptor antagonism with spironolactone decreases the incidence of AF in patients undergoing cardiothoracic surgery.[78]

Angiotensin Receptor Blockers

Clinical and experimental data support the notion that angiotensin-receptor blockers have similar effects as angiotensin-converting enzyme

Table 2
Drugs used as adjuvant therapy of atrial fibrillation and their proposed mechanism of action

Drugs	Proposed Mechanism of Action
ACE-I	Blockade of the RAAS
ARB	Inhibition of atrial remodeling Anti-inflammatory effect
Aldosterone	Inhibition of atrial fibrosis Anti-inflammatory effect
Omega-3 fatty acids	Unclear, may be direct antiarrhythmic effect
Steroids	Anti-inflammatory effect
Statins	Anti-inflammatory effect

Abbreviations: ACE-I, angiotensin-converting enzyme inhibitors; ARB, angiotensin-receptor blockers; RAAS, renin-angiotensin-aldosterone system.

inhibitors in affecting atrial structural remodeling and reducing atrial arrhythmias.[79,80] A retrospective analysis of two large randomized clinical trials, Valsartan Heart Failure Trial and Losartan Intervention for Endpoint Reduction in Hypertension, demonstrates that valsartan and losartan significantly reduced new-onset AF compared with the control groups, respectively, placebo and atenolol.[81,82] These findings were confirmed further in a prospective trial of hypertensive patients who had paroxysmal AF randomized to losartan or amlodipine, both in combination with amiodarone.[83] Also, treatment with irbesartan and amiodarone was found more effective than amiodarone alone in preventing recurrence of AF after electrical cardioversion.[84]

Conversely, the Candesartan in the Prevention of Relapsing Atrial Fibrillation trial did not show significant difference in maintenance of sinus rhythm after electrical cardioversion in patients treated with candesartan or placebo.[85]

Larger prospective trials are needed to test the efficacy of angiotensin-receptor blockers in adjunctive treatment of AF. The results of ongoing prospective trials, such as Angiotensin II-Antagonist in Paroxysmal Atrial Fibrillation trial using omesartan[86] and the Gruppo Italiano per lo Studio della Sopravvivenza nell'Infarto Miocardico–Atrial Fibrillation Trial using valsartan,[87] are eagerly awaited.

Further research is also investigating the role of angiotension II in contributing to a prothombotic state in atrial tissue. Increased atrial levels of angiotensin II have been shown to increase expression of vascular cell adhesion molecules, causing increased adhesion of inflammatory cells. This proinflammatory state has been hypothesized to contribute to atrial thrombus formation. The Atrial Fibrillation Clopidogrel Trial with Irbesartan for Prevention of Vascular Events is assessing whether angiotension II receptor antagonists may reduce the incidence of stroke in patients with AF.[88]

Aldosterone Antagonists

Although to date no clinical trial has evaluated the effect of aldosterone blockade in AF, in vitro experimental data suggest a beneficial effect. Spironolactone and its major metabolite, canrenoic acid, successfully inactivated the potassium channels HERG, hKv1.5, Kv4.3, and Kv7.1+mink, which generate the human IKur, Ito, and IKs currents when transfected in murine cell lines.[89] Prospective clinical trials testing the efficacy of aldosterone antagonists in AF are currently enrolling patients.[90]

MISCELLANEOUS AGENTS
Anti-Inflammatory Agents: Steroids and Statins

A largely unexplored field is the relationship between inflammation and AF. This seems of particular importance in postoperative states and in cases of myopericarditis. Some experimental models point to a role for steroids as anti-inflammatory agents. The use of prednisone at high doses in a canine model suppresses the expression of markers of inflammation and the onset and perpetuation of atrial flutter and AF.[91]

A recently published trial of patients undergoing coronary bypass graft surgery with or without aortic valve replacement found that perioperative use of corticosteroids decreased the incidence of postoperative AF.[92] The trial corroborated earlier findings from smaller studies,[93,94] but because of their adverse effects, more evidence is needed before the routine use of corticosteroids can be recommended.

Statins exhibit anti-inflammatory properties. Given the theory that AF is linked to inflammation, studies have begun to examine whether or not statins decrease the occurrence of AF.[95,96] In a small study of persistent AF, the use of statins was associated with a significant decrease in the risk for arrhythmia recurrence after successful cardioversion.[97] In an observational study in a large outpatient cardiology practice, statin therapy seemed protective against the development of AF.[98] Statin use has been associated with less AF after lung, esophageal, and coronary bypass surgery.[99,100]

To test whether pretreatment with statins may reduce postoperative AF, the Atorvastatin for Reduction of Myocardial Dysrhythmia After Cardiac Surgery study randomized 200 patients undergoing elective cardiac surgery with cardiopulmonary bypass to pretreatment with atorvastatin, 40 mg, or placebo daily, starting 7 days before surgery. Postoperative AF occurred in 35% of patients receiving atorvastatin compared with 57% in the placebo group.[101] A recent study of 124 patients undergoing elective off-pump coronary bypass surgery showed similar results with patients given atorvastatin, 20 mg daily, starting 3 days before surgery. The incidence of AF was 13% in the atorvastatin group versus 27% in the placebo group.[102] Larger-scale trials are needed to confirm these findings.

The Atorvastatin Therapy for the Prevention of Atrial Fibrillation trial is a prospective randomized, placebo-controlled study that is testing whether or not atorvastatin (80 mg daily) can reduce the recurrence rate of AF after elective electrical cardioversion compared with standard therapy.[103]

Table 3
Currently available drugs for treatment of atrial fibrillation according to the Vaughan-Williams classification, their mechanism of action, and their main adverse effects

Drug	Mechanism of Action	Main Adverse Effect
Class I		
Ia – Quinidine	Sodium channel blockade, delays phase 0 of action potential	Torsades de pointes, diarrhea, dyspepsia, hypotension
Ic – Flecanide	Sodium channel blockade, strongly delays phase 0 of action potential	Ventricular tachycardia, congestive heart failure, increased atrioventricular conduction
Ic – Propafenone	Sodium channel blockage, strongly delays phase 0 of action potential	Ventricular tachycardia, congestive heart failure, increased atrioventricular conduction
Class III		
Amiodarone	Multichannel blockade	Thyroid toxicity, pulmonary toxicity, hepatic toxicity, dyspepsia, QT prolongation, torsades de pointes (rare), hypotension, bradycardia
Sotalol	Potassium channel blockade (mainly I_{Kr}), β-receptor blockage	Torsades de pointes, congestive heart failure, bronchospasm
Dofetilide	Potassium channel blockade (mainly I_{Kr})	QT prolongation, torsades de pointes
Ibutilide	Potassium channel blockade (mainly I_{Kr}), activation of a slow, delayed I_{Na} current that occurs early during repolarization	QT prolongation, torsades de pointes

Omega-3 Fatty Acids

Incorporation of dietary omega-3 fatty acids into rabbit atrial tissue reduces stretch-induced susceptibility to AF.[104] In a study of patients who had paroxysmal atrial tachycardia and an implanted permanent pacemaker, daily intake of omega-3 fatty acids (1 g) reduced the number of episodes and total burden of atrial arrhythmia significantly.[105] Additionally, a recent trial randomized patients undergoing elective coronary bypass surgery to omega-3 fatty acids (2 g daily) or placebo.[106] Patients receiving omega-3 fatty acid had a significantly lower incidence of postoperative AF and a shorter hospital stay than those receiving placebo.

The Rotterdam study prospectively examined the relationship between dietary fish intake, long-chain omega-3 fatty acid supplementation, and the incidence of AF. After a mean follow-up of 6.4 years, neither omega-3 fatty acid nor dietary fish intake was linked to a lower incidence of AF.[107]

Given conflicting results in the current literature, large randomized control trials are needed to delineate better what effect, if any, omega-3 fatty acids have on AF. These trials are in progress.

SUMMARY

Many pharmacologic options are available for the treatment of AF. The results of large clinical trials, such as AFFIRM and RACE, suggest that controlling ventricular rates during AF is a valid approach. For symptomatic patients, sinus rhythm can be restored and maintained using pharmacologic or ablative therapy. The role of antiarrhythmic therapy after AF ablation remains unclear, because further research is needed in this area. **Table 3** lists the antiarrhythmic drugs currently available for use in patients who have AF. In addition to these drugs, several agents that target remodeling and inflammation can be used for prevention of AF or as adjunctive therapy. New and promising pharmacologic agents are under investigation. All of these approaches will increase the ability to control the increasing prevalence of AF, especially in the growing aging population.

REFERENCES

1. Go A, Hylek E, Phillips K, et al. Prevalence of diagnosed atrial fibrillation in adults: national implications for rhythm management and stroke

prevention. The anticoagulation and risk factors in atrial fibrillation study. JAMA 2001;285:2370–5.

2. Wyse DG, Waldo JP, DiMarco JM, et al. A comparison of rate control and rhythm control in patients with atrial fibrillation. N Engl J Med 2002;347:1825–33.

3. Van Gelder I, Hagens V, Bosker H, et al. A comparison of rate control and rhythm control in patients with recurrent persistent atrial fibrillation. N Engl J Med 2002;347:1834–40.

4. Chung MK, Shemanski L, Sherman DG, et al. Functional status in rate-versus rhythm control strategies for atrial fibrillation. J Am Coll Cardiol 2005;46:1891–9.

5. Roy D, Talajic M, Nattel S, et al. Rhythm control versus rate control for atrial fibrillation and heart failure. N Engl J Med 2008;358(25):2667–77.

6. Fuster V, Ryden LE, Cannom DS, et al. ACC/AHA/ESC 2006 guidelines for the management of patients with atrial fibrillation. J Am Coll Cardiol 2006;48(4):e149–246.

7. Naccarelli GV, Wolbrette DL, Bhatta L, et al. A review of clinical trials assessing the efficacy and safety of newer antiarrhythmic drugs in atrial fibrillation. J Interv Card Electrophysiol 2003;9:215–22.

8. Nattel S, Lionel HO. Controversies in atrial fibrillation. Lancet 2006;367:262–72.

9. Lafuente-Lafuente C, Mouly S, Longas-Tejero MA, et al. Antiarrhythmic drugs for maintaining sinus rhythm after cardioversion of atrial fibrillation. Arch Intern Med 2006;166:719–28.

10. Naccarelli GV, Wolbrette DL, Khan M, et al. Old and new antiarrhythmic drugs for converting and maintaining siuns rhythm in atrial fibrillation: comparative efficacy and results of trials. Am J Cardiol 2003;91(Suppl):15D–26D.

11. Roy D, Talajic M, Dorian P, et al. Amiodarone to prevent recurrence of atrial fibrillation. N Engl J Med 2000;342:913–20.

12. Singh BN, Singh SN, Reda DJ, et al. Amiodarone versus sotalol for atrial fibrillation. N Engl J Med 2005;352:1861–72.

13. Deedwania PC, Singh BN, Ellenbogen K, et al. Spontaneous conversion and maintenance of sinus rhythm by amiodarone in patients with heart failure and atrial fibrillation. Circulation 1998;98:2574–9.

14. Chimenti M, Cullen MT, Casadei G. Safety of long-term flecainide and propafenone in the management of patients with symptomatic paroxysmal atrial fibrillation: report from the Flecainide and Propafenone Italian Study Investigators. Am J Cardiol 1996;77(3):60A–75A.

15. Meinertz T, Lip GY, Lombardi F, et al. Efficacy and safety of propafenone sustained release in the prophylaxis of symptomatic paroxysmal atrial fibrillation (The European Rythmol/Rytmonorm Atrial Fibrillation Trial [ERAFT] Study). Am J Cardiol 2002;90(12):1300–6.

16. Pritchett ELC, Page RL, Carlson M, et al. Efficacy and safety of sustained-release propafenone (Propafenone SR) for patients with atrial fibrillation. Am J Cardiol 2003;92:941–6.

17. Torp-Pederson C, Mooler M, Block-Thomsen PE, et al. Dofetilide in patients with congestive heart failure and left ventricular dysfunction. N Engl J Med 1999;341:857–65.

18. Pedersen OD, Bagger H, Keller N, et al. Efficacy of Dofetilide in the treatment of atrial fibrillation-flutter in patients with reduced left ventricular function. Circulation 2001;104:292–6.

19. Singh S, Zoble RG, Yellen L, et al. Efficacy and safety of oral dofetilide in converting to and maintaining sinus rhythm in patients with chronic atrial fibrillation or atrial flutter. Circulation 2000;102:2385–90.

20. Greenbaum RA, Campbell TJ, Channer KS, et al. Conversion of atrial fibrillation and maintenance of sinus rhythm by dofetilide. The EMERALD (European and Australian Multicenter Evaluative Research on Atrial Fibrillation Dofetilide) Study. Circulation 1998;98:1633 [abstract].

21. Alboni P, Botto GL, Baldi N, et al. Outpatient treatment of recent-onset atrial fibrillation with the pill-in-the-pocket approach. N Engl J Med 2004;351:2384–91.

22. Boriani G, Diemberger I, Biffi M, et al. Pharmacological cardioversion of atrial fibrillation: current management and treatment options. Drugs 2004;64(24):2741–62.

23. Reiffel JA. Maintenance of normal sinus rhythm with antiarrhythmic drugs. In: Kowey P, Naccarelli G, editors. Atrial fibrillation. New York: Marcel Dekker; 2005. p. 195–217.

24. Goldstein RN, Stambler BS. New antiarrhythmic drugs for prevention of atrial fibrillation. Prog Cardiovasc Dis 2005;48(3):193–208.

25. Pecini R, Elming H, Pedersen OD, et al. New antiarrhythmic agents for atrial fibrillation and atrial flutter. Expert Opin Emerg Drugs 2005;10(2):311–22.

26. Sun W, Sarma JS, Singh BN. Electrophysiological effects of dronedarone (SR33589), a noniodinated benzofuran derivative, in the rabbit heart: comparison with amiodarone. Circulation 1999;100(22):2276–81.

27. Sun W, Sarma JS, Singh BN. Chronic and acute effects of dronedarone on the action potential of rabbit atrial muscle preparations: comparison with amiodarone. J Cardiovasc Pharmacol 2002;39(5):677–84.

28. Touboul P, Brugada J, Capucci A, et al. Dronedarone for prevention of atrial fibrillation: a dose-ranging study. Eur Heart J 2003;24(16):1481–7.

29. Singh BN, Connolly SJ, Crijins HJ, et al. Dronedarone for maintenance of sinus rhythm in atrial fibrillation or flutter. N Engl J Med 2007;357(10):987–99.

30. Davy JM, Herold M, Hoglund C, et al. Dronedarone for the control of ventricular rate in permanent atrial fibrillation: the efficacy and safety of dronedarone for the control of ventricular rate during atrial fibrillation (ERATO) study. Am Heart J 2008;156(3):527 e1–9.

31. Kober L, Torp-Pedersen C, McMurray JJ, et al. Increased mortality after dronedarone therapy for severe heart failure. N Engl J Med 2008;358(25):2678–87.

32. Hohnloser SH, Connolly SJ, Crijins HJ, et al. Rationale and design of ATHENA: a placebo-controlled, double-blind, parallel arm trial to assess the efficacy of dronedarone 400 mg for the prevention of cardiovascular hospitalization or death from any cause in patients with atrial fibrillation/atrial flutter. J Cardiovasc Electrophysiol 2008;19(1):69–73.

33. Coletta AP, Cleland JG, Cullington D, et al. Clinical trials update from Heart Rhythm 2008 and Heart Failure 2008: ATHENA, URGENT, INH study, HEART and CK-1827452. Eur J Heart Fail 2008; 10(9):917–20.

34. Gautier P, Guillemare E, Djandjighian L, et al. In vivo and in vitro characterization of the novel antiarrhythmic agent SSR149744C: electrophysiological, anti-adrenergic, and anti-angiotensin II effects. J Cardiovasc Pharmacol 2004;44(2):244–57.

35. Kowey PR, Aliot EM, Capuzzi A, et al. Placebo-controlled double-blind dose-ranging study of the efficacy and safety of SSR149744C in patients with recent atrial fibrillatin/flutter. Heart Rhythm 2007;4: S72 [abstract].

36. Double blind placebo controlled dose ranging study of the efficacy and safety of SSR149744c 300 or 600 mg for the conversion of atrial fibrillation/flutter (CORYFEE trial). Available at: http://www.clinicaltrials.gov. Trial identifier NCT00232310. Accessed November 14, 2008.

37. Raatikainen MJ, Napolitano CA, Druzgala P, et al. Electrophysiological effects of a novel, short-acting and potent ester derivative of amiodarone, ATI-2001, in guinea pig isolated heart. J Pharmacol Exp Ther 1996;277(3):1454–63.

38. Raatikainen MJ, Morey TE, Druzgala P, et al. Potent and reversible effects of ATI-2001 on atrial and atrioventricular nodal electrophysiological properties in guinea pig isolated perfused heart. J Pharmacol Exp Ther 2000;295(2):779–85.

39. Juhasz A, Bodor N. Cardiovascular studies on different classes of soft drugs. Pharmazie 2000; 55(3):228–38.

40. Morey TE, Seubert CN, Raatikainen MJ, et al. Structure-activity relationships and electrophysiological effects of short-acting amiodarone homologs in guinea pig isolated heart. J Pharmacol Exp Ther 2001;297(1):260–6.

41. Salata JJ, Brooks R. Pharmacology of azimilide dihydrochloride (NE-10064). Cardiovasc Drug Rev 1997;15:137–56.

42. Pritchett EL, Page RL, Connolly SJ, et al. Antiarrhythmic effects of azimilide in atrial fibrillation: efficacy and dose-response. Azimilide Supraventricular Arrhythmia Program 3 (SVA-3) Investigators. J Am Coll Cardiol 2000;36(3):794–802.

43. Camm AJ, Pratt CM, Schwartz PJ, et al. Mortality in patients after a recent myocardial infarction: a randomized, placebo-controlled trial of azimilide using heart rate variability for risk stratification. Circulation 2004;109(8):990–6.

44. Page RL. A-STAR and A-COMET trials (azimilide in atrial fibrillation). Europace 2002;3. [abstract] A-2.

45. Pritchett EL, Kowey P, Connolly S, et al. Antiarrhythmic efficacy of azimilide in patients with atrial fibrillation: maintenance of sinus rhythm after conversion to sinus rhythm. Am Heart J 2006;151(5):1043–9.

46. Lombardi F, Borggrefe M, Ruzyllo W, et al. Azimilide vs. placebo and sotalol for persistent atrial fibrillation: the A-COMET-II (Azimilide-CardiOversion MaintEnance Trial-II) trial. Eur Heart J 2006; 27(18):2224–31.

47. Kerr CR, Connolly SJ, Kowey P, et al. Efficacy of azimilide for the maintenance of sinus rhythm in patients with paroxysmal atrial fibrillation in the presence and absence of structural heart disease. Am J Cardiol 2006;98(2):215–8.

48. Connolly SJ, Schnell DJ, Page RL, et al. Dose-response relations of azimilide in the management of symptomatic, recurrent, atrial fibrillation. Am J Cardiol 2001;88:974–9.

49. Ravens U, Amos GJ, Li Q, et al. Effects of the antiarrhythmic agent tedisamil. Exp Clin Cardiol 1997; 2:231–6.

50. Hohnloser SH, Dorian P, Straub M, et al. Safety and efficacy of intravenously administered tedisamil for rapid conversion of recent-onset atrial fibrillation or atrial flutter. J Am Coll Cardiol 2004;44(1):99–104.

51. Beatch GN, Shinagawa K, Johnson B, et al. RSD1235 selectively prolongs atrial refractoriness and terminates AF in dogs with electrically remodeled atria. Pacing Clin Electrophysiol 2002;25:698 [abstract].

52. Beatch GN, Lin S-P, Hesketh JC, et al. Electrophysiological mechanism of RSD1235, a new atrial fibrillation converting drug. Circulation 2003;108:IV85 [abstract].

53. Ezrin AM, Grant SM, Bell G, et al. A dose-ranging study of RSD1235, a novel antiarrhythmic agent, in healthy volunteers. Pharmacologist 2002; 44(Suppl 1):A15 [abstract].

54. Roy D, Rowe BH, Stiell IG, et al. A randomized, controlled trial of RSD1235, a novel anti-arrhythmic agent, in the treatment of recent onset atrial fibrillation. J Am Coll Cardiol 2004;44(12):2355–61.

55. Roy D, Craig MP, Torp-Pederson C, et al. Vernakalant hydrochloride for rapid conversion of atrial fibrillation. Circulation 2008;117:1518–25.

56. Roy D, Pratt C, Juul-Moller S, et al. Efficacy and tolerance of RSD1235 in the treatment of atrial fibrillation or atrial flutter: results of a phase III, randomized, placebo-controlled, multicenter trial. J Am Coll Cardiol 2006;47:10A [abstract].

57. Kowey PR, Roy D, Pratt C, et al. Efficacy and safety of vernakalant hydrochloride injection for the treatment of atrial fibrillation after valvular or coronary bypass surgery. Circulation 2007;114 [abstract 2860].

58. Torp-Pederson C, Roy D, Pratt C, et al. Efficacy and safety of RSD1235 injection in the treatment of atrial fibrillation: combined analysis of two phase II trials. Eur Heart J 2006;27:887 [abstract].

59. A phase III superiority study of vernakalant versus amiodarone in subjects with recent onset atrial fibrillation (AVRO trial). Available at: http://www.clinicaltrials.gov. Trial identifier: NCT00668759. Accessed November 14, 2008.

60. Wirth KJ, Paehler T, Rosenstein B, et al. Atrial effects of the novel K(+)-channel-blocker AVE0118 in anesthetized pigs. Cardiovasc Res 2003;60(2):298–306.

61. Blaauw Y, Gogelein H, Tieleman RG, et al. "Early" class III drugs for the treatment of atrial fibrillation: efficacy and atrial selectivity of AVE0118 in remodeled atria of the goat. Circulation 2004;110(13):1717–24.

62. Goldstein RN, Khrestian C, Carlsson L, et al. Azd7009: a new antiarrhythmic drug with predominant effects on the atria effectively terminates and prevents reinduction of atrial fibrillation and flutter in the sterile pericarditis model. J Cardiovasc Electrophysiol 2004;15(12):1444–50.

63. Wu Y, Carlsson L, Liu T, et al. Assessment of the proarrhythmic potential of the novel antiarrhythmic agent AZD7009 and dofetilide in experimental models of torsades de pointes. J Cardiovasc Electrophysiol 2005;16(8):898–904.

64. Efficacy and safety of AZD7009 in the treatment of atrial fibrillation. Available at: http://www.clinicaltrials.gov. Trial identifier: NCT00255281. Accessed November 14, 2008.

65. Kaumann AJ, Sanders L, Brown AM, et al. A 5-HT receptor in human atrium. Br J Pharmacol 1990;100:879–85.

66. Grammer JB, Zeng X, Bosch RF, et al. Atrial L-type Ca2+-channel, beta-adrenorecptor, and 5-hydroxytryptamine type 4 receptor mRNAs in human atrial fibrillation. Basic Res Cardiol 2001;96(1):82–90.

67. Rahme MM, Cotter B, Leistad E, et al. Electrophysiological and antiarrhythmic effects of the atrial selective 5-HT(4) receptor antagonist RS-100302 in experimental atrial flutter and fibrillation. Circulation 1999;100(19):2010–7.

68. Xiao XD, Fuchs S, Campbell DJ, et al. Mice with cardiac-restricted ACE have atrial enlargement, cardiac arrhythmias and sudden death. Am J Pathol 2004;165:1019–32.

69. Boss CJ, Lip GY. Targeting the renin-angiotensin-aldosterone system in atrial fibrillation: from pathophysiology to clinical trials. J Hum Hypertens 2005;19:855–9.

70. Shi Y, Tardif JC, Nattel S. Enalapril effects on atrial remodeling and atrial fibrillation in experimental congestive heart failure. Cardiovasc Res 2002;54:456–61.

71. Pedersen OD, Bagger H, Kober L, et al. Trandolapril reduces the incidence of atrial fibrillation after acute myocardial infarction in patients with left ventricular dysfunction. Circulation 1999;100(4):376–80.

72. Vermes E, Tardif JC, Bourassa MG, et al. Enalapril decreases the incidence of atrial fibrillation in patients with left ventricular dysfunction: insight from the studies of left ventricular dysfunction (SOLVD) trials. Circulation 2003;107(23):2926–31.

73. L'Allier PL, Ducharme A, Keller PF, et al. Angiotensin-converting enzyme inhibition in hypertensive patients is associated with a reduction in the occurrence of atrial fibrillation. J Am Coll Cardiol 2004;44(1):159–64.

74. Anand K, Mooss AN, Hee TT, et al. Meta-analysis: inhibition of renin-angiotensin system prevents new-onset atrial fibrillation. Am Heart J 2006;152(2):217–22.

75. Healey JS, Baranchuk A, Crystal E, et al. Prevention of atrial fibrillation with angiotensin-converting enzyme inhibitors and angiotensin receptor blockers: a meta-analysis. J Am Coll Cardiol 2005;45:1832–9.

76. Salehian O, Healey J, Stambler B, et al. Impact of ramipril on the incidence of atrial fibrillation: results of the Heart Outcomes Prevention Evaluation Study. Am Heart J 2007;154(3):448–53.

77. Ueng KC, Tsai TP, Yu WC, et al. Use of enalapril to facilitate sinus rhythm maintenance after external cardioversion of long-standing persistent atrial fibrillation: results of a prospective and controlled study. Eur Heart J 2003;24(23):2090–8.

78. Renin-angiotension-aldosterone system (RAAS), inflammation, and post-operative atrial fibrillation. Available at: http://www.clinicaltrials.gov/ct/show/NCT00141778?order=1. November 14, 2008.

79. Nakashima H, Kumagai K, Urata H, et al. Angiotensin II antagonist prevents electrical remodeling in atrial fibrillation. Circulation 2000;101(22):2612–7.

80. Kumagai K, Nakashima H, Urata H, et al. Effects of angiotensin II type 1 receptor antagonist on electrical and structural remodeling in atrial fibrillation. J Am Coll Cardiol 2003;41(12):2197–204.

81. Maggioni AP, Latini R, Carson PE, et al. Valsartan reduces the incidence of atrial fibrillation in patients with heart failure: results from the Valsartan Heart Failure Trial (Val-HeFT). Am Heart J 2005;149(3):548–57.

82. Wachtell K, Lehto M, Gerdts E, et al. Angiotensin II receptor blockade reduces new-onset atrial fibrillation and subsequent stroke compared to atenolol: the Losartan Intervention for End Point Reduction in Hypertension (LIFE) study. J Am Coll Cardiol 2005;45(5):712–9.

83. Fogari R, Mugellini A, Destro M, et al. Losartan and prevention of atrial fibrillation recurrence in hypertensive patients. J Cardiovasc Pharmacol 2006;47(1):46–50.

84. Madrid AH, Bueno MG, Rebollo JM, et al. Use of irbesartan to maintain sinus rhythm in patients with long-lasting persistent atrial fibrillation: a prospective and randomized study. Circulation 2002;106(3):331–6.

85. Tveit A, Grundvold I, Olufsen M, et al. Candesartan in the prevention of relapsing atrial fibrillation. Int J Cardiol 2007;120(1):85–91.

86. Goette A, Breithardt G, Fetsch T, et al. Angiotension II antagonist in paroxysmal atrial fibrillation (ANTI-PAF) trial: rationale and study design. Clin Drug Investig. 2007;27(10):697–705.

87. Disertori M, Latini R, Maggioni AP, et al. Rationale and design of the GISSI-Atrial Fibrillation Trial: a randomized, prospective, multicentre study on the use of valsartan, an angiotensin II AT1-receptor blocker, in the prevention of atrial fibrillation recurrence. J Cardiovasc Med (Hagerstown) 2006;7(1):29–38.

88. Connolly S, Yusuf S, Budaj A, et al. Rationale and design of ACTIVE: the atrial fibrillation clopidogrel trial with irbesartan for prevention of vascular events. ACTIVE Investigators. Am Heart J 2006;151:1187–93.

89. Caballero R, Moreno I, Gonzalez T, et al. Spironolactone and its main metabolite, canrenoic acid, block human ether-a-go-go-related gene channels. Circulation 2003;107(6):889–95.

90. Spironolactone for paroxysmal atrial fibrillation. Available at: http://clinicaltrials.gov/ct2/show/NCT00689598. Accessed November 14, 2008.

91. Goldstein RN, Kyungmoo R, Van Wagoner DR, et al. Prevention of postoperative atrial fibrillation and flutter using steroids. Pacing Clin Electrophysiol 2003;26:1068 [abstract].

92. Halonen J, Halonen P, Jarvinen O, et al. Corticosteroids for the prevention of atrial fibrillation after cardiac surgery. JAMA 2007;297:1562–7.

93. Prasongsukarn K, Abel JG, Jamieson WR, et al. The effects of steroids on the occurrence of postoperative atrial fibrillation after coronary artery bypass grafting surgery: a prospective randomized trial. J Thorac Cardiovasc Surg 2005;130(1):93–8.

94. Halvorsen P, Raeder J, White PF, et al. The effect of dexamethasone on side effects after coronary revascularization procedures. Anesth Analg 2003;96(6):1578–83.

95. Kumagai K, Nakashima H, Saku K. The HMG-CoA reductase inhibitor atorvastatin prevents atrial fibrillation by inhibiting inflammation in a canine sterile pericarditis model. Cardiovasc Res 2004;62(1):105–11.

96. Shiroshita-Takeshita A, Schram G, Lavoie J, et al. Effect of simvastatin and antioxidant vitamins on atrial fibrillation promotion by atrial-tachycardia remodeling in dogs. Circulation 2004;110(16):2313–9.

97. Siu CW, Lau CP, Tse HF. Prevention of atrial fibrillation recurrence by statin therapy in patients with lone atrial fibrillation after successful cardioversion. Am J Cardiol 2003;92(11):1343–5.

98. Young-Xu Y, Jabbour S, Goldberg R, et al. Usefulness of statin drugs in protecting against atrial fibrillation in patients with coronary artery disease. Am J Cardiol 2003;92(12):1379–83.

99. Amar D, Zhang H, Heerdt PM, et al. Statin use is associated with a reduction in atrial fibrillation after noncardiac thoracic surgery independent of C-reactive protein. Chest 2005;128(5):3421–7.

100. Marin F, Pascual DA, Roldan V, et al. Statins and postoperative risk of atrial fibrillation following coronary artery bypass grafting. Am J Cardiol 2006;97(1):55–60.

101. Patti G, Chello M, Candura D, et al. Atorvastatin for reduction of myocardial dysrhythmia after cardiac surgery (ARMYDA-3). Circulation 2006;114:1455–61.

102. Young BS, Young KO, Kim JH, et al. The effects of atorvastatin on the occurrence of postoperative atrial fibrillation after off-pump coronary artery bypass grafting surgery. Am Heart J 2008;156:373 e9–373.e16.

103. Atorvastatin therapy for the prevention of atrial fibrillation (SToP-AF Trial). Available at www.clinicaltrials.gov. Accessed November 14, 2008.

104. Ninio DM, Murphy KJ, Howe PR, et al. Dietary fish oil protects against stretch-induced vulnerability to atrial fibrillation in a rabbit model. J Cardiovasc Electrophysiol 2005;16(11):1189–94.

105. Biscione F, Totteri A, De Vita A, et al. Effect of omega-3 fatty acids on the prevention of atrial arrhythmias. Ital Heart J 2005;6(1):53–9.

106. Calo L, Bianconi L, Colivicchi F, et al. N-3 Fatty acids for the prevention of atrial fibrillation after coronary artery bypass surgery: a randomized, controlled trial. J Am Coll Cardiol 2005;45(10):1723–8.

107. Brouwer IA, Heeringa J, Geleijnse JM, et al. Intake of very long-chain n-3 fatty acids from fish and incidence of atrial fibrillation. The Rotterdam Study. Am Heart J 2006;151(4):857–62.

Anticoagulation: Stroke Prevention in Patients with Atrial Fibrillation

Albert L. Waldo, MD

KEYWORDS

• Atrial fibrillation • Oral anticoagulation • Stroke risk

EPIDEMIOLOGY OF STROKE RISK

It is well recognized that during atrial fibrillation (AF), clots may form in the left atrium, which may embolize and cause ischemic stroke or systemic embolism. The presence of AF confers a fivefold increased risk for stroke.[1] Moreover, the prevalence of stroke in patients who have AF increases with age. The prevalence is less than 0.5% in patients younger than 60 years, but virtually doubles with each decade beginning with the seventh. Therefore, the prevalence of AF is 2% to 3% for patients in their 60s, 5% to 6% in their 70s, and 8% to 10% in their 80s.[1] The population-attributable risk also increases with age, so that it is 16.5% by the 70s and just more than 30%.by the 80s.[1] Thus, unsurprisingly, AF is the most common and important cause of stroke.

STROKE RISK STRATIFICATION SCHEMES FOR PATIENTS WHO HAVE ATRIAL FIBRILLATION

The risk for stroke varies among all patients who have AF. Based on a series of studies, the widely recognized risk factors are prior stroke or transient ischemic attack (TIA), hypertension, age of 75 years or older, heart failure and poor left ventricular function, and diabetes.[2,3] Other recognized stroke risk factors include mechanical prosthetic valve, mitral stenosis, coronary artery disease, age of 65 to 74 years, thyrotoxicosis, and female gender.[4] All of these factors are important when considering indications for oral anticoagulation. As incorporated into the American College of Cardiology/American Heart Association/European Society of Cardiology (ACC/AHA/ESC) 2006 revised Guidelines for the Management of Patients with Atrial Fibrillation, not all stroke risk factors have the same degree of association with stroke in patients who have AF.[4]

Several stroke risk stratification schemes for patients who have AF are available. One that has gained great favor is the CHADS2 scheme.[5] Based on analysis of 1773 patients in the National Registry of Atrial Fibrillation, it uses most of the accepted stroke risk factors to assess individual patient risk. The C stands for recent congestive heart failure, the H for hypertension, the A for age 75 or older, the D for diabetes, and the S for prior stroke or TIA. Each category is assigned one point except stroke or TIA, which gets two because of its high association with subsequent stroke. The adjusted stroke rate per 100 patient years increases as the CHADS2 score increases (**Fig. 1**).

The Framingham risk score[6] uses five steps to predict the 5-year risk for stroke in patients who have AF (**Fig. 2**). The steps consider age, gender, systolic blood pressure, diabetes, and prior stroke or TIA, and assign points depending on these factors. The points from steps 1 through 5 are added, and then the predicted 5-year stroke risk for each individual in the absence of anticoagulation therapy is determined from a table. This strategy may help in weighing available therapeutic options and even enable patients to understand the need for anticoagulation therapy.

A version of this article originally appeared in *Medical Clinics of North America*, volume 92, issue 1. Supported in part by Grant R01 HL38408 from the United States Public Health Service, National Institutes of Health, National Heart, Lung and Blood Institute, Bethesda, Maryland, and Grant BRTT/WCI TECH 05-066 from the Ohio Wright Center of Innovations, a Third Frontier program from The State of Ohio, Columbus, OH. Division of Cardiovascular Medicine, Department of Medicine, Case Western Reserve University/University Hospitals of Cleveland Case Medical Center, 11100 Euclid Avenue, MS LKS 5038, Cleveland, OH 44106-5038, USA
E-mail address: albert.waldo@case.edu

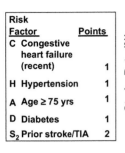

Risk Factor	Points
C Congestive heart failure (recent)	1
H Hypertension	1
A Age ≥ 75 yrs	1
D Diabetes	1
S_2 Prior stroke/TIA	2

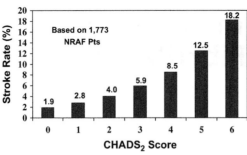

Fig. 1. Key AF stroke risk factors: CHADS2 risk stratification scheme. NRAF, National Registry of Atrial Fibrillation. (*Data from* Gage BF, Waterman AD, Shannon W, et al. Validation of clinical classification schemes for predicting stroke: results from a national registry of atrial fibrillation. JAMA 2001;285:2864–70.)

PROPHYLAXIS AGAINST STROKE
Warfarin Therapy

Many clinical trials have shown warfarin's remarkable efficacy in reducing stroke risk in patients who have AF. As shown overwhelmingly almost 15 years ago in a meta-analysis[3] of five randomized, controlled clinical trials comparing warfarin and placebo in patients who had AF (Copenhagen Atrial Fibrillation Aspirin and Anticoagulation [AFASAK],[7] Stroke Prevention in Atrial Fibrillation [SPAF],[8] Boston Area Anticoagulation Trial for Atrial Fibrillation [BAATAF],[9] Canadian Atrial Fibrillation Anticoagulation [CAFA],[10] and Stroke Prevention in Nonrheumatic Atrial Fibrillation [SPINAF],)[11] the intention-to-treat analysis showed that patients taking warfarin had a 68% risk reduction in stroke compared with those taking placebo ($P < .001$).[3]

An on-treatment analysis of these same trials showed an 83% risk reduction for stroke in patients taking warfarin compared with placebo.[12]

These and subsequent data established warfarin's therapeutic range as an international normalized ratio (INR) between 2 and 3, with a target INR of 2.5 to provide efficacy and safety.

Despite warfarin's well-demonstrated efficacy as prophylaxis against stroke in patients who have AF, many problems impact its use. These disadvantages include a narrow therapeutic range (INR 2–3), an unpredictable and patient-specific dose response, delayed onset and offset of action, need for anticoagulation monitoring, slow reversibility when that may be necessary, and many drug–drug and drug–food interactions that affect INR levels.[13] Drug interactions with warfarin are common and include virtually all anti-inflammatory drugs, most antibiotics, many diuretics, phenytoin, prednisone, thyroid hormone replacement, tamoxifen, alcohol, and statins.[13] Many foods also interact, including those high in vitamin K (eg, green, leafy vegetables; kiwi), high-dose vitamin C, vitamin E, cranberries, and licorice.[13]

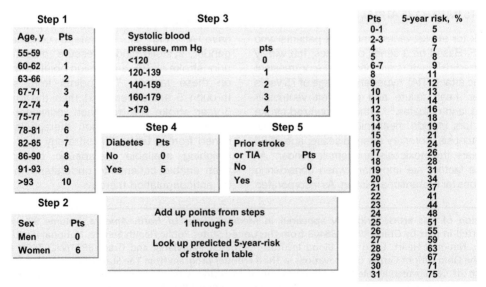

Fig. 2. Framingham risk score for predicting the 5-year risk of stroke in patients who have AF. (*Data from* Wang TJ, Massaro JM, Levy D, et al. A risk score for predicting stroke or death in individuals with new-onset atrial fibrillation in the community: the Framingham Heart Study. JAMA 2003;290:1049–105).

Furthermore, warfarin has a narrow therapeutic range, because once the INR falls below 2, the odds ratio for stroke rises steeply (eg, an INR of 1.7 doubles this risk) (**Fig. 3**).[14] When the INR rises to more than 3, it does not enhance the therapeutic efficacy, but increases the risk for bleeding, with major hemorrhage and intracranial hemorrhage the two greatest concerns. An INR up to 3.5 (target 3.0) is acceptable and indicated for patients who have a mechanical heart valve. The incidence of intracranial hemorrhage is flat,[15,16] varying between 0.3 and 0.6 per 100 person years when the INR is between 1.5 and approximately 3.5 (see **Fig. 3**), and is also remarkably flat until patient age is 80 years or older. No difference is seen in occurrence of intracerebral hemorrhage or subdural hematoma.[16] These data help to show the therapeutic target and range for the INR.

In view of the recognized difficulties in administrating warfarin, the U. S. Food and Drug Administration approved safety labeling revisions to advise about the need for individualization of warfarin therapy to minimize the risk for bleeding.[13] The most serious risks associated with anticoagulant therapy with warfarin are hemorrhage in any tissue or organ and, less frequently (incidence <0.1%), necrosis or gangrene of skin or other tissues. The risk for bleeding is highest during treatment initiation and with higher doses. Risk factors include a high intensity of anticoagulation (INR $\geq$ 4), age 65 years or older, high variability of INRs, history of gastrointestinal bleeding, hypertension, cerebrovascular disease, serious heart disease, anemia, malignancy, trauma, renal insufficiency, concomitant drugs, and long duration of warfarin therapy.

This safety relabeling appropriately emphasizes the need to individualize treatment with warfarin because of a low therapeutic index and potential effects from interaction with other drugs or foods, especially dietary vitamin K intake. Regular monitoring of the INR, usually at least monthly, is recommended for all patients. Those at high risk for bleeding may benefit from more frequent monitoring, careful dose adjustments to achieve the desired INR, and, when possible, shorter duration of therapy. To minimize the risk for bleeding, patients should be advised to avoid initiating or discontinuing other medications, including salicylates, and should be wary of other over-the-counter medications and herbal products. Maintaining a balanced diet with a consistent amount of vitamin K is advised. Drastic changes in diet (eg, eating large amounts of green leafy vegetables) and consumption of cranberry juice or its products should be avoided.

Despite the recognized indications for warfarin use and its clear efficacy in stroke prevention, warfarin therapy remains underused.[17] Most studies indicate use between 40% and 60% in patients who have AF and risk factors for stroke. Additionally, although the risk for stroke notably increases with increasing age, the use of warfarin decreases as patients get older,[17] with elderly persons using warfarin the least. In this latter group, a principle reason seems to be fear of an intracranial hemorrhage. Although whether to use warfarin must be decided on a case-by-case basis, the risks for potential intracranial hemorrhage or major bleeding usually are outweighed significantly by the risks for stroke or systemic embolus, so that often warfarin therapy is warranted.[18,19]

Aspirin

Aspirin as prophylaxis against stroke is controversial in patients who have AF and stroke risks.

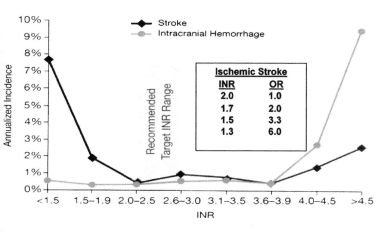

Fig. 3. Annualized incidence of stroke or intracranial hemorrhage according to international normalized ratio (INR). Also included is the odds ratio (OR) for ischemic stroke in patients who have AF based on their INR. (*Data from* Hylek E, Skates S, Sheehan M, et al. An analysis of the lowest effective intensity of prophylactic anticoagulation for patients with nonrheumatic atrial fibrillation. N Engl J Med 1996;335:540–6; and Hylek EM, Go AS, Chang Y, et al. Effect of intensity of oral anticoagulation on stroke severity and mortality in atrial fibrillation. N Engl J Med 2003;349:1019–26.)

Meta-analysis of studies comparing aspirin with placebo suggest a relative risk reduction of approximately 22% with use of aspirin.[20] This is driven in large part, however, by data from one clinical trial, the SPAF I study (**Fig. 4**). Only these data indicate that aspirin is significantly better than placebo, but these results should be examined closely (see **Fig. 4**).[21] SPAF I was a National Institutes of Health–sponsored trial that randomized patients who had AF to treatment with warfarin, aspirin, or placebo (group I) or, for those who had a relative or absolute contraindication to warfarin, to aspirin versus placebo (group II). In group I, of 206 patients in the aspirin arm, only one event occurred, whereas 18 events occurred among 211 patients in the placebo arm, resulting in a relative risk reduction of 94% for aspirin ($P < .001$). No other data have confirmed these results, suggesting that they are outliers. Moreover, in group II, 25 events occurred among 346 patients in the aspirin arm and 26 events among 357 patients in the placebo arm, giving aspirin a relative risk reduction of 8% ($P = .75$). The aspirin versus placebo data from groups I and II were pooled, resulting in a 42% ($P = .02$) relative risk reduction for aspirin. The confidence intervals of the pooled data are wide, however, because of the disparate nature of the data reported. Thus, this relative risk reduction should be considered unreliable.

Other data suggest that aspirin is less effective than desirable. Unlike warfarin, aspirin was never shown to affect mortality in patients who have AF.[22] In addition, the SPAF III trial[23] evaluated the benefit of an adjusted dose of warfarin (INR, 2–3; target 2.5) versus low-intensity, fixed-dose warfarin (INR, 1.2–1.5) plus aspirin in patients who had AF at high risk for stroke (ie, patients who had one or more of the following risk factors: female gender and age of 75 years; impaired left ventricular function; systolic blood pressure greater than 160 mm Hg; or prior thromboembolism).[24] The investigators reasoned that warfarin was more effective than aspirin as prophylaxis against stroke, but there was concern about excess and serious bleeding in patients receiving warfarin. The hope was that combining aspirin (324 mg daily) with a fixed but low dose of warfarin to achieve an INR between 1.2 and 1.5 would provide effective stroke prevention but avoid the bleeding risks associated with adjusted-dose warfarin administered to achieve an INR between 2 and 3.

However, the trial was stopped early (after a mean follow-up of 1.1 years) because the event rate in patients undergoing combination therapy was 7.9% per year versus an event rate on adjusted-dose warfarin of 1.9% per year ($P = .001$) (**Fig. 5**).[23] Moreover, no significant difference was seen in major bleeding and intracranial hemorrhage rates between the groups. Slightly more major bleeding and intracranial hemorrhage was seen in the group receiving aspirin plus fixed low-dose warfarin compared with the group receiving adjusted-dose warfarin (see **Fig. 5**). Furthermore, the annual event rate of stroke began to increase in the adjusted-dose warfarin group as soon as the INR fell below 2; whereas the incidence of stroke decreased as the INR approached 2 in the group receiving combination aspirin and fixed low-dose warfarin (**Fig. 6**) Additionally, SPAF III had a low–stroke-risk patient cohort (patients who had AF who had no high risk factors for stroke) in a nonrandomized, aspirin-only arm of this trial. In these patients, just a history of hypertension conferred a 3.6% risk for stroke or systemic embolism per year.[24]

Additional data indicate the problems with aspirin therapy compared with warfarin therapy. Hylek and colleagues[14] studied a cohort of 13,559

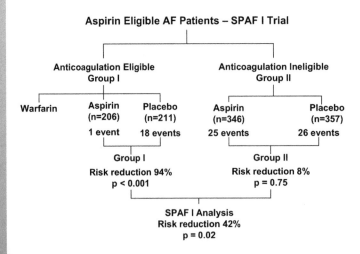

Aspirin Eligible AF Patients – SPAF I Trial

Anticoagulation Eligible
Group I

Anticoagulation Ineligible
Group II

Warfarin

Aspirin
(n=206)

1 event

Placebo
(n=211)

18 events

Aspirin
(n=346)

25 events

Placebo
(n=357)

26 events

Group I
Risk reduction 94%
p < 0.001

Group II
Risk reduction 8%
p = 0.75

SPAF I Analysis
Risk reduction 42%
p = 0.02

Fig. 4. Analysis of the data from the SPAF I trial in patients taking aspirin compared with placebo. (*Data from* The SPAF Investigators. A differential effect of aspirin on prevention of stroke in atrial fibrillation. J Stroke Cerebrovasc Dis 1993;3:181–8.)

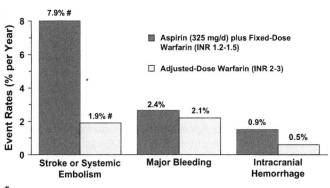

Fig. 5. Analysis of the SPAF III data in the high-risk patient cohort. (*Data from* Israel CW, Gronefeld G, Ehrlich JR, et al. Long-term risk of recurrent atrial fibrillation as documented by an implantable monitoring device: implications for optimal patient care. J Am Coll Cardiol 2004;43:47–52.)

#p = 0.0001

patients who had nonvalvular AF who experienced 596 ischemic strokes. Among these patients, 32% were on warfarin, 27% were undergoing aspirin therapy, and 42% were on neither warfarin nor aspirin therapy. The investigators compared the severity of neurologic deficit at discharge and the early and 30-day mortality rates in patients who had a stroke while receiving warfarin (with an INR ≥ 2 or < 2), aspirin, or no antithrombotic therapy. Patients taking aspirin or warfarin but who had an INR of less than 2 had a 2.6- to 3-fold increase in the severity of the stroke, including early (in-hospital) fatality or stroke resulting in total dependence, compared with patients who had an INR of greater than or equal to 2. Similarly, the 30-day mortality rate was approximately 2.5 times greater in patients taking aspirin or who had an INR less than 2 if taking warfarin compared with those

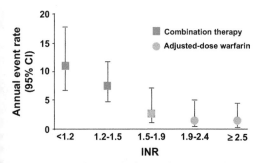

Fig. 6. SPAF III relative risk for stroke or systemic embolism in adjusted-dose warfarin and combination therapy cohorts. Event rates for ischemic stroke for systemic embolism based on the INR in SPAF III patients in the combination therapy (*square*) and adjusted-dose warfarin therapy (*circle*) groups. (*Data from* The SPAF Investigators. Adjusted-dose warfarin versus low-intensity, fixed dose warfarin plus aspirin for high-risk patients with atria fibrillation: Stroke Prevention in Atrial Fibrillation III randomized clinical trial. Lancet 1996;348:633–8.)

who had an INR greater than or equal to 2. In short, these data showed that warfarin with an INR greater than or equal to 2 not only reduced the frequency of ischemic stroke but also reduced the severity and risk for death from stroke compared with aspirin.

Data from the Birmingham Atrial Fibrillation Treatment of the Aged (BAFTA) study,[25] a trial of warfarin versus aspirin therapy for stroke prevention in an elderly (age ≥75 years, mean 82) community with AF, add still more to the limits of the effectiveness of aspirin. In this elderly patient population, for the combined primary end point of fatal or nonfatal disabling stroke or significant arterial embolism, patients taking warfarin experienced significantly fewer events than patients taking aspirin (P = .007; hazard ratio, 0.48). Not only did the data show warfarin was significantly better than aspirin in stroke prevention (P = .003; relative risk reduction, 46%) and disabling nonfatal strokes (P = .005; relative risk reduction, 33%), but also no difference was seen in the incidence of hemorrhagic stroke (P = .83) or subdural hemorrhage (P = .65) between the groups. In the absence of contraindications, these data clearly support the use of warfarin over aspirin for people older than 75 years who have AF.

The meta-analysis performed in 2002 (perhaps a bit out of date) by van Walraven and colleagues[26] provides useful way to think about risks versus benefits of prophylaxis with warfarin or aspirin. Their meta-analysis concludes that treating 1000 patients who have AF for 1 year with warfarin instead of aspirin would prevent 23 ischemic strokes but cause nine additional major bleeds, including two hemorrhagic strokes. Thus, in patients who have AF and stroke risk factors, the risk for stroke or systemic embolism is significant. However, the risks for bleeding also must be taken into account, although in most patients, the risk for stroke outweighs the risk for bleeding. Therefore, warfarin therapy should be administered in patients who have AF and are at high risk for stroke.

For patients who have AF and are not at high risk for stroke or systemic embolism, administration of warfarin seems to make the most sense unless it is contraindicated, although the Guidelines for the Management of Atrial Fibrillation offer aspirin or warfarin as options for therapy.[4] In sum, in patients at risk for stroke caused by AF, anticoagulation with warfarin (INR, 2–3; target, 2.5) reduces stroke rate and mortality, and also reduces morbidity associated with stroke if the latter occurs. Aspirin has considerably less, if not just minimal, effect on stroke rate and severity, and no demonstrated effect on mortality associated with stroke.

Emerging New Anticoagulants

The problems associated with the use of warfarin and the limited efficacy of aspirin in stroke prevention in patients who have AF highlight the unmet need for new, safe, and effective oral anticoagulants. Several promising agents are under active clinical study,[27] including dabigatran, a direct thrombin inhibitor (the RE-LY trial[27]); apixaban, a factor Xa inhibitor (the ARISTOTLE trial[27]); and rivaroxaban (the ROCKET-AF trial[27]), also a factor Xa inhibitor. These three trials are ongoing, and, in fact, the RE-LY trial stopped recruiting subjects in December, 2007. Therefore, whether these agents, which do not require anticoagulation monitoring and have little-to-no interaction with other drugs and food, will earn a place in the therapeutic armamentarium will be known in the very near future.

AMERICAN HEART ASSOCIATION/AMERICAN COLLEGE OF CARDIOLOGY/EUROPEAN SOCIETY OF CARDIOLOGY 2006 GUIDELINES ON RISK FACTORS FOR STROKE AND STROKE PREVENTION IN ATRIAL FIBRILLATION

The ACC/AHA/ESC 2006 revised Guidelines for the Management of Patients with Atrial Fibrillation[4] have divided risk factors for stroke into three groups (Table 1). High-risk factors include prior stroke, TIA, or thromboembolism; mitral stenosis; or presence of a prosthetic mechanical heart valve. Moderate risk factors include age older than 75 years, hypertension, heart failure, left ventricular ejection fraction less than or equal to 0.35, or diabetes mellitus. A third category might be called low risk, but is formally labeled less-validated or weaker risk factors, including female gender, age 65 to 74 years, coronary artery disease, and thyrotoxicosis.

In the presence of these risk factors, various recommendations for antithrombotic therapy have

been made (see Table 1).[4] For patients who have any high risk factor for stroke, oral anticoagulation with warfarin therapy (range 2–3; target 2.5) is recommended. Similarly, oral anticoagulation with warfarin is recommended for patients who have two or more moderate stroke risk factors, whereas aspirin (81 or 324 mg) or oral anticoagulation with warfarin is recommended for patients who have one moderate risk factor. Aspirin (81 or 324 mg) or oral anticoagulation is recommended for patients who have less validated or weaker risk factors. For patients younger than 60 years, aspirin (81 or 324 mg) or no therapy is recommended. For patients who have no risk factors who are 60 to 65 years of age, aspirin (81 or 324 mg) or oral anticoagulation with warfarin is recommended. The indications for antithrombotic therapy are no different for persistent, permanent, or paroxysmal AF.

OTHER CONSIDERATIONS

Although these guidelines were designed carefully, some concerns exist. Data supporting the use of aspirin in patients who have stroke risk factors are wanting. The guidelines suggest that in patients older than 75 years who have risk factors for stroke but no history of stroke, and for whom no concern for bleeding exists, administering warfarin to achieve an INR of 1.6 to 2.5 with a target of 2 should be considered.[4] As the data reported by Hylek and colleagues[15] show, lowering the INR below 2 does not decrease the incidence of intracranial hemorrhage. However, it reduces the efficacy of warfarin therapy, causing that the odds ratio for stroke to increase dramatically (see Fig. 3). Thus, this IIc recommendation of the guidelines is questionable.

Managing anticoagulation interruptions is important. In general, the average weekly risk for stroke in the absence of oral anticoagulation is low but not zero. The highest risk is believed to be in patients who have mechanical heart valves or history of stroke.[4] In patients for whom the oral anticoagulation must be stopped for a procedure, bridging the interruption with unfractionated heparin or low molecular weight heparin therapy is recommended.[4] Thus, heparin or low molecular weight heparin therapy would be administered in lieu of warfarin through the day before the procedure, and then stopped. Warfarin or bridging with heparin usually is reinstated at a safe time after the procedure.

CARDIOVERSION

The question of adequate anticoagulation to prevent stroke in association with cardioversion has been standardized for a while, and has not changed with the 2006 revised ACC/AHA/ESC

Table 1
American Heart Association/American College of Cardiology/European Society of Cardiology 2006 revised guidelines for antithrombotic therapy based on stroke risk

Less Validated or Weaker Risk Factors	Moderate Risk Factors	High Risk Factors
Rx: ASA or OAC	Rx: 1 risk factor—ASA or OAC; ≥2 risk factors—OAC	Rx: OAC
Female gender Age 65–74 y Coronary artery disease Thyrotoxicosis	Age > 75 y Hypertension Heart failure LVEF ≤ 0.35 Diabetes mellitus	Prior stroke, TIA, or embolism Mitral stenosis Mechanical heart valve

Abbreviations: ASA, aspirin; LVEF, left ventricular ejection fraction; OAC, oral anticoagulation with warfarin; RF, stroke risk factor; Rx, therapy.

Data from Fuster V, Ryden LE, Cannom DS, et al. ACC/AHA/ESC 2006 Guidelines for the management of patients with atrial fibrillation: a report of the American College of Cardiology/American Heart Association Task Force on Practice Guidelines and the European Society of Cardiology Committee for Practice Guidelines (Writing Committee to revise the 2001guidelines for the management of patients with atrial fibrillation). J Am Coll Cardiol 2006;48:854–906.

guidelines (**Box 1**).[4] It is based on data and consensus. If AF is known to have been present for fewer than 48 hours, cardioversion may proceed without any anticoagulation. If AF has been present 48 hours or more, however, cardioversion raises the risk for embolism, with a 1% to 5% risk for emboli occurring within hours to weeks after cardioversion in the absence of anticoagulation. However, anticoagulation well before and after cardioversion greatly reduces this risk. Therefore, if AF has been present for two or more days or for an unknown period, the guidelines state that the INR should be between 2 and 3 for 3 weeks consecutively before cardioversion, and for at least 4 weeks after restoring and maintaining normal sinus rhythm.

If AF is present for two or more days in the absence of warfarin therapy with an INR in the therapeutic range, and if the clinician wants to perform a cardioversion, two options are available. One option is to perform a transesophageal echocardiogram in the presence of therapeutic heparin administration. If no thrombus is present, anticoagulation with heparin (unfractionated or low molecular weight) is continued through the cardioversion and as a bridge to achieving a therapeutic INR on warfarin, when the heparin is stopped. The warfarin is continued, maintaining an INR in the therapeutic range for at least 1 month after successful cardioversion. If chronic warfarin therapy is indicated, it is continued. If it is not indicated, the warfarin is stopped. If a thrombus is present at precardioversion transesophageal echocardiography, however, anticoagulation with an INR between 2 and 3 for 3 days consecutively is recommended, followed by reevaluation. The second option is simply to provide oral anticoagulation with warfarin, and, after achieving an INR in

the therapeutic range for 3 weeks consecutively, then perform the cardioversion. Again, if long-term warfarin therapy is not indicated, it may be stopped after 1 month; otherwise, it is continued long-term. The ACUTE study[28] shows that the two approaches (transesophageal echocardiography with heparin before cardioversion or 3 consecutive weeks of an INR in the therapeutic range on warfarin) have no important difference in terms of morbidity and mortality.

Risk factors for stroke in AF do not apply to these rules. Thus, if patients have no risk factor for stroke and ordinarily would not need warfarin long-term, patients still should be anticoagulated before cardioversion if AF has been present for 48 or more hours or an unknown duration. The main reason is that an approximately 25% incidence of atrial stunning (absence of atrial contraction) exists after cardioversion for patients who have had AF for 48 or more hours.[29] The stunning may last up to 1 month, although most often it lasts only for hours or days after sinus rhythm is restored.[29] During this period of stunning is when the milieu that predisposes to left atrial clots is believed to still be present. Thus, clots may form in the left atrium during sinus rhythm. For patients who do not have a need for long-term anticoagulation, ordinarily the anticoagulation would be stopped after 1 month of therapy.

ISSUES IN LONG-TERM USE OF ORAL ANTICOAGULATION

What about continuation of warfarin therapy for patients who have AF and risk factors for stroke who achieve and seem to maintain sinus rhythm? Data from the Atrial Fibrillation Follow-Up Investigation of Rhythm Management (AFFIRM)[30,31] and

<table>
<tr><td>

Box 1
Elective cardioversion of atrial fibrillation anticoagulation: standards for use of anticoagulation in connection with cardioversion of atrial fibrillation

Cardioversion seems to increase risk for embolism

Anticoagulation well before and after greatly reduces risk

For use of anticoagulation, risk factors for stroke in AF do not apply

Standard guidelines for electrical or drug cardioversion

INR 2 to 3 for weeks before cardioversion and INR 2 to 3 for 4 weeks after normal sinus rhythm (continue warfarin beyond 4 weeks if stroke risk factors present)

If AF less than 2 days' duration, may proceed without AC

If transesophageal echocardiography performed and no thrombus; anticoagulation just before and 4 weeks after cardioversion

Thrombus present; anticoagulation with INR 2 to 3 for 3 weeks and reevaluate

Data from Fuster V, Ryden LE, Cannom DS, and colleagues ACC/AHA/ESC 2006 guidelines for the management of patients with atrial fibrillation: a report of the American College of Cardiology/American Heart Association Task Force on Practice Guidelines and the European Society of Cardiology Committee for Practice Guidelines (Writing Committee to revise the 2001 guidelines for the management of patients with atrial fibrillation). J Am Coll Cardiol 2006;48:854–906.

</td></tr>
</table>

sinus rhythm and maintained it for at least 1 month, warfarin therapy could be stopped. This was worrisome because of the known tendency for AF to recur, but was requested by the study sites because they believed it would have a negative impact on patient recruitment to the study. The result was that patients in the rhythm control arm, initially more than 90% of patients took warfarin in the first 4 months after randomization. But by the end of year 1, this dropped to just under 80%, and by years 2 to 5, only approximately 70% were taking warfarin in the rhythm control arm. In the rate control arm, in which failure to use warfarin was a protocol violation, more than 90% of patients were taking warfarin through year 4, although by year 5, only approximately 85% were taking warfarin. Furthermore, throughout the AFFIRM study's 3.5-year average follow-up, only 84% of the rate control group and 52% of the rhythm control group remained continuously on warfarin. At the end of the AFFIRM trial, when the relationships among ischemic stroke, INR, and the presence of AF in the rate-versus-rhythm–control arms were examined (**Table 2**), the incidence of ischemic stroke was not significantly different between the arms (*P* = .79). However, 57% of the patients in the rhythm control arm who had a stroke were not taking warfarin. Although documented only partly in this trial, these patients probably experienced recurrence of AF, and much of it was likely asymptomatic.[33,34] Another 22% of patients who had a stroke in the rhythm control arm had an INR of less than 2, again emphasizing the importance of maintaining the INR in the therapeutic range. Additionally, in the rate control arm, 33% of patients who had a stroke were not taking warfarin, which was a protocol violation, emphasizing the difficulty of keeping patients on warfarin therapy even though its use is clearly indicated. Moreover, 36% of patients who had a stroke in the rate control arm also had an INR of less than 2, again emphasizing the importance of maintaining the INR

the Comparison of Rate Control and Rhythm Control in Patients with Recurrent Persistent Atrial Fibrillation (RACE)[32] trials are most instructive in this regard. In the AFFIRM trial, if a patient achieved

Table 2
The relationship between ischemic stroke, international normalization ratio, and presence or absence of atrial fibrillation

	Rate Control, n (%)	Rhythm Control, n (%)
Ischemic stroke	77 (5.5)[a]	80 (7.1)[a]
INR $\geq$ 2	23 (31)	16 (21)
INR < 2	27 (36)	17 (22)
Not taking warfarin	25 (33)	44 (57)
AF at time of event	42 (69)	25 (37)

[a] Event rates derived from Kaplan-Meier analysis (*P* = .79).
　Data from Wyse DG, Waldo AL, DiMarco JP, et al. A comparison of rate control and rhythm control in patients with recurrent persistent atrial fibrillation. N Engl J Med 2002;347:1825–33.

in the therapeutic range. Similar data were reported in the RACE trial.[31]

In patients who have AF, an estimated 10% to 30% of all AF cases are totally asymptomatic and up to 70% of patients who have symptomatic AF are believed to also have symptomatic episodes.[33] The risk for stroke in symptomatic and asymptomatic AF is similar,[4] and therefore asymptomatic AF requires not only ventricular rate control but also adherence to anticoagulation guidelines.

In addition, Israel and colleagues[34] examined the incidence of asymptomatic AF in patients who had a history of AF and also had an implanted pacemaker with excellent stored memory capacity and the ability to detect atrial arrhythmias. In 38% of patients who experienced AF recurrences, the AF was asymptomatic and lasted more than 48 hours, and 16% of them did so even after documentation of freedom from AF for 3 months. The implication is that success rates of maintaining continuous sinus rhythm in patients who have a history of AF often are grossly overestimated. And for patients who have AF and risk factors for stroke, the data suggest they should undergo warfarin therapy indefinitely, even when sinus rhythm seems to have been restored and maintained.

LONG-TERM ANTICOAGULATION AFTER RADIOFREQUENCY ABLATION OF ATRIAL FIBRILLATION

What should be done about long-term anticoagulation for patients who undergo apparently successful ablation to cure AF has yet to be determined. The hope is that these patients truly would be cured, so that the need for anticoagulation to prevent stroke resulting from AF is no longer present. These patients have an uncertain but real incidence of asymptomatic AF recurrence, however; both early and late after the ablation.[35] A difficulty in assessing long-term warfarin need in these patients is the absence of long-term data to give perspective, not only on the incidence of recurrence of AF beyond the 2- to 3-month "blanking period," when AF recurrence may not indicate failure of the procedure, but also on the incidence of stroke in the absence of anticoagulation therapy, especially in patients who have risk factors for stroke. In this sense, whether enough data exist even to reach an informed consensus must be considered.

For patients who do not have stroke risk factors (which is currently probably most of those who undergo apparently successful ablation of AF), consensus exists that after the blanking period,

further anticoagulation with warfarin is not necessary.[36–38] What should be done, then, for patients who have stroke risk factors? Data from small studies suggest that the stroke incidence is low, but the incidence of AF recurrence, manifest and asymptomatic, is uncertain. Moreover, data indicate a late AF recurrence (beyond the first year postablation) of at least 5%.[39,40] In addition, data suggest that not only does AF recurrence indicate the need for warfarin therapy in patients who have stroke risks, but also, as a consequence of radiofrequency ablation to cure AF, some patients experience up to a 30% reduction of left atrial transport function. The latter may predispose to thromboembolic events despite the presence of sinus rhythm.[40]

Because of these considerations and the absence of long-term, randomized, controlled trial data, the Heart Rhythm Society/European Heart Rhythm Association/European Cardiac Arrhythmia Society Expert Consensus Statement on Catheter and Surgical Ablation of Atrial Fibrillation[37] generally does not recommend discontinuation of warfarin therapy postablation in patients who have a CHADS2 score of 2 or more. It also recommends warfarin for all patients for at least 2 months after an AF ablation procedure. Whether to use warfarin for more than 2 months after the ablation should be decided based on patient risk factors for stroke. The Venice Chart International Consensus Document on Atrial Fibrillation[38] makes similar recommendations; the only real difference is that they recommend warfarin be given for at least 3 to 6 months after the ablation procedure.

OVERVIEW AFTER RADIOFREQUENCY ABLATION OF ATRIAL FIBRILLATION

The following is the author's considered overview for patients who have risk factors for stroke.

(1) For patients who require antiarrhythmic drug therapy after radiofrequency ablation to suppress AF recurrence (ie, despite radiofrequency ablation, cure has not been obtained, but successful therapy seemingly is obtained with the addition of antiarrhythmic drug therapy that was not successful before the ablation), warfarin therapy to maintain an INR in the therapeutic range should be continued long-term.

(2) For patients in whom no clinically manifest episodes of AF have been documented 2 months after ostensibly successful radiofrequency ablation to cure AF, warfarin therapy should be maintained for a minimum of 1 year, when

continued use of warfarin therapy should be reconsidered.

(3) For patients who have any documented recurrence of AF after the blanking period, warfarin therapy should be maintained for at least 1 year and then reconsidered.

(4) If asymptomatic AF does occur, warfarin therapy should be maintained long-term.

(5) A recommendation concerning continuation of warfarin therapy beyond 1 year postablation in patients who have stroke risks must be couched in uncertainties and considered on an individual basis. If no apparent AF recurrence has occurred, termination of warfarin therapy may be acceptable, with the understanding that the chance for late recurrence of AF, although likely to be low, is present, with the attendant risks. If patients experience AF recurrence, continued long-term warfarin therapy is recommended.

REFERENCES

1. Wolf PA, Abbott RD, Kannel WB. Atrial fibrillation: a major contributor to stroke in the elderly. The Framingham Study. Arch Intern Med 1987;147: 1561–4.

2. Stroke Prevention in Atrial Fibrillation Investigators. Predictors of thromboembolism in atrial fibrillation: I. Clinical features of patients at risk. Ann Intern Med 1992;116:1–5.

3. Atrial Fibrillation Investigators. Risk factors for stroke and efficacy of antithrombotic therapy in atrial fibrillation: analysis of pooled data from five randomized controlled trials. Arch Intern Med 1994;154:1449–57.

4. Fuster V, Ryden LE, Cannom DS, et al. ACC/AHA/ESC 2006 guidelines for the management of patients with atrial fibrillation: a report of the American College of Cardiology/American Heart Association Task Force on Practice Guidelines and the European Society of Cardiology Committee for Practice Guidelines (Writing Committee to revise the 2001 guidelines for the management of patients with atrial fibrillation). J Am Coll Cardiol 2006;48:854–906.

5. Gage BF, Waterman AD, Shannon W, et al. Validation of clinical classification schemes for predicting stroke: results from a national registry of atrial fibrillation. JAMA 2001;285:2864–70.

6. Wang TJ, Massaro JM, Levy D, et al. A risk score for predicting stroke or death in individuals with new-onset atrial fibrillation in the community: the Framingham Heart Study. JAMA 2003;290:1049–56.

7. Petersen P, Boysen G, Godtfredsen J, et al. Placebo-controlled, randomized trial of warfarin and aspirin for prevention of thromboembolic complications in chronic atrial fibrillation. The Copenhagen AFASAK Study. Lancet 1989;1:175–8.

8. Stroke Prevention in Atrial Fibrillation Investigators. Stroke prevention in atrial fibrillation study: final results. Circulation 1991;84:527–39.

9. The Boston Area Anticoagulation Trial for Atrial Fibrillation Investigators. The effect of low-dose warfarin on the risk of stroke in patients with nonrheumatic atrial fibrillation. N Engl J Med 1990;323:1505–11.

10. Connolly S, Laupacis A, Gent M, et al. Canadian Atrial Fibrillation Anticoagulation (CAFA) Study. J Am Coll Cardiol 1991;18:349–55.

11. Ezekowitz M, Bridgers S, James K, et al. Warfarin in the prevention of stroke associated with nonrheumatic atrial fibrillation. N Engl J Med 1992;327: 1406–12.

12. Albers GW, Sherman DG, Gress DR, et al. Stroke prevention in nonvalvular atrial fibrillation: a review of prospective randomized trials. Ann Neurol 1991; 30:511–8.

13. Anticoagulant coumadin tablets (warfarin sodium tablets, USP crystalline). In: Physicians desk reference, 62nd edition, 2008; Thomson PDR, Montvale (NJ); 3457–63.

14. Hylek E, Skates S, Sheehan M, et al. An analysis of the lowest effective intensity of prophylactic anticoagulation for patients with nonrheumatic atrial fibrillation. N Engl J Med 1996;335:540–6.

15. Hylek EM, Go AS, Chang Y, et al. Effect of intensity of oral anticoagulation on stroke severity and mortality in atrial fibrillation. N Engl J Med 2003;349: 1019–26.

16. Fang MC, Chang Y, Hylek EM, et al. Advanced age anticoagulation intensity and risk for intracranial hemorrhage among patients taking warfarin for atrial fibrillation. Ann Intern Med 2004;141:745–52.

17. Waldo AL, Becker RC, Tapson VF, et al. Steering Committee. Hospitalized patients with atrial fibrillation and a high risk of stroke are not being provided with adequate anticoagulation. J Am Coll Cardiol 2005;46:1729–36.

18. Fang MC, Go AS, Hylek EM, et al. Age and the risk of warfarin-associated hemorrhage: the anticoagulation and risk factors in atrial fibrillation study. J Am Geriatr Soc 2006;54:1231–6.

19. Garcia D, Hylek E. Stroke prevention in elderly patients with atrial fibrillation. Lancet 2007;370:460–1.

20. Hart R, Benavente O, McBridge R, et al. Antithrombotic therapy to prevent stroke in patients with atrial fibrillation: a meta-analysis. Ann Intern Med 1999; 131:492–501.

21. The SPAF Investigators. A differential effect of aspirin on prevention of stroke in atrial fibrillation. J Stroke Cerebrovasc Dis 1993;3:181–8.

22. Cleland JGF, Kaye GC. Only warfarin has been shown to reduce stroke risk in patients with atrial fibrillation. Br Med J 2001;323:233.

23. The SPAF Investigators. Adjusted-dose warfarin versus low-intensity, fixed dose warfarin plus aspirin for high-risk patients with atria fibrillation: Stroke Prevention in Atrial Fibrillation III Randomized clinical trial. Lancet 1996;348:633–8.

24. The SPAF III Writing Committee for the Stroke Prevention in Atrial Fibrillation Investigators. Patients with nonvalvular atrial fibrillation at low risk of stroke during treatment with aspirin. JAMA 1998;279:1273–7.

25. Mont J, Hobbs FDR, Fletcher K, et al. Warfarin versus aspirin for stroke prevention in an elderly community population with atrial fibrillation (the Birmingham Atrial Fibrillation Treatment of the Aged Study). Lancet 2007;370:493–503.

26. van Walraven C, Hart RG, Singer DE, et al. All anticoagulants vs aspirin in nonvalvular atrial fibrillation: an individual patient meta-analysis. JAMA 2002;288:2441–8.

27. Turpie AGG. New oral anticoagulants in atrial fibrillation. Eur Heart J 2007;29:155–65.

28. Klein AL, Grimm RA, Murray RD, et al. Use of transesophageal echocardiography to guide cardioversion in patients with atrial fibrillation. N Engl J Med 2001;344:1420–41.

29. Thamilarasan M, Klein AL. Transesophageal echocardiography (TEE) in atrial fibrillation. Cardiol Clin 2000;18:819–31.

30. Wyse DG, Waldo AL, DiMarco JP, et al. A comparison of rate control and rhythm control in patients with recurrent persistent atrial fibrillation. N Engl J Med 2002;347:1825–33.

31. Sherman DG, Kim SJ, Boop BS, et al. The occurrence and characteristics of stroke events in the AFFIRM study. Arch Intern Med 2005;105:1185–91.

32. van Gelder IC, Hagens VE, Bosker HA, et al. A comparison of rate control and rhythm control in patients with recurrent persistent atrial fibrillation. N Engl J Med 2002;347:1834–40.

33. Rho RW, Page RL. Asymptomatic atrial fibrillation. Prog Cardiovasc Dis 2005;48:79–87.

34. Israel CW, Gronefeld G, Ehrlich JR, et al. Long-term risk of recurrent atrial fibrillation as documented by an implantable monitoring device: implications for optimal patient care. J Am Coll Cardiol 2004;43:47–52.

35. Martinek M, Aichinger J, Nesser HJ, et al. New insights into long-term follow-up of atrial fibrillation ablation: full disclosure by an implantable pacemaker device. J Cardiovasc Electrophysiol 2007;18:818–23.

36. Waldo AL. Guidelines for anticoagulation of atrial fibrillation: is it time for an update? In: Raviele A, editor. Cardiac arrhythmias 2005. Italy: Springer-Verlag Italia; 2006. p. 169–76.

37. Calkins H, Brugada J, Packer DL, et al. HRS/EHRA/ECAS Expert consensus statement on catheter and surgical ablation of atrial fibrillation: recommendations for personnel, policy, procedures and follow-up. A report of the Heart Rhythm Society (HRS Task Force on Catheter and Surgical Ablation of Atrial Fibrillation). Heart Rhythm 2007;4:816–61.

38. Natale A, Raviele A, Arentz T, et al. Venice Chart international consensus document on atrial fibrillation ablation. J Cardiovasc Electrophysiol 2007;18:560–80.

39. Pappone C, Rosario S, Augello G, et al. Mortality, morbidity, and quality of life after circumferential pulmonary vein ablation for atrial fibrillation. Outcomes from a controlled, nonrandomized long term study. J Am Coll Cardiol 2003;42:185–97.

40. Oral H, Chugh A, Ozaydin M, et al. Risk of thromboembolic events after percutaneous left atrial radiofrequency ablation of atrial fibrillation. Circulation 2006;114:759–65.

The Role of Pacemakers in the Management of Patients with Atrial Fibrillation

Gautham Kalahasty, MD[a],*, Kenneth Ellenbogen, MD[a,b]

KEYWORDS

- Pacemaker • Implantable cardioverter defibrillator
- Atrial fibrillation • Sinus node dysfunction
- Atrioventricular junction ablation

This article reviews the wide range of implantable device–based therapies (mainly pacemakers) that are being used in the management of atrial fibrillation (AF), atrial flutter, and atrial tachycardia (AT). Pacemakers have an important and evolving role in the management of some patients with AF. The frequency of their use relative to other non-pharmacologic strategies has increased over time as the incidence and prevalence of AF increase, especially in the elderly. In fact, almost all the increase in pacemaker implantation rates has been for the indication of sinus node dysfunction (SND). The clinical burden of AF in the elderly population is staggering. In the groups aged 70 to 79 years and 80 to 89 years, the prevalence of AF is at least 4.8% and 8.8%, respectively. By 2050, it is estimated that 50% of the patients with AF are going to be more that 80 years old.[1] **Box 1** summarizes the most common strategies that have been used for device-based management of patients with AF. The goals of this article are first to review the evolution of the important current paradigms of pacing as they relate to AF and then to discuss how pacemakers are used in the specific subpopulations of patients with AF.

The most common indication for pacemaker implantation in the United States is for SND. AF is a primary feature of SND in many patients. In effect, understanding the role of pacemakers in the management of AF requires an understanding of the role of pacemakers in SND. Pacemaker implantation practice patterns in the United States vary from those in Europe. Dual-chamber (rather than single-chamber) pacemakers are usually implanted in the United States for patients who have sick sinus syndrome and paroxysmal AF even if there is no AV conduction abnormality at the time of implantation. In one study, the incidence of developing AV block was 8.4% over a period of 34 months.[2] In a European study of patients who received a single-chamber (AAI) pacemaker for sick sinus syndrome, there was a 1.7% annual incidence of AV block.[3] Because the incidence of AV block is not insignificant, in the United States, patients who have paroxysmal AF and sick sinus syndrome almost universally receive dual-chamber pacemakers. With careful patient selection, however, the incidence of development of AV block can be as low as 0.6%.[4] Thoughtful pacemaker programming and careful pacemaker mode selection with the goal of maintaining "physiologic pacing" are critical.

In the current American College of Cardiology (ACC)/American Heart Association (AHA)/Heart Rhythm Society (HRS) guidelines, AF is described as permanent or chronic if it is long standing (eg,

A version of this article originally appeared in *Medical Clinics of North America*, volume 92, issue 1.
[a] Division of Cardiology, Department of Internal Medicine, Virginia Commonwealth University, PO Box 980053, Richmond, VA 23298–0053, USA
[b] Cardiac Electrophysiology, Department of Internal Medicine, Virginia Commonwealth University, Richmond, VA, USA
* Corresponding author.
E-mail address: gkalahasty@mcvh-vcu.edu (G. Kalahasty).

Box 1
Device-related applications for the management of atrial fibrillation

Rate control

Pacing to facilitate the use of rate-lowering agents

Pacing in chronic AF

Pacing for rate regularization

Pacing in conjunction with AV node ablation or modification

Rhythm control or maintenance of sinus rhythm

Pacing to facilitate the use of antiarrhythmic medication

Pacing to maintain or promote sinus rhythm

Algorithms to promote sinus rhythm

Multisite pacing (dual site, biatrial)

Novel site pacing

Pacing or defibrillation to terminate AF

Box 2
Potential adverse effects of ventricular pacing right ventricle in sinus node dysfunction

Ventricular dyssynchrony

Altered cardiac hemodynamics attributable to loss of "atrial kick"

Atrial proarrhythmia

Ventricular proarrhythmia

Increased valvular regurgitation

Adverse electrical remodeling of the atria promoting AF

Pacemaker syndrome

---

longer than 1 year) and if cardioversion has failed or has been foregone. AF is called persistent if it lasts more than 7 days regardless of whether cardioversion is needed to restore sinus rhythm; it is considered paroxysmal if episodes of AF terminate spontaneously.[5] Pacemakers have applications in each of these clinical types of AF.

PHYSIOLOGIC PACING

An appreciation of the role of pacemakers in the management of AF (especially in the context of SND) requires an understanding of the evolution of the meaning of "physiologic pacing" and optimal pacing modalities. The function of a pacemaker is to approximate normal cardiac function as much as possible. Therefore, careful mode selection (eg, AAI, VVI, DDI, DDD) and proper programming (eg, AV delay, hysteresis, mode switch rates) are needed to optimize the beneficial effects and minimize the potentially detrimental effects of pacing. Although "demand" ventricular pacemakers have been in clinical use since the 1960s, and although it seems intuitive that dual-chamber pacing would be superior to ventricular demand pacing, the body of clinical data needed to support this conclusion took almost 20 years to accumulate. The benefits of dual-chamber AV synchronous pacing in patients with SND and paroxysmal AF are now widely accepted. More recently, the potentially adverse effects of ventricular pacing (synchronous or asynchronous) have been recognized and are summarized in **Box 2**. Some of

these effects are not unique to dyssynchronous pacing but may occur with dual-chamber pacing and are discussed elsewhere in this article. Even ventricular proarrhythmia (ventricular tachycardia and ventricular fibrillation) has been described with single-chamber ventricular and dual-chamber pacing.[6] Ventricular remodeling, hemodynamic parameters, quality-of-life (QOL) measures, and clinical end points (eg, incidence of AF, stroke risk, congestive heart failure [CHF], mortality) have all been investigated. In terms of the incidence of AF, the data from the large clinical trials supporting physiologic pacing are fairly compelling. In terms of the other clinical end points, such as QOL, stroke risk, and mortality, however, the data are not entirely consistent and continue to evolve. Hemodynamic studies have demonstrated that AV synchrony improves stroke volume and cardiac output and reduces right atrial pressure and pulmonary-capillary wedge pressures. A significant number of patients who receive a single-chamber ventricular (VVI) pacemaker for sick sinus syndrome develop pacemaker syndrome, consisting of such symptoms as fatigue, palpitations, and chest pain. These symptoms resolve after patients receive atrioventricular (AV) synchronous pacing.[7,8] When comparisons are made within an individual patient testing different pacing modes rather than between patients, dual-chamber synchronous pacing is strongly preferred to single-chamber ventricular pacing.[9]

Table 1 summarizes the key clinical findings in the eight major randomized studies that have demonstrated the benefits of AV synchronous pacing or atrial-based pacing. These trials have collectively enrolled nearly 9000 patients. Although it was a small study with limited power, the Danish study was the first randomized prospective study to support the concept that selection-specific pacing modalities could improve outcomes in patients

Table 1
Clinical Trials in Pacing

Trial	Year	Average Follow-Up (years)	Design	Key Findings
Danish (Andersen and colleagues)[4]	1994	5.5	AAI versus VVI in 225 patients with SSS	At long-term follow-up (mean of 5.5 years), the incidence of paroxysmal AF and chronic AF was reduced in the AAI group. Overall survival, heart failure, and thromboembolic events were reduced with atrial-based pacing.
PASE[7]	1998	2.5	Single-blind assignment of VVIR or DDDR mode in 407 patients with SSS, AV block, and other indications	Patients with SSS showed a trend toward a lower incidence of AF and all-cause mortality (AF: 19% versus 28%, $P = .06$; mortality: 12% versus 20%, $P = .09$). QOL was not different between the two pacing modes. Twenty-six percent of patients developed pacemaker syndrome when paced in the VVIR mode
Mattioli and colleagues[54]	1998	2.0	VVI/VVIR versus AAI/DDD/DDDR/VDD pacing in patients with AV block (n = 100) and SSS (n = 110)	Incidence of AF was 10% at 1 year, 23% at 2 years, and 31% at 5 years. An increase in the incidence of chronic AF was observed in patients with SSS in the VVI/VVIR arm.
Canadian Trial of Physiologic Pacing (CTOPP)[10]	2000	6.0	2568 patients randomized to ventricular pacing (VVIR) versus physiologic pacing (DDDR or AAIR) for any appropriate indication	The annual rate of AF was less with physiologic pacing. No difference was observed in stroke or cardiovascular death between the two groups. There was a 27% reduction in the annual rate of progression to chronic AF.
Mode Selection in Sinus-Node Dysfunction Trial (MOST)[11]	2002	4.5	2010 patients with sinus node dysfunction (only) randomized to VVIR versus DDDR programming; more than 50% had prior AF	AF was reduced in patients randomized to physiologic pacing. No difference in mortality and stroke rates was observed between pacing modes. Thirty-one percent of patients crossed over from the VVIR to the DDDR mode, 49% of which was attributable to pacemaker syndrome.
Pacemaker Atrial Tachycardia (PAC-ATACH)[13]	2001	2.0	198 patients with sinus node dysfunction and a history of atrial arrhythmias randomized to DDDR pacing or VVIR pacing	Abstract only; full report remains to be published. Mortality was lower in the dual-chamber group. (3.2% versus 6.8%; $P = .007$) There was no difference in the AF recurrence rate.
United Kingdom Pacing and Cardiovascular Events (UKPACE)[12]	2002	4.6	2021 patients, aged >70 years randomly assigned to three arms: DDD (50%), VVIR (25%), and VVI 25%)	There was no difference in all-cause mortality, rate of stroke, or incidence of AF between the dual-chamber group and ventricular pacing group.
Search Atrioventricular Extension and Managed Ventricular Pacing for Promoting Atrioventricular Conduction (SAVEPACe)[17]	2007	1.7	530 patients in DDD mode and 535 patients in AAI←→DDD mode for symptomatic sinus node dysfunction; nearly an equal number of patients in both groups (38%) had paroxysmal AF	Persistent AF occurred in 12.7% of patients in the conventional pacing group and 7.9% of patients in the minimal ventricular pacing group.

with sick sinus syndrome (SSS).[4] Another study, the Pacemaker Selection in the Elderly (PASE) trial, did not show a difference in the QOL scores between those patients programmed to the VVIR versus DDDR mode; however, up to 45% of patients with SSS who were in VVIR mode developed pacemaker syndrome.[7] The Canadian Trial of Physiologic Pacing (CTOPP) showed a clear benefit for physiologic pacing in terms of reducing the incidence of AF, but it did not demonstrate a preferential advantage in patients with SSS. In addition, the CTOPP study demonstrated a higher rate of perioperative complications in those patients who received a dual-chamber pacemaker compared with those who received a single-chamber device (9.0% versus 3.5%, respectively). The risk for AF was lower for physiologic pacing (21.5%) than for ventricular pacing (27.1%).[10] The power of the Mode Selection in Sinus-Node Dysfunction Trial (MOST) may have been compromised because of the high rate of crossover from VVI mode to DDD mode. Nevertheless, this trial, contrary to the CTOPP study, showed improvements in QOL scores after reprogramming to a dual-chamber mode.[11] The United Kingdom Pacing and Cardiovascular Events (UKPACE) trial is remarkable for its negative results. Patients received single-chamber (VVI or VVIR) pacemakers or dual-chamber pacemakers for AV block. Patients with permanent AF or paroxysmal AF that was present for more than 3 months were excluded from the trial. There was no benefit from dual-chamber pacing modes over single-chamber modes in terms of stroke rate or AF.[12] The Pacemaker Atrial Tachycardia (PAC-ATACH) trial is the only trial to demonstrate a mortality benefit for dual-chamber pacing compared with ventricular pacing; however, the results of that trial have been presented only in abstract form.[13] A recent meta-analysis by Healey and colleagues[14] pooled data from five of these trials (Danish, PASE, CTOPP, MOST, and UKPACE) to detect clinically significant outcomes that the individual trials were not powered to detect. The combined data from these trials represent 35,000 patient-years of follow-up and demonstrated that although the incidence of AF was less with atrial-based pacing compared with ventricular-only pacing, there was no significant benefit in terms of all-cause mortality. Despite the reduced incidence of AF, there was no significant reduction in the risk for stroke.

In a secondary analysis of the MOST data, two additional important findings were reported. Increasing proportions of ventricular pacing were found to be associated with an increasing incidence of AF during VVIR and DDDR pacing. Also, greater percentages of ventricular pacing were associated with a greater risk for hospitalization for heart failure.[11] If ventricular pacing occurred more than 40% of the time, there was a twofold increase in the risk for developing CHF. This study suggests that the relative benefits of AV synchronous pacing compared with ventricular only pacing are attributable to the deleterious effects of right ventricular (RV) pacing rather than to the presumed advantages of AV synchronous pacing. The CTOPP and MOST studies had relatively few patients with true atrial only–based pacing (AAI) without the confounding effect of ventricular pacing. In the MADIT II study, patients who received an implantable cardioverter defibrillator (ICD) had higher survival rates but also demonstrated a trend toward increased rates of CHF; 73 patients (14.9%) in the conventional therapy group and 148 in the defibrillator group (19.9%) were hospitalized with heart failure ($P = .09$).[15] In the Dual Chamber and VVI Implantable Defibrillator (DAVID) trial, a composite end point of time to death and first hospitalization for CHF was compared in patients who had ICDs programmed to receive dual-chamber pacing (DDDR-70) or ventricular backup pacing (VVI-40).[16] At 1 year, 83.9% of the patients in the VVI-40 group were free from the composite end point compared with 73.3% of patients in the DDDR-70 group. Hospitalization for CHF occurred in 13.3% of VVI-40 patients compared with 22.6% of DDD-70 patients, trending in favor of the VVI-40 group. Although the DAVID study looked only at an ICD population, it has had a major impact on the programming of dual-chamber pacemakers. By highlighting the deleterious effects of RV pacing, it underscores the importance of mode selection in patients with SND and paroxysmal AF. The programmed parameters of a pacemaker or ICD should promote minimal ventricular pacing.

All major pacemakers have features that allow for maximization of the AV delay to promote intrinsic ventricular depolarization. Algorithms even exist that allow the dual-chamber pacemaker to change from single-chamber atrial-based pacing (AAIR) to dual-chamber AV sequential pacing (DDDR) automatically. When selected, the device operates in an AAIR mode until AV block occurs and then instantly changes to a DDDR mode (**Fig. 1**). In a study by Sweeney and colleagues (Search Atrioventricular Extension and Managed Ventricular Pacing for Promoting Atrioventricular Conduction [SAVE PACe]),[17] there was a 40% relative risk reduction in the development of persistent AF as compared with conventional dual-chamber pacing for patients with SND and normal left ventricular (LV) function. There was no difference in mortality between the two groups.

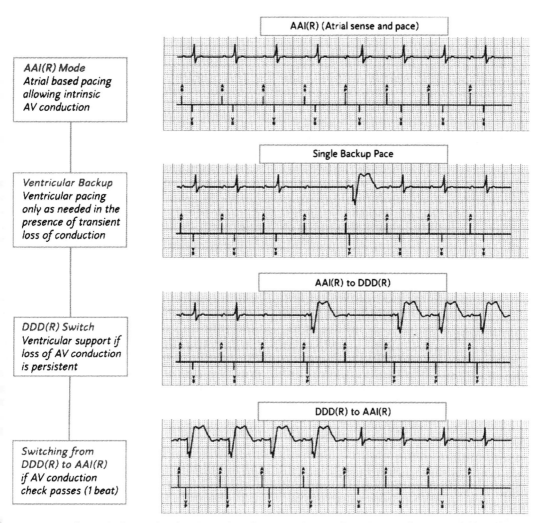

AAI(R) (Atrial sense and pace)

AAI(R) Mode
Atrial based pacing allowing intrinsic AV conduction

Single Backup Pace

Ventricular Backup
Ventricular pacing only as needed in the presence of transient loss of conduction

AAI(R) to DDD(R)

DDD(R) Switch
Ventricular support if loss of AV conduction is persistent

DDD(R) to AAI(R)

Switching from DDD(R) to AAI(R) if AV conduction check passes (1 beat)

Fig. 1. Managed ventricular pacing (MVP; Medtronic, Inc., Minneapolis, Minnesota) is an atrial-based pacing mode that significantly reduces unnecessary right ventricular pacing by primarily operating in an AAIR pacing mode while providing the safety of a dual-chamber backup mode if necessary. As shown in the figure, the algorithm allows for a single blocked beat before a back-up ventricular paced beat is delivered. Mode switch occurs only if two blocked beats occur. Two sequential blocked beats cannot occur because of back-up ventricular pacing.

Data from the MADIT II and DAVID studies only involved patients with severe LV dysfunction. This raises the question as to whether or not the detrimental effects of RV pacing (in terms of heart failure and mortality) are seen in patients with lesser degrees of LV dysfunction or normal LV function. There are limited data with which to answer this question. If physiologic pacing can be thought of as the pacing mode that most closely mimics normal cardiac physiology while yielding the best outcomes with the least detrimental effects, it seems that atrial-based pacing that promotes intrinsic conduction and minimizes RV apical pacing (in patients with no cardiac resynchronization therapy

[CRT] indications) is the mode of choice. AV synchrony alone is not adequate.

PACEMAKER DIAGNOSTICS

Pacemaker diagnostics not only can provide insight into the burden of AF but can reveal the presence of asymptomatic AF that was not previously suspected.[18] Routine interrogation of a pacemaker implanted for SND may reveal episodes of AF that have been stored in the memory as mode switch episodes or atrial high-rate episodes. "Mode switch" refers to a programmable function allowing the pacemaker to change from a dual-chamber pacing mode (DDD) to a nontracking mode (DDI or

VVI). This feature is available in all current pacemakers and ICDs. Once selected, it is an automatic function and does not require office-based reprogramming. An atrial arrhythmia that meets a programmed duration (a few seconds) and rate (usually 160 beats per minute [bpm]) results in a mode switch event and an entry into the log. When the atrial arrhythmia terminates, dual-chamber pacing is resumed. Mode switching prevents rapid ventricular pacing in response to the tracking of rapid atrial rhythms. The frequency and duration of atrial arrhythmias, including AF and atrial flutter, can be recorded and stored. Most current pacemakers are capable of storing intracardiac electrograms, sometimes allowing the clinician to distinguish between AF, AT, and atrial flutter. Some older devices are only capable of reporting the number and duration of mode switch episodes without storing any associated electrograms. In these cases, an event monitor may be needed to document the atrial arrhythmias. Overall, the false-positive detection of AF is reported at approximately 2.9%.[19] In contrast, the results of the Balanced Evaluations of Atrial Tachyarrhythmia in Stimulated Patients (BEATS) study showed that ATs could occur in 54% of patients with stored electrograms compared with only 15% of patients screened by surface electrocardiograms and 24-hour Holter monitors.[20] Artifact and oversensing of atrial or far field ventricular events can result in inappropriate mode switch episodes. Stored data should be reviewed and interpreted by someone who is knowledgeable in the interpretation of intracardiac electrograms. Capucci and colleagues[21] demonstrated that patients with device-monitored AF for longer than 24 hours had an increased risk for embolic events. Identification of appropriate mode switches can have a significant impact on the management of patients in terms of initiation of anticoagulation, perhaps reducing the risk for future thromboembolic events. All major manufacturers of pacemakers and ICDs have the capability of some form remote monitoring. Remote monitoring frequency and alerts can be individualized to meet the needs of the each patient and each physician.

Fig. 2 shows the interrogation report from a dual-chamber pacemaker. It was implanted for symptomatic sinus bradycardia in a 73-year-old patient not previously known to have AF. During the 1 month after implantation, the patient had 186 episodes of atrial high rates, 4 of which were longer than 1 minute in duration. The longest mode switch episode lasted almost 6 hours. These episodes were asymptomatic. Based on these findings, the initiation of warfarin sodium was discussed with the patient and the dose of the beta-blocker was increased. Fig. 3 shows an example of a stored

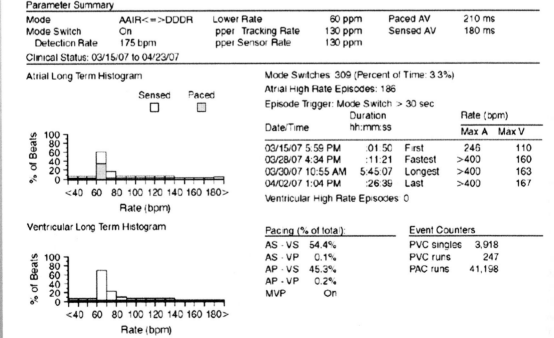

Fig. 2. Arrhythmia summary report from a dual-chamber pacemaker (Adapta Dual Chamber Pacemaker Medtronic, Inc., Minneapolis, Minnesota).

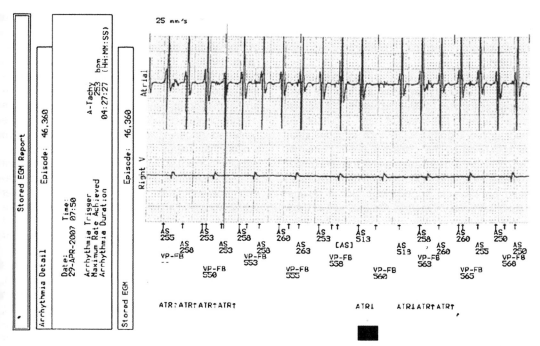

Fig. 3. Example of stored electrograms (EMGs) from an appropriate mode switch episode. The atrial channel shows a rapid irregular atrial rate with a maximum atrial rate of 253 bpm.

electrogram of an atrial tachyarrhythmia resulting in an appropriate mode switch.

In addition to mode switch events, pacemaker diagnostics can provide other important information. Rate histograms can provide insight into the adequacy of the rate response and suggest the need for more a sensitive sensor setting to provide appropriate chronotropic support in a patient with AF and a slow ventricular rate. Rate histograms can help to assess the adequacy of rate control in patients with AF. It is also important to know the percentage of ventricular pacing in patients with intact AV conduction. The practice of maximizing the AV delay to promote intrinsic AV conduction is supported by data from the DAVID, MADIT II, and MOST studies.

Chronic or Permanent Atrial Fibrillation

It is not uncommon for patients with chronic AF to require a permanent pacemaker. Over time, these patients may develop a slow ventricular response resulting in symptomatic bradycardia. Progressively slower conduction is often the result of age-related degeneration of the conduction system. Because this process is gradual, some elderly patients do not readily recognize or complain of the symptoms of exercise intolerance, dyspnea on exertion, and easy fatigability that can accompany bradycardia and chronotropic

incompetence. Physicians and patients frequently dismiss these nonspecific symptoms as a natural consequence of aging. In addition, comorbid conditions may be present, which can result in similar symptoms confounding the diagnosis of SSS. Therefore, a Holter monitor or event monitor may be needed to obtain true symptom-rhythm correlation. A single-chamber rate-responsive pacemaker (VVIR) can provide symptom relief and improve functional capacity.

Bradycardia may also be an unavoidable consequence of the medications used to prevent a rapid ventricular response associated with AF. Beta-blockers, calcium channel blockers, and digoxin are used to control rapid ventricular rates during AF but can result in intermittent symptomatic bradycardia or long pauses that can lead to syncope or presyncope. Of note, pauses up to 2 to 3 seconds during sleep are not unusual and are not solely an indication for pacing. Instead, this bradycardia is just a function of the relatively high vagal tone that is present during sleep. Dosage adjustment of medications or the use of beta-blockers with intrinsic sympathomimetic activity (ISA) can sometimes mitigate the bradycardia or pauses but can also result in suboptimal rate control when a patient is active and awake. A pacemaker is indicated to facilitate the use of medications that are considered essential and for which there are no other suitable alternatives. Typically, pacemakers in these patients are programmed to VVI or VVIR mode with a lower rate of 60 bpm. Pharmacologic therapy prevents extreme tachycardia.

Whatever the indication, a rate-responsive pacemaker can also provide an appropriate chronotropic response to the patient's physiologic needs. Current pacemakers use a variety of sensor-driven algorithms to increase the heart rate according to the patient's needs. The two most common sensors are accelerometers (based on movement) and minute ventilation monitors (based on thoracic impedance). Some devices can use both in combination. Optimal use of these devices requires routine office-based follow-up and reprogramming.

Regulation of Atrioventricular Nodal Conduction by Pacing

During AF, the rapid ventricular rate and irregular ventricular response contribute to deleterious hemodynamic effects. Irregular ventricular response can result in decreased cardiac output and increased wedge pressure independent of mean rate.[22] It has also been shown that cycle length variability has more influence on ventricular performance at faster heart rates. Ventricular pacing can result in concealed conduction into the AV node and His-Purkinje system, resulting in slowing of AV conduction. Algorithms have been developed that result in pacing slightly faster than the mean ventricular rate but with more regular ventricular response. Despite the expected benefits, the clinical trials that studied regularization algorithms yielded mixed and somewhat disappointing results. In the AF Symptoms Study, the effect of ventricular rate regularization on the end points of QOL, AF symptoms, and exercise capacity was evaluated. The investigators reported that ventricular rate regulation had a positive impact on reported symptoms, particularly palpitations, but did not have a significant impact on overall QOL or functional capacity.[23] Based on these studies, ventricular pacing during chronic rapid AF using regularization algorithms cannot be considered an alternative to atrioventricular junction (AVJ) ablation.

Atrioventricular Junction Ablation

It is not possible to achieve typical heart rate targets in many patients with chronic or paroxysmal AF with medical therapy alone. A resting heart rate of 80 bpm or less, 24-hour Holter average of 100 bpm or less, and heart rate of 120 bpm or less with modest activity are reasonable empiric goals for rate control but should be individualized based on symptoms. For patients in whom pharmacologic

therapy cannot reach the desired rate targets and for whom there are no other alternatives, ablation of the AVJ and pacemaker implantation is the preferred strategy. Although more commonly used in patients with chronic AF, it is also performed in select patients with paroxysmal AF and in whom antiarrhythmic drugs (AADs) do not provide adequate rhythm control or in whom AF ablation is not the preferred option. These patients should receive a dual-chamber pacemaker with mode switch capability to maintain AV synchrony when the patient is in sinus rhythm. Otherwise, a standard single-chamber ventricular rate-responsive pacemaker is all that is need in patients with preserved LV function and chronic AF.

The benefits of AVJ ablation and pacemaker implantation are significant and were summarized in a meta-analysis covering 21 studies that included 1181 patients.[24] Echocardiographic parameters, such as ejection fraction (EF), have been shown to improve, as have the number of office visits, hospital admissions, and the New York Heart Association (NYHA) functional capacity. QOL measures, such as QOL scores, activity level, exercise intolerance, symptom frequency and severity, were also improved.[24]

Despite the expected advantages, there are some serious disadvantages that should be considered and explained to patients. The most obvious is that the procedure, unlike medications, is generally irreversible and renders the patient pacemaker dependent for life. The procedure itself is generally of low risk, nearly 100% successful, and usually not technically difficult. Patients are exposed to a small risk for thromboembolic events if their anticoagulation is stopped for the ablation procedure. There is a small risk for vascular complications, such as hematoma and pseudoaneurysm formation. A recurrence rate of 5% necessitating repeat ablation has been reported. Although practice patterns vary widely, there is growing evidence that pacemaker implantation and pacemaker generator replacements can be performed safely while patients are on therapeutic doses of coumadin.[25,26] Most importantly, AVJ ablation does not obviate the need for long-term anticoagulation. AV synchrony is not preserved, and in those patients with significant diastolic dysfunction, the expected symptomatic improvement may be lessened by the loss of the "atrial kick."

There was a concern that patients are at risk for sudden death after AVJ ablation and pacemaker implantation. Based on reported survival data, the risks for sudden death and total mortality are 2% to 6% at 1 year, respectively. Long-term (6 years) mortality is similar in patients undergoing pacing and ablation compared with continued medical therapy, however.[27] The increased risk is thought to be attributable to bradycardia-dependent arrhythmias (torsades de pointes). Programming the lower rate of the pacemaker at 80 to 90 bpm for the first month has been shown to minimize this risk.[28] Another concern is the risks associated with lead dislodgement in these patients, who are usually pacemaker dependent. Because of these concerns, many physicians implant the pacemaker several weeks in advance of the ablation procedure. The use of a CRT device or standard RV pacing device in patients with significant LV dysfunction is discussed elsewhere in this review.

Paroxysmal or Persistent Atrial Fibrillation

The results of the Atrial Fibrillation Follow-up Investigation of Rhythm Management (AFFIRM) trial do not apply to every subset of patients with AF; therefore, rhythm control remains an appropriate strategy in many patients with paroxysmal AF.[29] Such factors as symptoms, QOL, and the interplay between AF and comorbidities are important considerations when selecting a rhythm control strategy over a rate control strategy. For example, patients with diastolic dysfunction or valvular heart disease, such as aortic or mitral stenosis, do not tolerate AF and require aggressive rhythm control. Some patients are also at risk for developing CHF or tachycardia-induced cardiomyopathy. Despite their limited efficacy and potential for side effects, including proarrhythmia, AADs play an important role in the treatment of AF. Symptomatic bradycardia and bradycardia-dependent polymorphic ventricular tachycardia (VT) have been reported with sotalol, propafenone, and, rarely, with amiodarone. These medications can also exacerbate AV conduction disease, which is sometimes seen in patients with SND. Pauses seen immediately after termination of AF may also be prolonged by these drugs. Pacemakers can be used to facilitate the use of these medications.

There has been a great deal of interest in preventing AF in patients with paroxysmal AF by the use of device-based algorithms designed to address two aspects of the pathophysiology of AF: triggers and substrate. Clinical and experimental data suggest that AF may be triggered by atrial premature complexes (APCs). The atria of some patients may be more susceptible to AF because of inhomogeneous atrial refractoriness. These patients sometimes have atrial myopathy and often have atrial remodeling and enlargement. Overdrive pacing, multisite pacing (dual and biatrial), and alternate site pacing are device-based strategies designed to reduce AF burden by addressing these pathophysiologic mechanisms.

The Atrial Pacing Periablation for the Prevention of AF (PA³) trial was the first to examine the effect of pacing on the frequency and duration of AF in patients with medically refractory AF who were also being considered for AVJ ablation and pacemaker implantation.[30] These patients did not otherwise have a bradycardia indication for pacemaker implantation. This study showed that atrial rate-adaptive pacing does not prevent paroxysmal AF recurrence or reduce the frequency or duration of AF. The duration of this study was short term (3 months), and no specific overdrive pacing algorithms were used.

Overdrive pacing algorithms seek to reduce APCs and prevent pauses and bradycardia. Fixed-rate atrial pacing alone (lower rate of 70 bpm) has been shown to have no effect on AF burden. The major device manufacturers have algorithms that attempt to reduce AF recurrence and overall AF burden. The dynamic atrial overdrive algorithm (DAO; St. Jude Medical, Sylmar, California) is one example that has been shown to achieve a modest reduction in symptomatic AF burden[31] and has been given US Food and Drug Administration (FDA) labeling for this indication. The effect of this algorithm on total AF burden is unknown. Overall, several other pacing algorithms have been studied in a relatively small number of patients yielding, at best, inconsistent results on the effect on AF burden. Therefore, the clinical utility of these algorithms is limited.

Multisite atrial pacing involves placement of one lead in the high right atrium and another lead near the coronary sinus ostium (dual site) or into the coronary sinus to pace the left atrium (biatrial). Small nonrandomized studies show conflicting results in terms of reducing AF burden.[32,33] A prolonged P wave duration (>120 milliseconds) may be a necessary condition for multisite pacing to be beneficial compared with single-site pacing.[34] Larger clinical trials have not demonstrated a significant AF burden reduction. In one study, dual-site right atrial pacing reduced the recurrence risk for AF compared with standard pacing only in those patients treated with AADs.[35] Biatrial pacing seems to have a limited routine clinical application when used acutely in postoperative patients. A meta-analysis involving eight studies enrolling 776 patients reported a significant reduction in the risk for developing AF in patients after heart surgery who received temporary biatrial pacing using two epicardial wires.[36]

The premise of alternate-site atrial pacing is that more uniform interatrial conduction can be achieved by pacing at the interatrial septum. The resultant decrease in heterogeneity of atrial refractoriness is expected to reduce AF burden. Pacing can be done from the high atrial septum (Bachmann's bundle) or the low atrial septum (near the coronary sinus os). The Atrial Septal Pacing Efficacy Clinical Trial (ASPECT) is a small study that demonstrated no reduction in AF burden with septal or Bachmann's bundle pacing sites compared with traditional right atrial appendage pacing sites, even when combined with atrial pacing algorithms.[37] Other studies have yielded conflicting results in a relatively small number of patients. The variability in results may be attributable to the difficulty in confirming the location or positioning the lead near Bachmann's bundle.

In summary, there are not enough long-term clinical data to support the recommendation of overdrive pacing algorithms, multisite pacing, or alternate-site pacing as a primary indication for pacemaker implantation in the management of AF. The results of some of the available studies have likely been confounded by the presence of ventricular pacing. In fact, data from the MOST suggest that for every 1% increase in ventricular pacing, there is a 1% decline in the benefit of dual-chamber atrial-based pacing in terms of AF.

Cardiac Resynchronization Therapy and Atrial Fibrillation

CRT, also known as biventricular pacing, is an important treatment modality in patients who have moderate and advanced CHF. The current ACC/AHA/HRS guidelines indicate that patients with a left ventricular ejection fraction (LVEF) less than or equal to 35%, sinus rhythm, and NYHA class III or ambulatory class IV symptoms despite recommended optimal medical therapy and who have cardiac dyssynchrony (currently defined as a QRS duration greater than 120 milliseconds) should receive CRT. Many patients who are candidates for CRT also have a history of paroxysmal or chronic AF. In patients who were candidates for CRT defibrillators (CRT-Ds), a history of paroxysmal AF is associated with as much as a 25% incidence of AF within the first 6 months from the time of implantation. Patients with a CRT indication are also at high risk for developing AF. The prevalence and incidence of AF increases with increasing severity of heart failure.[38] The risk for AF may be as high as 50% in patients who have class IV CHF.[39] In fact, either condition is known to predispose to the other condition. There are several issues to examine when considering the benefits of CRT in patients who have chronic and paroxysmal AF.

First, in those patients with existing CRT devices, what are the hemodynamic and clinical impacts of the development of AF? The effects parallel those that are seen in patients who have heart failure but do not have a CRT device. The most immediate effect on AF of biventricular pacing is the loss of AV synchrony, possibly leading to decompensated heart failure. In one small study of acute hemodynamics, systolic function as measured by dP/dT was worse in patients who had heart failure with RR-irregularity and rapid ventricular rates (120 bpm) but was better when ventricular rates were regular at approximately 120 bpm or when ventricular rates were in the normal range (80 bpm).[40] The timing of ventricular pacing is based on sensed or paced atrial events. AV synchrony can be maintained only during sinus rhythm. Most CRT devices have algorithms that promote biventricular pacing even during AF, despite the loss of AV synchrony. These algorithms are imperfect, and despite device-reported biventricular pacing of greater than 90%, clinical benefits are less certain. This is attributable to variable degrees of fusion between the intrinsic conduction and the paced ventricular complex. Furthermore, these algorithms tend to result in pacing rates that are, on average, faster than during intrinsic conduction (up to the programmed upper pacing rate), raising the concern of tachycardia-induced cardiomyopathies.

Does CRT reduce the likelihood of developing AF? As in patients with normal LV function, the benefits of biventricular pacing in patients with a CRT device in terms of the reduction of AF burden are mixed and uncertain. In a small cohort study, the annual incidence of AF was 2.8% in the CRT group and 10.2% in the control group ($P = .025$).[41] Analysis of data from the Cardiac Resynchronization in Heart Failure Trial did not show that the incidence of AF was affected by CRT, however.[42] Most studies do not show any benefit of CRT pacing on the incidence of AF.

What is the effect of chronic AF on CRT benefit? Large-scale clinical trial data elucidating the benefits of CRT in patients with AF are limited. The Multisite Stimulation in Cardiomyopathies (MUSTIC) study reported on a small number of patients with chronic AF who received a CRT device. Patients in the sinus rhythm group and the AF group showed improvements in heart failure class, in the 6-minute walk test results, and in the need for hospitalization.[43] The improvement was greater in the sinus rhythm group. In a recent prospective observational study, the benefit of CRT in patients who had heart failure with AF was similar to that seen in patients who had heart failure without AF, even at 3 years of follow-up.[44] In a study by Molkoek and colleagues,[45] patients with normal sinus rhythm and with chronic AF derived benefit from CRT. Heart failure class, QOL score, and exercise capacity were improved in both groups. In the group with AF, those who had a previous AVJ ablation derived the most benefit. Those patients who had not previously had an AVJ ablation did not show an improvement in QOL scores at 6 months. There were more nonresponders in the AF group than in the sinus group (36% versus 20%; *P*<.05). The Atrioventricular Junction Ablation Followed by Resynchronization Therapy in Patients with CHF and AF (AVERT-AF) study is a prospective, randomized, double-blind, multi-center trial that is going to test the hypothesis that AVJ ablation followed by biventricular pacing significantly improves exercise capacity and functional status as compared with pharmacologic rate control in patients with chronic AF and depressed EF, regardless of rate or QRS duration. Enrollment is scheduled to be completed in 2008.[46]

Another unresolved issue is the timing of implantation of a CRT-D device versus a standard pacemaker relative to AVJ ablation. Given that there can be an improvement of the LVEF in some patients after AVJ ablation, some practitioners implant a standard dual-chamber pacemaker in patients with borderline LVEF (30%–35%). The EF is then re-evaluated after a specific period of time (ie, 6 months), and the need for a CRT device is determined.[47] Others elect to implant a CRT-D or CRT pacemaker without defibrillation capability (CRT-P) at initial implantation to avoid the need for another procedure within a relatively short period.

A CRT-P is a consideration in patients with a more preserved EF. The Post Atrioventricular Nodal Ablation Evaluation (PAVE) trial has provided some important insights into the type of pacing that is best in this group of patients. This trial compared chronic biventricular pacing with RV-only pacing in patients undergoing AVJ ablation for the management of AF with rapid ventricular rates. The mean LVEF was 46% ± 16% in the two groups. The mean LVEF in the RV pacing group was 45% at the onset of the study and 41% at 6 months (*P*<.05).[48] There are no guidelines for the use of a CRT-P in patients with moderate LV dysfunction who are undergoing AVJ ablation.

Atrial Therapies

Some implantable devices are capable of delivering electrical therapy to manage AF and atrial flutter. These therapies include antitachycardia pacing with burst and ramp pacing in the atrium, high-frequency (50 Hz) burst pacing, and atrial defibrillation. All three have been successfully used in terminating ATs and atrial flutter.

Pacing therapies are more suitable for relatively slow AT with a regular cycle length. They are not well suited for AF. AF has been known to organize into atrial flutter or AT that may be more susceptible to pace termination, however. There is no evidence that 50-Hz burst pacing has any significant efficacy in terminating AF or in reducing the overall burden of AF in humans. There are conflicting data with respect to the effect that these therapies have on the overall burden of AF. In the ATTEST trial, prevention and termination algorithms were tested prospectively and failed to show a reduction in AF burden.[49] In another prospective trial, atrial therapies resulted in a reduction of AT burden from a mean of 58.5 to 7.8 hours per month. This study enrolled patients with a standard ICD indication and atrial tachyarrhythmias.[50]

Stand-alone implantable atrial defibrillators are not used clinically and are not currently marketed in the United States. ICDs with atrial defibrillation capability have been developed, but their use is limited by the painful nature of the shock. The pain threshold for an atrial defibrillation shock is far less than the threshold for successful AF. The ADSAS 2 study demonstrated that premedication with oral midazolam has been effective in mitigating some of the perceptions of pain.[51] This option can only be used in select highly motivated patients.

Currently, there are no guidelines that advocate using devices with these features as a primary means to manage ATs. Most physicians use these features as adjunctive therapy in patients with other standard indications for pacemakers or ICDs. Overall, they have limited utility.

SUMMARY

The role of pacemakers in the management of patients with AF and in the prevention of AF has been extensively studied. Based on well-designed prospective clinical trials, only a few of these strategies can be recommended for routine clinical use in related subpopulations. From the available studies, several key considerations are apparent:

1. The definition of physiologic pacing has evolved. It is no longer enough to maintain AV synchrony with a dual-chamber atrial-based pacemaker. A single-chamber ventricular-based pacemaker should be avoided in patients with paroxysmal AF and SND. When possible, intrinsic AV conduction should be promoted to minimize the deleterious effects of RV pacing. Therefore, mode selection is important (AAI ← → DDD, DDI, or DDD with long AV delays). Unresolved questions include the

maximum hemodynamically acceptable AV delay and the optimal site for RV pacing.[52]

2. In appropriate patients, pacemaker implantation and AVJ ablation provide clinical and mortality benefits. The procedure should be considered in any patient with suboptimal rate control and in any patient who is at risk for developing or has developed tachycardia-mediated cardiomyopathy. Although this procedure is most often done in patients with chronic AF, it is also appropriate for some patients with paroxysmal AF.

3. The benefits of pacing in patients with a CRT device may be maximized in those patients with AF who have undergone AVJ ablation. In patients with chronic AF who are receiving a CRT device, AVJ ablation can be recommended if adequate rate control to allow LV pacing cannot be achieved by medical therapy. This issue is unresolved in patients with paroxysmal AF who receive a CRT device.

4. Pacing in chronic AF to promote ventricular rate regularization has limited clinical value, and careful attention should be paid to overall adequacy of rate control. An average ventricular rate greater than the upper pacing limit may lead to tachycardia-mediated cardiomyopathy and signals the need for more aggressive rate control or AVJ ablation.

5. Pacing algorithms that attempt to prevent AF have limited value. As a sole indication, they are not widely accepted or recommended as a primary indication for pacemaker implantation in patients with paroxysmal or persistent AF.[53]

6. Multisite and novel site pacing strategies do not have broad clinical applications at this time. An exception is the use of short-term multisite pacing at the time of cardiac surgery.

REFERENCES

1. Go AS, Hylek EM, Phillips KA, et al. Prevalence of diagnosed atrial fibrillation in adults. JAMA 2001;285:2370–5.

2. Sutton R, Kenny RA. The natural history of sick sinus syndrome. Pacing Clin Electrophysiol 1986;9(6 Pt 2):1110–4.

3. Kristensen L, Nielsen JC, Pedersen AK, et al. AV block and changes in pacing mode during long-term follow-up of 399 consecutive patients with sick sinus syndrome treated with an AAI/AAIR pacemaker. Pacing Clin Electrophysiol 2001;24(3):358–65.

4. Andersen HR, Nielsen JC, Thomsen PE, et al. Long-term follow-up of patients from a randomized trial of atrial versus ventricular pacing for sick sinus syndrome. Lancet 1997;350:1210–6.

5. Fuster V, Ryden LE, Asinger RW, et al. ACC/AHA/ESC 2006 a report of the American College of Cardiology/American Heart Association Task Force on Practice Guidelines and the European Society of Cardiology Committee for Practice Guidelines (Writing Committee to Revise the 2001 Guidelines for the Management of Patients with Atrial Fibrillation). J Am Coll Cardiol 2006;48:854–906.

6. Sweeney MO, Ruetz LL, Belk P, et al. Bradycardia pacing-induced short-long-short sequences at the onset of ventricular tachyarrhythmias: a possible mechanism of proarrhythmia? J Am Coll Cardiol 2007;50(7):614–22.

7. Lamas GA, Orav J, Stambler BS, et al. for the Pacemaker Selection in the Elderly Investigators. Quality of life and clinical outcomes in elderly patients treated with ventricular pacing as compared with dual chamber pacing. N Engl J Med 1998;338:1097–104.

8. Lamas GA, Lee KL, Sweeney MO, et al. Ventricular pacing or dual-chamber pacing for sinus-node dysfunction. N Engl J Med 2002;346:1854–62.

9. Sulke N, Chamber J, Dritsas A, et al. A randomized double blind crossover comparison of four rate-responsive pacing modes. J Am Coll Cardiol 1991;17:696–706.

10. Connolly SJ, Kerr CR, Gent M, et al. Effects of physiologic pacing versus ventricular pacing on the risk of stroke and death due to cardiovascular causes. N Engl J Med 2000;342:1385–91.

11. Sweeney MO, Hellkamp AS, Ellenbogen KA, et al. Adverse effect of ventricular pacing on heart failure and atrial fibrillation among patients with normal baseline QRS duration in a clinical trial of pacemaker therapy for sinus node dysfunction. Circulation 2003;107:2932–7.

12. Toff WD, Skehan JD, deBono DP, et al. The United Kingdom Pacing and Cardiovascular Events Trial [UK Pacing Clinical Electrophysiology]. Heart 1997;78:221–3.

13. Wharton JM, Sorrentino RA, Campbell P, et al. Effects of pacing modality on atrial tachyarrhythmia recurrence in the tachycardia-bradycardia syndrome preliminary results of the Pacemaker Atrial Tachycardia Trial. [abstract]. Circ 1998;98:I-494.

14. Healey JS, William TD, Gervasio LA, et al. Cardiovascular outcomes with atrial-based pacing compared with ventricular pacing: meta-analysis of randomized trials, using individual patient data. Circulation 2006;114:11–7.

15. Moss AJ, Zareba W, Hall WJ, et al. Prophylactic implantation of a defibrillator in patients with myocardial infarction and reduced ejection fraction. N Engl J Med 2002;346:877–83.

16. Wilkoff BL, Cook JR, Epstein AE, et al. Dual-chamber pacing or ventricular backup pacing in patients with an implantable defibrillator: the Dual Chamber

and VVI Implantable Defibrillator (DAVID) trial. JAMA 2002;288(24):3115–23.

17. Sweeney MO, Bank AJ, Nsah E, et al. Minimizing ventricular pacing to reduce atrial fibrillation in sinus-node disease: the Search AV Extension and Managed Ventricular Pacing for Promoting Atrioventricular Conduction (SAVE PACE) trial. N Engl J Med 2007;357(10):1000–8.

18. Israel CW, Barold SS. Pacemaker systems as implantable cardiac rhythm monitors. Am J Cardiol 2001;88:442–5.

19. Fitts SM, Hill MR, Mehra R, et al. High rate atrial tachycardia detections in implantable pulse generator: low incidence of false-positive detections. The PA Clinical Trial Investigators. Pacing Clin Electrophysiol. 2000;23(7):1080–6.

20. Israel CW, Neubauer H, Olbrich HG, et al. Incidence of atrial tachyarrhythmia in pacemaker patients: results from the Balanced Evaluations of Atrial Tachyarrhythmia in Stimulated Patients (BEATS) study. Pacing Clin Electrophysiol 2006; 29(6):582–8.

21. Capucci A, Santini M, Padeletti L, et al. Monitor atrial fibrillation duration predicts arterial embolic events in patients suffering from bradycardia and atrial fibrillation implanted with antitachycardia pacemakers. J Am Coll Cardiol 2005;46(10):1913–20.

22. Popovic ZB, Mowrey KA, Zhang Y, et al. Slow rate during AF improves ventricular performance by reducing sensitivity to cycle length irregularity. Am J Physiol Heart Circ Physiol 2002;283:H2706–13.

23. Tse HF, Newman D, Ellenbogen KE, et al. Effects of ventricular rate regularization pacing on quality of life and symptoms in patients with atrial fibrillation (Atrial Fibrillation Symptoms Mediated by Pacing to Mean Rates [AF SYMPTOMS study]). Am J Cardiol 2004;94(7):938–41.

24. Wood MA, Brown-Mahoney C, Kay GN, et al. Clinical outcomes after ablation and pacing therapy for atrial fibrillation: a meta-analysis. Circ 2000;101:1138–44.

25. Giudici MC, Paul DL, Bontu P, et al. Pacemaker and implantable cardioverter defibrillator implantation without reversal of warfarin therapy. Pacing Clin Electrophysiol 2004;27(3):359–60.

26. al-Khadra AS. Implantation of pacemakers and implantable cardioverter defibrillators in orally anticoagulated patients. Pacing Clin Electrophysiol 2003; 26(1 Pt 2):511–4.

27. Ozean C, Jahangir A, Friedman PA, et al. Long-term survival after ablation of the atrioventricular node and implantation of a permanent pacemaker in patients with atrial fibrillation. N Engl J Med 2001;334: 1043–51.

28. Geelen P, Brugada J, Andries E, et al. Ventricular fibrillation and sudden death after radiofrequency catheter ablation of the atrioventricular junction. Pacing Clin Electrophysiol 1997;20:343–8.

29. Wyse DG, Waldo AL, DiMarco JP, et al. for the Atrial Fibrillation Follow-Up Investigation of Rhythm Management (AFFIRM) Investigators. A comparison of rate control and rhythm control in patients with atrial fibrillation. N Engl J Med 2002;347(23): 1825–33.

30. Gillis AM, Wyse DG, Connolly SJ, et al. Atrial pacing periablation for prevention of paroxysmal atrial fibrillation. Circ 1999;99(19):2553–8.

31. Carlson MD, Ip J, Messenger J, et al. A new pacemaker algorithm for the treatment of atrial fibrillation: results of the Atrial Dynamic Overdrive Pacing Trial (ADOPT). J Am Coll Cardiol 2003; 42(4):627–33.

32. Delfaut P, Saksena S, Prakash K, et al. Long-term outcome of patients with drug-refractory atrial flutter and fibrillation after single- and dual-site right atrial pacing for arrhythmia prevention. J Am Coll Cardiol 1998;32:1900–8.

33. Levy T, Walker S, Rex S, et al. No incremental benefit of multisite atrial pacing compared with right atrial pacing in patients with drug refractory paroxysmal atrial fibrillation. Heart 2001;85(1):48–52.

34. Leclercq JF, De Sisti A, Fiorello P, et al. Is dual site better than single site atrial pacing in the prevention of atrial fibrillation? Pacing Clin Electrophysiol 2000; 23:2101–7.

35. Saksena S, Prakash A, Ziegler P, et al. Improved suppression of recurrent atrial fibrillation with dual-site right atrial pacing and antiarrhythmic drug therapy. J Am Coll Cadriol 2002;40(6):1140–50.

36. Daoud EG, Snow R, Hummel JD, et al. Temporary atrial epicardial pacing as prophylaxis against atrial fibrillation after heart surgery: a meta-analysis. J Cardiovasc Electrophysiol 2003;14(2):127–32.

37. Padeletti L, Purerfellner H, Adler SW, et al. Combined efficacy of atrial septal lead placement and atrial pacing algorithms for prevention of paroxysmal atrial tachyarrhythmia. J Cardiovasc Electrophysiol 2003;14(11):1189–95.

38. Saxon LA, Greenfield RA, Cradnall BG, et al. Results of the multicenter RENEWAL 3 AVT clinic study of cardiac resynchronization defibrillator therapy in patients with paroxysmal atrial fibrillation. J Cardiovasc Electrophysiol 2006;17(5):520–5.

39. Shinbane JS, Wood MA, Jensen DN, et al. Tachycardia-induced cardiomyopathy: a review of animal models and clinical studies. J Am Coll Cardiol 1997;29(4):709–15.

40. Melenovsky V, Hay I, Fetics BJ, et al. Functional impact of rate irregularity in patients with heart failure and atrial fibrillation receiving cardiac resynchronization therapy. Eur Heart J 2005;26(7):705–11.

41. Fung J, Yu CM, Chan J, et al. Effects of cardiac resynchronization therapy on the incidence of atrial fibrillation in patients with poor left ventricular systolic function. Am J Cardiol 2005;96:728–31.

42. Hoppe UC, Casares JM, Eiskjaer H, et al. Effect of cardiac resynchronization on the incidence of atrial fibrillation in patients with severe heart failure. Circulation 2006;114(1):18–25.

43. Cazeau S, Leclercq C, Lavergne T, et al. Effects of multisite biventricular pacing in patients with heart failure and intraventricular conduction delay. N Engl J Med 2001;344(12):873–80.

44. Delnoy PP, Ottervanger JP, Luttikhuis HO, et al. Comparison of usefulness of cardiac resynchronization therapy in patients with atrial fibrillation and heart failure versus patients with sinus rhythm and heart failure. Am J Cardiol 2007;99:1252–7.

45. Molkoek SG, Bax JJ, Bleeker GB, et al. Comparison of response to cardiac resynchronization therapy in patients with sinus rhythm versus chronic atrial fibrillation. Am J Cardiol 2004;94(12):1506–9.

46. Hamdan MH, Freedman RA, Gilbert EM, et al. Atrioventricular Junction Ablation Followed by Resynchronization Therapy in Patients with Congestive Heart Failure and Atrial Fibrillation (AVERT-AF) study design. Pacing Clin Electrophysiol 2006;29(10):1081–8.

47. Bruce G, Friedman PA. Device-based therapies for atrial fibrillation. Curr Treat Options in Cardiovasc Med 2005;7:359–70.

48. Doshi RN, Daoud EG, Fellows C, et al. Left ventricular-based cardiac stimulation Post AV Nodal Ablation Evaluation (the PAVE study). J Cardiovasc Electrophysiol 2005;16(11):1160–5.

49. Lee MA, Weachter R, Pollak S, et al. The effect of atrial pacing therapies on atrial tachyarrhythmia burden and frequency: results of a randomized trial in patients with bradycardia and atrial tachyarrhythmias. J Am Coll Cardiol 2003;41:1926–32.

50. Friedman PA, Dijkman B, Warman EN, et al. Atrial therapies reduce atrial arrhythmia burden in defibrillator patients. Circ 2001;104:1023–8.

51. Boodhoo L, Mitchell A, Ujhelyi M, et al. Improving the acceptability of the atrial defibrillator: patient-activated cardioversion versus automatic night cardioversion with and without sedation (ADSAS 2). Pacing Clin Electrophysiol 2004;27:910–7.

52. Barold SS, Herweg B. Right ventricular outflow tract pacing: not ready for prime-time. J Interv Card Electrophysiol. 2005;13(1):39–46.

53. Knight BP, Gersh BJ, Carlson MD, et al. Role of permanent pacing to prevent atrial fibrillation: science advisory from the American Heart Association Council on Clinical Cardiology (Subcommittee on Electrocardiography and Arrhythmias) and the Quality of Care and Outcomes Research Interdisciplinary Working Group, in collaboration with the Heart Rhythm Society. Circ 2005;111(2):240–3.

54. Mattioli AV, Castellani ET, Vivoli D, et al. Prevalence of atrial fibrillation and stroke in paced patients without prior atrial fibrillation: a prospective study. Clin Cardiol 1998;21(2):117–22.

Atrial Fibrillation in Patients with Implantable Defibrillators

Rahul Sakhuja, MD, MPP[a], Ashok J. Shah, MD[b], Mary Keebler, MD[a], Ranjan K. Thakur, MD, MPH[b],*

KEYWORDS

- Atrial fibrillation • Defibrillator • ICD
- Sudden cardiac death • Review

The interrelation between implantable cardioverter defibrillators (ICDs) and atrial fibrillation (AF) is becoming increasingly relevant. AF affects more than 2 million Americans and 6 million in Europe. In the United States alone, the prevalence is expected to increase to 5.6 million by 2050.[1] Since the initial US Food and Drug Administration approval in 1985, ICDs have evolved to become standard therapy in patients at high risk for sudden cardiac death (SCD). ICDs have been shown to reduce SCD in patients with ventricular arrhythmias (secondary prevention) and in those at high risk for ventricular arrhythmias (primary prevention).[2–4] The number of ICD implants continues to grow; currently, 70,000 ICDs are implanted in the United States on yearly basis.[5] The recipients of these devices are generally older adults who have heart disease. It is well known that the incidence and prevalence of AF also increase with age. In addition, given the aging of the population and the adoption of more aggressive approaches to cardiovascular disease, this overlap is likely to continue to increase. AF in the ICD population leads to special problems, such as the delivery of inappropriate ICD therapies, and offers special opportunities for assessing therapy effectiveness because the patient's AF burden can be assessed more accurately.

OVERLAPPING EPIDEMIOLOGY

Many of the factors that predispose people to AF are the same risk factors that put them at risk for SCD. Therefore, it stands to reason that these subgroups that are most affected by AF are the same groups that might benefit most from ICD therapy. **Fig. 1** demonstrates the many associations and overlapping features that connect AF and ICD therapy. In addition to many common risk factors, there are some direct associations, which are discussed elsewhere in this article.

Age

Increasing age predisposes patients to AF and SCD. AF clearly increases with advancing age. In fact, AF doubles in incidence with each decade of age, afflicting up to 10% of patients older than the age of 80 years.[1,6,7] Similarly, subanalyses of major primary and secondary prevention ICD trials in addition to meta-analyses have all shown preserved efficacy of ICDs in the elderly.[2,3,8–11] Substudies of the Multicenter Automatic

[a] Massachusetts General Hospital, Division of Cardiology, 55 Fruit Street, Boston, MA 02114, USA
[b] Thoracic Cardiovascular Institute, Sparrow Health System, Michigan State University, 405 West Greenlawn, Suite 400, Lansing, MI 48910, USA
* Corresponding author. Thoracic and Cardiovascular Institute, Sparrow Health System, Michigan State University, 405 West Greenlawn, Suite 400, Lansing, MI 48910, USA.
E-mail address: thakur@msu.edu (R.K. Thakur).

Cardiol Clin 27 (2009) 151–161
doi:10.1016/j.ccl.2008.09.014
0733-8651/08/$ – see front matter © 2009 Elsevier Inc. All rights reserved.

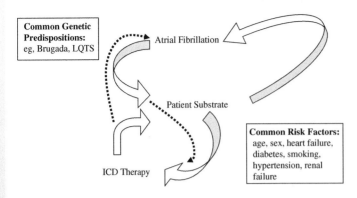

Fig. 1. There is a complex interplay between AF and SCD, with direct effects as well as common risk factors and similar genetic underpinnings.

Defibrillator Implantation Trial (MADIT)-II demonstrated that not only is the efficacy similar in patients older than 75 years of age, but it might even be greater.[12,13]

Gender

Men are generally at higher risk for atrial and ventricular arrhythmias. There is a male predominance in the risk for AF, adjusted for confounders.[1,7] As of yet, this remains unexplained. Data also suggest that ICDs may be more beneficial in men as compared with women. At baseline, a Multicenter Unsustained Tachycardia Trial (MUSTT) substudy demonstrated that women have less inducibility of sustained ventricular tachycardia (VT).[14] A meta-analysis investigating the impact of gender on survival among patients with defibrillators for primary prevention also suggested a greater benefit among men.[15]

Heart Failure

Heart failure (HF) is one of the most significant factors for patients at risk for SCD and AF. AF can be found in up to 40% of patients who have symptomatic HF.[16] Conversely, one quarter of patients with AF have HF. After adjustment, HF was associated with a 4.5- to 6-fold increase risk for AF.[1,7] Similarly, greater than 99% of ICD recipients have HF attributable to severe LV dysfunction (left ventricular ejection fraction ≤35%).[17] In the largest and most recent randomized controlled trial (RCT), patients who had New York Heart Association (NYHA) class IV HF had a 46% reduction in the risk for death with an ICD. This is in contrast to a nonsignificant reduction in risk among NYHA class II patients.[9] Of note, this trend has not been replicated in all the other large RCTs.[8,18]

Fig. 2 demonstrates the cycle in which AF begets HF, which, in turn, increases the burden of AF. This cycle ultimately increases the risk for SCD as well.

Other Cardiovascular Risk Factors

Many of the cardiovascular risk factors for AF are also risk factors for ventricular arrhythmias and SCD. Of the major cardiovascular risk factors, diabetes is a significant predictor of AF.[1,7] Other cardiovascular risk factors, such as smoking and renal failure, also predispose patients to AF.[1,7] Although there are few published data on the relationship between these cardiovascular risk factors and the efficacy of ICDs, the data available suggest that these same risk factors increase the risk for SCD. For instance, suboptimal glycemic control, smoking, and renal failure have all been associated with increased risk for ventricular arrhythmias.[19–21] Therefore, in patients who already have an indication for ICD, these subgroups (eg, smokers, diabetics, patients who have renal failure) may derive greater benefit from ICDs. Quantifying the extent of benefit derived from ICD therapy in these populations is an area in which further investigation is required, however.

The role of hypertension in the overlapping epidemiology is more complex. Although hypertension is clearly a strong independent risk factor for AF, its influence on the effectiveness of ICDs is less straightforward.[1,7] A subanalysis of MADIT-I demonstrated an inverse relation between systolic and diastolic blood pressure and ICD efficacy. That is, among patients with "higher" blood pressures (systolic blood pressures of ≥130 mm Hg or diastolic blood pressures of ≥80 mm Hg), with a higher risk for SCD, the efficacy of an ICD is attenuated.[22]

Patients with Channelopathies (Long QT Syndrome, Brugada Syndrome)

The association between repolarization channelopathies of the ventricular myocardium and AF has recently become more clear. The prevalence of AF in patients with long QT syndrome (LQTS) and Brugada syndrome is significantly higher than the

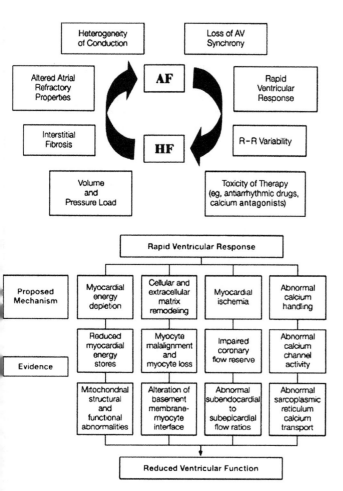

Fig. 2. Mechanisms: AF begets HF, and HF begets AF. This cycle is similar for SCD. (*From* Maisel WH, Stevenson LW. Atrial fibrillation in heart failure: epidemiology, pathophysiology, and rationale for therapy. Am J Cardiol 2003;91(Suppl 1):5D; with permission.)

background incidence of lone AF in the same, often young, age group (**Fig. 3**).[23,24]

Brugada syndrome is classically characterized in relation to its propensity for SCD attributable to ventricular arrhythmias. Therefore, ICDs are indicated for patients who have Brugada syndrome.[25] The arrhythmogenic substrate may not be restricted to the ventricles, however, and may

also be present in the atria. Atrial arrhythmias are being increasingly recognized in patients who have Brugada syndrome, the most common of which is AF. One of the largest studies is a retrospective evaluation from 14 centers of 220 patients with ICDs who had Brugada syndrome. In this study, 10% (23 of 220) of patients had AF.[26] AF was an important cause of inappropriate

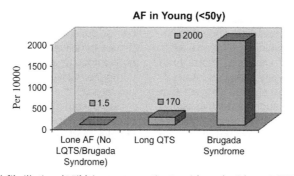

Fig. 3. Prevalence of atrial fibrillation (AFib) in young patients with and without LQTS and Brugada syndrome.

ICD shocks in these patients. One study reported that the number of inappropriate shocks exceeded the number of appropriate shocks (14.5% vs 10%).[27]

Similarly, patients who have LQTS are at considerable risk for SCD, with indication for an ICD. In LQTS, the potassium and sodium channels are thought to be defective in the atria and ventricles. A recent study reported an incidence of AF of 1.7% among patients who are gene-positive for LQTS. This is significantly greater than the baseline risk of 0.1% in an otherwise similar comparison group.[23]

Although the excess burden of AF in these patients who have channelopathies is quite clear, the therapeutic options are less so. Most cardiac ion channel disorders, which predispose to familial AF, shorten the action potential duration (APD). Sotalol may prolong the APD through potassium channel blockade, which would be particularly unsafe in patients who have LQTS. Reports of harm with amiodarone may further limit medical management in these subsets of patients.[23] Therefore, catheter ablation targeting pulmonary venous triggers might have a more prominent role in these subsets of patients and may even be considered primary therapy. One study showed that AF ablation in patients with paroxysmal AF and electrocardiograms consistent with Brugada syndrome was safe and effective.[28]

IMPACT OF ATRIAL FIBRILLATION ON PATIENTS WITH IMPLANTABLE CARDIOVERTER DEFIBRILLATORS

Although there is clear overlap in risk factors that predispose patients to AF and SCD, whether AF is independently associated with an increased risk for death in patients at risk for SCD is debated. It does not appear, however, that the presence of AF reduces the efficacy of ICDs.[29,30]

Atrial Fibrillation as an Independent Risk Factor for Mortality in Patients who have Implantable Cardioverter Defibrillators

Among patients who have congestive HF in general, AF has not been consistently shown to increase mortality. In the Framingham cohort, AF is an independent marker of increased mortality in patients who have structurally diseased hearts.[31] In addition, data from large studies suggest that patients who have HF and supraventricular tachyarrhythmias in general, and AF in particular, have an increased rate of HF exacerbation, an increased rate of hospitalization for HF, and an increased rate of death.[32] Other large studies confirmed these findings however, the survival

benefits from restoration and maintenance of sinus rhythm were offset by adverse effects of antiarrhythmic drugs (ie digoxin).[33] Furthermore, additional smaller studies did not identify AF as an independent predictor of mortality.[34,35]

Specific data on the additional risk for AF in patients with ICDs are limited and similarly conflicting. From the Antiarrhythmic Versus Implantable Defibrillators (AVID) registry, patients who present initially with life-threatening ventricular arrhythmias and have a history of AF or atrial flutter are at increased risk for death (HR = 1.20; 95% confidence interval [CI] = 1.03–1.40). Of note, given that the patients were not randomized, there were many significant differences in baseline characteristics between the patient groups. Insofar as such an analysis can adequately adjust for these differences, the data suggest that a history of AF or atrial flutter is an independent risk factor for mortality.[29] A substudy of predictors of VT or ventricular fibrillation (VF) occurrence in patients who had ICDs also confirmed this association.[36]

In a substudy of MADIT-II, 102 (8%) of the patients who had AF at baseline were evaluated for the combined risk for HF hospitalization and death. First, there was no significant difference in the incidence of inducible VT between patients with AF and sinus rhythm at study baseline. Second, after adjustment, mortality was no longer significantly higher in patients with AF at baseline (hazard ratio [HR] = 1.54, 95% CI: 0.85–2.87). The combined end point of HF hospitalization and death, however, occurred significantly more frequently in patients with AF even after adjustment (HR = 1.68, 95% CI: 1.02–2.75; **Fig. 4**). Of the patients with newly detected AF (58 patients [6%]), multivariate regression analysis demonstrated an increased risk for combined HF hospitalization and death in comparison to patients with sinus rhythm.[30] Further study, such as a meta-analysis, might clarify the effect of AF on mortality in patients with ICDs.

Inappropriate Shocks and Atrial Fibrillation

Despite the proven benefit of ICDs, inappropriate shocks remain a problem in a significant number of patients. Inappropriate shocks are shock therapies delivered by an ICD for the treatment of nonventricular arrhythmias. Inappropriate shocks comprise 12% to 30% of all shock therapies delivered.[37–42]

Supraventricular tachyarrhythmia is the most common independent predictor of inappropriate shocks, and of these, AF is the most frequent type (44%–51%).[37–42] Sinus tachycardia is the second most common cause of inappropriate shocks, which occur more commonly in patients

A

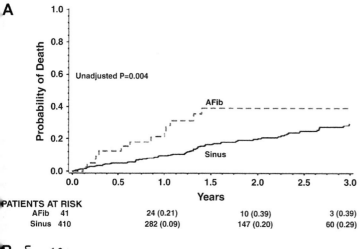

PATIENTS AT RISK

AFib	41	24 (0.21)	10 (0.39)	3 (0.39)
Sinus	410	282 (0.09)	147 (0.20)	60 (0.29)

B

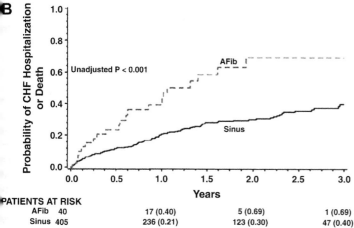

PATIENTS AT RISK

AFib	40	17 (0.40)	5 (0.69)	1 (0.69)
Sinus	405	236 (0.21)	123 (0.30)	47 (0.40)

Fig. 4. In a MADIT-II substudy, AF significantly increased mortality (A) and the cumulative probability of congestive heart failure (CHF) hospitalization or death compared to patients in sinus rhythm at baseline (B). Difference in mortality abated after controlling for age, NYHA class, blood urea nitrogen (BUN) level, and use of beta-blockers, however. (*From* Zareba W et al. Implantable cardioverter-defibrillator therapy and risk of congestive heart failure or death in MADIT II patients with atrial fibrillation. Heart Rhythm 2006; 3:633; with permission.)

with primary prevention ICDs.[39] Smoking and diastolic hypertension have been implicated as risk factors for inappropriate shocks as well.[40–42] Rare causes include device malfunction, lead failure, and oversensing of myopotentials or T waves.[37]

Ultimately, inappropriate shocks have all the adverse consequences of ICD shocks without any of the proven benefit. Moreover, patients who receive multiple inappropriate therapies experience a diminished quality of life. Some even experience psychologic symptoms, including "phantom shocks."[43,44] In addition, ICD shocks can incite dangerous arrhythmias. Finally, inappropriate ICD shocks cause premature battery depletion, which may render devices less cost-effective.[45] Ultimately, in the MADIT-II study, inappropriate therapies were associated with an increased probability of death.[30,46] These data stress the importance of reducing inappropriate shocks.

Principle strategies for inappropriate shock reduction include antiarrhythmic drugs and several

different device-based detection or discrimination enhancements. Earlier generation devices were hindered by atrial undersensing during long blanking periods and atrial oversensing of R waves during short blanking periods. This led to difficulty in diagnosing ventricular tachyarrhythmias in the setting of AF with rapid ventricular rates. To minimize inappropriate shocks from AF, newer single-chamber devices use enhanced detection criteria, such as R-R interval stability, abrupt onset of tachyarrhythmia, QRS morphology, and sustained duration. In addition to these technical advancements, dual-chamber devices also include comparisons of atrial and ventricular rates. Earlier clinical reports differ on the additional benefit of a dual-chamber device.[47] A meta-analysis comparing single-chamber with dual-chamber arrhythmia discrimination algorithms suggests that dual-chamber arrhythmia discrimination is associated with a further reduction of inappropriately treated episodes. Other reports also support this finding.[48–51]

Nevertheless, despite device improvements, inappropriate ICD therapy continues to be a problem and there is room for further improvement. For instance, among all episodes of VT, 3% occur during underlying AF. In patients with known paroxysmal AF, 18% of ventricular arrhythmias in the VF zone occur during AF.[52] Disabling discrimination of supraventricular from ventricular arrhythmias in the VF zone avoids undersensing of true VT or VF at the cost of an increased likelihood of inappropriate shocks. Enabling discrimination in the VF zone may delay or disable appropriate treatment, which is unacceptable. More work is needed to improve on current strategies.

Recent strategies to reduce the burden of inappropriate shocks include home-based monitoring and catheter ablation. Home-based monitoring of devices elucidates silent episodes of AF, breakthrough AF episodes on drugs, and previously unobserved atrial undersensing and VT. With easy and frequent availability of updates from the device's memory, allowing for early device reprogramming and appropriate medication adjustment can help to reduce the incidence of inappropriate shocks.[53] Atrioventricular node ablation in patients with drug refractory AF can eliminate rapid ventricular response-generated inappropriate shocks. Loss of atrial kick may not be desirable in some patients, however, specifically those with hypertrophic cardiomyopathy and severe diastolic dysfunction. If drug therapy is not effective in preventing recurrences of atrial fibrillation, and recurrent shocks and AV node ablation are deemed undesirable, left atrial catheter ablation (pulmonary vein isolation with or without linear lesions) might be considered as an alternative. While such a strategy has not been proven effective in ICD patients with recurrent shocks, the benefit of left atrial catheter ablation recently has been demonstrated in a randomized trial of patients who have drug-resistant atrial fibrillation and congestive heart failure.[54]

IMPACT OF IMPLANTABLE CARDIOVERTER DEFIBRILLATORS ON PATIENTS WITH ATRIAL FIBRILLATION

Data are limited on the efficacy of ICDs in patients with AF. In the MADIT-II substudy, the cumulative 2-year probability of AF was 7%. Among patients with AF, ICD therapy reduced the 2-year mortality rate from 39% in 41 conventionally treated patients to 22% in 61 ICD-treated patients (HR = 0.51), which was not statistically significant (P = .079). In this study, there was also no difference in the combined end point of HF hospitalization or death at 2 years among patients with AF treated with ICD therapy versus conventional therapy (69% versus 59%; Fig. 5).[30]

Although clinical reports of AF in patients who have ICDs are common, reports of ICD shocks inducing AF are rare. These reports suggest that defibrillation shocks within a threshold of "atrial vulnerability" are more likely to induce AF. It seems that defibrillations at greater than this threshold of vulnerability, which are now more common, are less likely to induce AF.[55] This might explain why there have been fewer reports of inducing AF with the more recent generations of ICDs. Timing shock delivery to the atrial cycle seems to be of marginal or no benefit in the prevention of shock-induced AF.[56] Notably, external cardioversion (ECV) can induce AF with high recurrence rates in patients with an established history of AF, but it bears no prognostic significance.[57] Also, epicardial leads may predispose patients to AF more so than endocardial leads, although the data are sparse.[58]

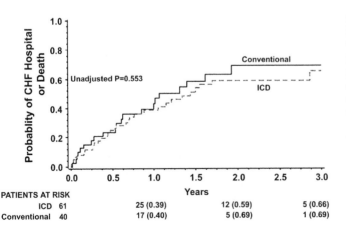

PATIENTS AT RISK

ICD	61	25 (0.39)	12 (0.59)	5 (0.66)
Conventional	40	17 (0.40)	5 (0.69)	1 (0.69)

Fig. 5. Cumulative probability of combined end point of congestive heart failure (CHF) hospitalization or death in MADIT-II patients with AF by: implantable ICD versus conventional therapy. (*From* Zareba W et al. Implantable cardioverter-defibrillator therapy and risk of congestive heart failure or death in MADIT II patients with atrial fibrillation. Heart Rhythm 2006;3:634; with permission.)

Conversely, AF is sometimes considered as a trigger for ventricular arrhythmia. Multiple reports have consistently identified an association between AF and appropriate ICD therapy, however, suggesting such a relation.[59,60] Mechanistically, irregular ventricular excitation with AF in diseased hearts leads to inhomogeneous repolarization, and thus to a higher vulnerability predisposing to sustained ventricular arrhythmias. In fact, short-long-short sequences could be proarrhythmic irrespective of underlying rhythm. The electrophysiologic mechanism seems to be irregular rather than rapid ventricular activation, with a high incidence of short-long-short sequences preceding ventricular tachyarrhythmias.[61]

Finally, these devices can also be used to record and follow the incidence and burden of AF. Using these devices for treatment on the other hand, atrial overdrive pacing to reduce the incidence of AF, has not yet been proven.[62]

DRUGS IN PATIENTS WITH ATRIAL FIBRILLATION AND IMPLANTABLE CARDIOVERTER DEFIBRILLATORS

To reduce the burden of inappropriate shocks and the need for appropriate therapies, many medical regimens have been tried. Up to 70% of patients with ICDs are also maintained on antiarrhythmic drugs for atrial or ventricular arrhythmia suppression.[63]

Antiarrhythmic Drugs and Implantable Cardioverter Defibrillator Shocks

Despite beta-blockade, up to 40% of patients still experience shocks in their first year.[63] Amiodarone and sotalol are most commonly used to suppress shocks. Amiodarone significantly reduces inappropriate and appropriate shocks relative to class I antiarrhythmics and beta-blockade alone.[64,65] Although sotalol significantly reduced the risk for a first shock compared with placebo, the risk reduction was not significant when compared with beta-blockers (HR = 0.61, 95% CI: 0.37–1.01).[64,66] All these drugs have relatively high discontinuation rates ($\sim$20%), however. Amiodarone, in particular, is associated with adverse pulmonary and thyroid events.[64,67]

A recent prospective observational study investigated the association between statin therapy and inappropriate shocks in patients with AF or atrial flutter. Of the 1445 patients treated with statins and ICDs, there was a significant reduction in inappropriate shocks (HR 0.47, 95% CI: 0.35–0.64).[68] This finding must be interpreted within the limitations of a nonrandomized study. A randomized

controlled study to evaluate the effects of statin therapy is needed.

Antiarrhythmic Drugs and Defibrillation Threshold

The efficacy of ICDs for terminating ventricular tachyarrhythmias is contingent on an adequate safety margin for defibrillation energy, commonly referred to as the defibrillation threshold (DFT). Antiarrhythmic drugs used to suppress AF, namely amiodarone and sotalol, have variable effects on DFTs. Amiodarone, the most effective anti-AF drug raises the DFT with chronic use ($\geq$6 weeks) by virtue of its Na+ channel-blocking property (although acute intravenous loading can reduce the DFT). Sotalol, dofetilide, ibutilide, and class II beta-blockers reduce the DFT.[69] The proarrhythmic nature of class IC drugs in patients with LV dysfunction limits their use; except for propafenone, these drugs raise the DFT in nonrandomized studies.[70]

The Optimal Pharmacological Therapy in Cardioverter Defibrillator Patients (OPTIC) substudy is one of the few RCTs looking at clinical outcomes in relation to the effects of antiarrhythmic drugs on DFTs. This study demonstrated that patients on beta-blockade had a decrease in mean DFT over time, which is often seen independent of beta-blockade. Consistent with prior studies, amiodarone increased the DFT and sotalol decreased the DFT. Importantly, this study demonstrated that in the era of modern device systems, the magnitude of the increase in the DFT with amiodarone is unlikely to be clinically significant.[71] Currently, the need for routine DFT reassessment after instituting antiarrhythmic drug therapy remains debated.

Anticoagulation in Patients with Implantable Cardioverter Defibrillators

Anticoagulation is advocated in patients who have AF with major predictors of stroke based on the $CHADS_2$ scoring system. Implantable cardioverter-defibrillators do not alter the decision to anticoagulate a patient or not. Moreover, anticoagulation protocols are not specific for patients with AF who have ICDs.

Anticoagulation for the evaluation of the DFT in patients with AF should be treated analogously to direct-current cardioversion in patients with AF. The risk for thromboembolism is assumed to be the same. There is even a potential for stroke from spontaneous (device-mediated) appropriate and inappropriate shocks in patients with subtherapeutic anticoagulation. Therefore, patients with ICDs and AF need to be anticoagulated as per the guidelines before and after undertaking DFT testing.[72]

With regard to anticoagulation at the time of implantation, it remains common practice to postpone device implantation until the international normalized ratio (INR) has normalized. Data are mixed regarding the benefit of reversing anticoagulation even at the time of implantation. The largest study is an observational study of 1025 patients followed prospectively over a 4-year period. Nearly 50% of the patients underwent device implantation (pacemakers and ICDs) without reversal of anticoagulation (mean INR = 2.6, range: 1.5–6.9). There was no significant difference in complication rates between the two groups (13 of 470 patients in the anticoagulated group, 21 of 555 patients in the "nonanticoagulated" group).[73] Another widely cited, small study revealed that there were significantly more pocket hematomas among patients who received warfarin plus intravenous heparin. There was no difference in outcome or complication rate among a subset of 49 patients randomized to receive heparin 6 versus 24 hours post-implant. The only stroke occurred in a patient on warfarin alone.[74]

CARDIOVERSION

As shown, the increasing rate of ICD implantation and AF is occurring in similar patient populations. One approach to management has been maintenance of sinus rhythm because of concern for higher morbidity and possible mortality in this population. Moreso in patients with CRT-Ds, AF may reduce the efficacy of the device.[75] External and internal cardioversion are alternatives to pharmacotherapy to restore sinus rhythm in these high-risk patients.

External Cardioversion

The use of ECV has long been a cause for concern in patients with ICDs because of the potential for adverse effects on the device generator or leads. These concerns are mainly based on reports before the 1990s.[76] More recently, a prospective randomized comparison of biphasic versus monophasic shock energy application in a group of 44 patients with implanted devices demonstrated that cardioversion was safe after excluding patients with known sensing abnormalities. There was no difference in response to biphasic versus monophasic shock energy. Currently, the guidelines suggest that ECV is safe in patients with ICDs. The recommendation remains to check devices before and after cardioversion. Studies

suggesting that this may not be necessary are small and inconclusive.[77]

Implantable Atrial Defibrillators

Implantable dual-chamber cardioverter defibrillators, with the capacity for atrial sensing and cardioversion for atrial arrhythmias, continue to be an active area of research. Several devices have been developed with atrial cardioversion and ventricular defibrillation capacity and are being tested in the United States and abroad. Results of their overall efficacy are mixed.[78,79] Of note, some data suggest that when episodes are treated quickly with an atrial defibrillator, the time between episodes is lengthened and the burden is reduced.[80] An important limitation of atrial defibrillators, however, is that few patients can tolerate the therapy. The pain threshold for defibrillation shocks is quite low. An internal shock less than 1 J is similarly uncomfortable to those of higher energy.[81] Further technical improvements and appropriate patient selection are still required to improve the potential benefits of such devices.

SUMMARY

AF is common in patients who have implantable defibrillators and presents some unique challenges and opportunities. AF burden can be assessed more accurately, allowing for evaluation of therapy efficacy (drugs or ablation). It remains to be shown whether home monitoring of defibrillators to detect and treat AF more quickly can reduce cardiovascular and stroke end points. The goals of therapy remain the same—reduction of symptoms (including HF exacerbation and inappropriate ICD therapies) by controlling rate or rhythm and anticoagulation for stroke prophylaxis.

REFERENCES

1. Kannel WB, Benjamin EJ. The status of the epidemiology of atrial fibrillation. Med Clin North Am 2008; 92(1):17–40.
2. Moss AJ, Zareba W, Hall WJ, et al. Prophylactic implantation of a defibrillator in patients with myocardial infarction and reduced ejection fraction. N Eng J Med 2002;346:877–83.
3. Buxton AE, Lee KL, Fisher JD, et al. A randomized study of the prevention of sudden death in patients with coronary artery disease. N Engl J Med 1999; 341:1882–90.
4. The Antiarrhythmic versus Implantable Defibrillators (AVID) Investigators. A comparison of antiarrhythmic-drug therapy with implantable cardioverter defibrillators in patients resuscitated from near-fata

ventricular arrhythmias. N Engl J Med 1997;337: 1576–83.

5. Zhan C, Baine WB, Sedrakyan A, et al. Cardiac device implantation in the United States from 1997 through 2004: a population-based analysis. J Gen Intern Med 2008;23(Suppl 1):13–19.

6. Go AS, Hylek EM, Phillips KA, et al. Prevalence of diagnosed atrial fibrillation in adults: national implications for rhythm management and stroke prevention: the Anticoagulation and Risk Factors in Atrial Fibrillation (ATRIA) study. JAMA 2001; 285(18):2370–5.

7. Benjamin EJ, Levy D, Vaziri SM, et al. Independent risk factors for atrial fibrillation in a population-based cohort: the Framingham Heart study. JAMA 1994; 271:840–4.

8. Moss AJ, Hall WJ, Cannom DS, et al. Improved survival with an implanted defibrillator in patients with coronary artery disease at high risk for ventricular arrhythmia. Multicenter Automatic Defibrillator Implantation Trial Investigators (MADIT). N Engl J Med 1996;335:1933–40.

9. Kadish A, Dyer A, Daubert JP, et al. Prophylactic defibrillator implantation in patients with nonischemic dilated cardiomyopathy (DEFINITE). N Engl J Med 2004;350:2151–8.

10. Bardy GH, Lee KL, Mark DB, et al. Amiodarone or an implantable cardioverter-defibrillator for congestive heart failure. N Engl J Med 2005;352:225–37.

11. Lee DS, Green LD, Liu PP, et al. Effectiveness of implantable defibrillators for preventing arrhythmic events and death: a meta-analysis. J Am Coll Cardiol 2003;41(9):1573–82.

12. Huang DT, Sesselberg HW, McNitt S, et al. Improved survival associated with prophylactic implantable defibrillators in elderly patients with prior myocardial infarction and depressed ventricular function: a MADIT-II substudy. J Cardiovasc Electrophysiol 2007;18(8):833–8.

13. Goldenberg I, Moss AJ. Treatment of arrhythmias and use of implantable cardioverter-defibrillators to improve survival in elderly patients with cardiac disease. Clin Geriatr Med 2007;23(1):205–19.

14. Russo AM, Stamato NJ, Lehmann MH, et al. Influence of gender on arrhythmia characteristics and outcome in the Multicenter Unsustained Tachycardia Trial. J Cardiovasc Electrophysiol 2004;15(9):993–8.

15. Henyan NN, White CM, Gillespie EL, et al. The impact of gender on survival amongst patients with implantable cardioverter defibrillators for primary prevention against sudden cardiac death. J Intern Med 2006;260(5):467–73.

16. Stevenson WG, Stevenson LW. Atrial fibrillation in heart failure. N Engl J Med 1999;341:910–1.

17. Goldberger Z, Lampert R. Implantable cardioverter-defibrillators: expanding indications and technologies. JAMA 2006;295(7):809–18.

18. Zareba W, Piotrowicz K, McNitt S, et al. Implantable cardioverter-defibrillator efficacy in patients with heart failure and left ventricular dysfunction. Am J Cardiol 2005;95(12):1487–91.

19. Chen-Scarabelli C, Scarabelli TM. Suboptimal glycemic control, independently of QT interval duration, is associated with increased risk of ventricular arrhythmias in a high-risk population. PACE 2006;29(1):9–14.

20. Goldenberg I, Moss AJ, McNitt S, et al. Cigarette smoking and the risk of supraventricular and ventricular tachyarrhythmias in high risk cardiac patients with implantable cardioverter defibrillators. J Cardiovasc Electrophysiol 2006;17(9):937–9.

21. Herzog CA, Li Shuling, Weinhandl ED, et al. Survival of dialysis patients after cardiac arrest and the impact of cardioverter defibrillators. Kidney Int 2005; 68:818–25.

22. Goldenberg I, Moss AJ, McNitt S, et al. Inverse relationship of blood pressure levels to sudden cardiac mortality and benefit of the implantable cardioverter-defibrillator in patients with ischemic left ventricular dysfunction. J Am Coll Cardiol 2007;49(13): 1427–33.

23. Johnson JN, Tester DJ, Perry J, et al. Prevalence of early-onset atrial fibrillation in congenital long QT syndrome. Heart Rhythm 2008;5:704–9.

24. Babai Bigi MA, Aslani A, Shahrzad S. Clinical predictors of atrial fibrillation in Brugada syndrome. Europace 2007;9:947–50.

25. Francis J, Antzelevich C. Atrial fibrillation and Brugada syndrome. J Am Coll Cardiol 2008;51:1149–53.

26. Sacher F, Probst V, Iesaka Y, et al. Outcome after implantation of a cardioverter-defibrillator in patients with Brugada syndrome: a multi-centre study. Circulation 2006;114(22):2317–24.

27. Park DW, Nam GB, Rhee KS, et al. Clinical characteristics of Brugada syndrome in a Korean population. J Am Coll Cardiol 2002;40:1437–44.

28. Yamada T, Yoshida Y, Tsuboi N, et al. Efficacy of pulmonary vein isolation in paroxysmal atrial fibrillation patients with a Brugada electrocardiogram. Circ J 2008;72(2):281–6.

29. Wyse DG, Love JC, Yao Q, et al. Atrial fibrillation: a risk factor for increased mortality—an AVID registry analysis. J Interv Card Electrophysiol 2001;5: 267–73.

30. Zareba W, Steinberg JS, McNitt S, et al. Implantable cardioverter-defibrillator therapy and risk of congestive heart failure or death in MADIT II patients with atrial fibrillation. Heart Rhythm 2006;3:631–7.

31. Benjamin EJ, Wolf PA, D'Agostino RB, et al. Impact of atrial fibrillation on the risk of death: the Framingham Heart study. Circulation 1998;98:946–52.

32. Dries DL, Exner DV, Gersh BJ, et al. Atrial fibrillation is associated with an increased risk for mortality and heart failure progression in patients with asymptomatic and symptomatic left ventricular systolic

dysfunction: a retrospective analysis of the SOLVD trials. J Am Coll Cardiol 1998;32:695–703.

33. Mathew J, Hunsberger S, Fleg J, et al. Incidence, predictive factors, and prognostic significance of supraventricular tachyarrhythmias in congestive heart failure. Chest 2000;118:914–22.

34. Crijns HJ, Tjeerdsma G, de Kam PJ, et al. Prognostic value of the presence and development of atrial fibrillation in patients with advanced chronic heart failure. Eur Heart J 2000;21:1238–45.

35. Carson PE, Johnson GR, Dunkman WB, et al. The influence of atrial fibrillation on prognosis in mild to moderate heart failure: the V-HeFT studies. Circulation 1993;87(Suppl VI):VI102–10.

36. Klein G, Lissel C, Fuchs AC, et al. Predictors or VT/VF-occurrence in ICD patients: results from the PROFIT-study. Europace 2006;8(8):618–24.

37. Klein RC, Raitt MH, Wilkoff BL, et al. Analysis of implantable cardioverter defibrillator therapy in the Antiarrhythmics Versus Implantable Defibrillators (AVID) trial. J Cardiovasc Electrophysiol 2003;14:940–8.

38. Sweeney MO, Wathen MS, Volosin K, et al. Appropriate and inappropriate ventricular therapies, quality of life, and mortality among primary and secondary prevention implantable cardioverter defibrillator patients: results from the Pacing Fast VT Reduces Shock Therapies (PainFREE Rx II) trial. Circulation 2005;111:2898–905.

39. Daubert JP, Zareba W, Cannom DS, et al. Inappropriate implantable cardioverter-defibrillator shocks in MADIT II: frequency, mechanisms, predictors, and survival impact. J Am Coll Cardiol 2008;51:1357–65.

40. Theuns DAMJ, Klootwijk AP, Simoons ML, et al. Clinical variables predicting inappropriate use of implantable cardioverter-defibrillator in patients with coronary heart disease or nonischemic dilated cardiomyopathy. Am J Cardiol 2005;95:271–4.

41. Alter P, Waldhans S, Plachta E, et al. Complications of implantable cardioverter defibrillator therapy in 440 consecutive patients. Pacing Clin Electrophysiol 2005;28:926–32.

42. Wilkoff BL, Hess M, Young J, et al. Differences in tachyarrhythmia detection and implantable cardioverter defibrillator therapy by primary or secondary prevention indication in cardiac resynchronization therapy patients. J Cardiovasc Electrophysiol 2004;15:1002–9.

43. Larsen G, Hallstrom A, McAnulty J, et al. Cost-effectiveness of the implantable cardioverter-defibrillator versus antiarrhythmic drugs in survivors of serious ventricular arrhythmias: results of the Antiarrhythmics Versus Implantable Defibrillators (AVID) economic analysis study. Circulation 2002;105(17):2049–57.

44. Mark DB, Anstrom KJ, Sun JL, et al. Quality of Life with Defibrillator Therapy or Amiodarone in Heart Failure. N Eng J Med 2008;359:999–1008.

45. Schron EB, Exner DV, Yao Q, et al. Quality of life in the Antiarrhythmics Versus Implantable Defibrillators trial: impact of therapy and influence of adverse symptoms and defibrillator shocks. Circulation 2002;105(5):589–94.

46. Poole JE, Johnson GW, Hellkamp AS, et al. Prognostic importance of defibrillator shocks in patients with heart failure. N Eng J Med 2008;359:1009–17.

47. Theuns DAMJ, Klootwijk AP, Goedhart DM, et al. Prevention of inappropriate therapy in implantable cardioverter-defibrillators: results of a prospective randomized study of tachyarrhythmia detection algorithms. J Am Coll Cardiol 2004;44:2362–7.

48. Theuns DAMJ, Rivero-Ayerza M, Boersma E, et al. Prevention of inappropriate therapy in implantable defibrillators: a meta-analysis of clinical trials comparing single-chamber and dual-chamber arrhythmia discrimination algorithms. Int J Cardiol 2008;125:352–7.

49. Swerdlow CD, Cannom DS. Supraventricular tachycardia–ventricular tachycardia discrimination algorithms in implantable cardioverter defibrillators state-of-the-art review. J Cardiovasc Electrophysiol 2001;12:606–12.

50. Friedman PA, McClelland RL, Bamlet WR, et al. Dual-chamber versus single-chamber detection enhancements for implantable defibrillator rhythm diagnosis: the Detect Supraventricular Tachycardia study. Circulation 2006;112(25):2871–9.

51. Wilkoff BL, Williamson BD, Stern RS, et al. Strategic programming of detection and therapy parameters in implantable cardioverter-defibrillators reduces shocks in primary prevention patients: results from the PREPARE study. J Am Coll Cardiol 2008;52(7):541–50.

52. Stein K, Hess M, Hannon C, et al. Simultaneous atrial and ventricular tachyarrhythmias in defibrillator recipients: does AF beget VF?. [abstract]. J Am Coll Cardiol 1999;22:115A.

53. Schoenfeld MH, Compton SJ, Mead RH, et al. Remote monitoring of implantable cardioverter defibrillators: a prospective analysis. Pacing Clin Electrophysiol 2004;27:757–63.

54. Khan MN, Jais PJ, Cummings J, et al. Pulmonary vein isolation for atrial fibrillation in patients with heart failure. NEJM 2008;359:1778–85.

55. Florin TJ, Weiss DN, Peters RW, et al. Induction of atrial fibrillation with low-energy defibrillator shocks in patients with implantable cardioverter defibrillators. Am J Cardiol 1997;80(7):960–2.

56. Jones GK, Johnson G, Troutman C, et al. Incidence of atrial fibrillation following ventricular defibrillation with transvenous lead system in man. J Cardiovasc Electrophysiol 1992;3(5):411–7.

57. Brembilla-Perrot B, Beurrier D, Houriez P, et al. Significance of external cardioversion induced atrial

tachyarrhythmias. Pacing Clin Electrophysiol 2003; 26(11):2111–5.

58. Katz A, Evans JJ, Fogel RI, et al. Atrial fibrillation/flutter induced by implantable ventricular shocks: difference between epicardial and endocardial energy delivery. J Cardiovasc Electrophysiol 1997;8(1):35–41.

59. Rienstra M, Smit MD, Nieuwland W, et al. Persistent atrial fibrillation is associated with appropriate shocks and heart failure in patients with left ventricular dysfunction treated with an implantable cardioverter defibrillator. Am Heart J 2007;153:120–6.

60. Stein KM, Euler DE, Meher R, et al. Do atrial tachyarrhythmias beget ventricular tachyarrhythmias in defibrillator patients? J Am Coll Cardiol 2002;40(2): 335–40.

61. Gronefeld GC, Mauss O, Li YG, et al. Association between atrial fibrillation and appropriate implantable cardioverter defibrillator therapy: results from a prospective study. J Cardiovasc Electrophysiol 2000;11(11):1208–14.

62. Padeletti L, Muto C, Maounis T, et al. Atrial fibrillation in recipients of cardiac resynchronization therapy devices: 1-year results of the randomized MASCOT trial. Am Heart J 2008;156(3):520–6.

63. Bollmann A, Husser D, Cannom DS. Antiarrhythmic drugs in patients with implantable cardioverter-defibrillators. Am J Cardiovasc Drugs 2005;5(6):371–8.

64. Connolly SJ, Dorian P, Roberts RS, et al. Optimal pharmacological therapy in cardioverter defibrillator patients. I. Comparison of beta-blockers, amiodarone plus beta-blockers, or sotalol for prevention of shocks from implantable cardioverter defibrillators: the OPTIC study: a randomized trial. JAMA 2006; 295:165–71.

65. The CASCADE Investigators. Cardiac arrest in Seattle: conventional versus amiodarone drug evaluation (CASCADE study). Am J Cardiol 1991;67(7):578–84.

66. Pacifico A, Hohnloser SH, Williams JH, et al. Prevention of implantable-defibrillator shocks by treatment with sotalol: d,l-Sotalol Implantable Cardioverter-Defibrillator Study Group. N Engl J Med 1999;340(24): 1855–62.

67. Lee CH, Nam GB, Park HG, et al. Effects of antiarrhythmic drugs on inappropriate shocks in patients with implantable defibrillators. Circ J 2008;72: 102–5.

68. Bhavnani SP, Coleman CI, White CM, et al. Association between statin therapy and reductions in atrial fibrillation or flutter and inappropriate shock therapy. Europace 2008;10:854–9.

69. Page RL. Effects of antiarrhythmic medication on implantable cardioverter-defibrillator function. Am J Cardiol 2000;85:1481–5.

70. Stevens SK, Haffajee CI, Naccarelli GV, et al. Effects of oral propafenone on defibrillation and pacing thresholds in patients receiving implantable cardioverter-defibrillators. Propafenone Defibrillation Threshold Investigators. J Am Coll Cardiol 1996; 28(2):418–22.

71. Hohnloser SH, Dorian P, Roberts R, et al. Effect of amiodarone and sotalol on ventricular defibrillation threshold: the Optimal Pharmacological Therapy in Cardioverter Defibrillator Patients (OPTIC) trial. Circulation 2006;114:104–9.

72. Fuster V, Ryden LE, Cannom DS, et al. ACC/AHA/ ESC 2006 guidelines for the management of patients with atrial fibrillation: a report of the American College of Cardiology/American Heart Association Task Force on practice guidelines and the European Society of Cardiology Committee for practice guidelines (Writing Committee to Revise the 2001 Guidelines for the Management of Patients with Atrial Fibrillation) developed in collaboration with the European Heart Rhythm Association and the Heart Rhythm Society. J Am Coll Cardiol 2006;48:149–246.

73. Giudici MC, Barold SS, Paul DL, et al. Pacemaker and implantable cardioverter defibrillator implantation without reversal of warfarin therapy. PACE 2004;27:358–60.

74. Michaud GF, Pelosi F, Noble MD, et al. A randomized trial comparing heparin initiation 6 h or 24 h after pacemaker or defibrillator implantation. J Am Coll Cardiol 2000;35(7):1915–8.

75. Gasparini M, Auricchio A, Regoli F, et al. Four-year efficacy of cardiac resynchronization therapy on exercise tolerance and disease progression: the importance of performing atrioventricular junction ablation in patients with atrial fibrillation. J Am Coll Cardiol 2006;48:734–43.

76. Levine PA. Effect of cardioversion and defibrillation on implanted cardiac pacemakers. In: Barold SS, editor. Modern cardiac pacing. Mount Kisco (NY): Futura Publ. Co; 1985. p. 875–86.

77. Manegold JC, Israel CW, Ehrlich JR, et al. External cardioversion of atrial fibrillation in patients with implanted pacemaker or cardioverter-defibrillator systems: a randomized comparison of monophasic and biphasic shock energy application. Eur Heart J 2007;28:1731–8.

78. Gradaus R, Seidl K, Korte T, et al. Reduction of ventricular tachyarrhythmia by treatment of atrial fibrillation in ICD patients with dual-chamber implantable cardioverter/defibrillators capable of atrial therapy delivery: the REVERT-AF study. Europace 2007; 9(7):534–9.

79. Geller JC, Reek S, Timmermans C, et al. Treatment of atrial fibrillation with an implantable atrial defibrillator—long term results. Eur Heart J 2003;24:2083–9.

80. Levy S, Ricard P, Lau CP, et al. Multicenter low energy transvenous atrial defibrillation (XAD) trial results in different subsets of atrial fibrillation. J Am Coll Cardiol 1997;29(4):750–5.

81. Dosdall DJ, Ideker RE. Intracardiac atrial defibrillation. Heart Rhythm 2007;4:S51–56.

Catheter Ablation of Atrial Fibrillation

Thomas D. Callahan IV, MD[a], Luigi Di Biase, MD[a,b],
Rodney Horton, MD[c], Javier Sanchez, MD[c],
Joseph G. Gallinghouse, MD[c], Andrea Natale, MD, FACC, FHRS[c,d,e,f],*

KEYWORDS

- Catheter ablation • Atrial fibrillation
- Pulmonary veins • Atrioventricular node ablation
- Antiarrhythmic drugs • Rate control • Rhythm control

Atrial fibrillation is a common arrhythmia associated with significant morbidity, including angina, heart failure, and stroke. Medical therapy remains suboptimal, with significant side effects and toxicities, and a high recurrence rate. Catheter ablation or modification of the atrioventricular node with pacemaker implantation provides rate-control, but exposes patients to the hazards associated with implantable devices and does nothing to reduce the risk for stroke. Pulmonary vein antrum isolation offers a nonpharmacologic means of restoring sinus rhythm, thereby eliminating the morbidity of atrial fibrillation and the need for anti-arrhythmic drugs.

Atrial fibrillation is a common arrhythmia associated with significant morbidity. It is the most common sustained arrhythmia and affects millions of Americans. The lifetime risk for development of atrial fibrillation is estimated at one in four for persons older than 40 years.[1] Atrial fibrillation contributes to the development of angina, heart failure, and stroke, with an estimated stroke risk of 3% to 5% per year in untreated individuals.[2,3] Furthermore, analysis of Framingham data suggests the mortality rate in patients who have atrial fibrillation is increased 1.5- to 2-fold compared with the general population.[4,5] Medical therapy for atrial fibrillation remains suboptimal and plagued by significant toxicities and frequent side effects and

intolerance. Recurrence rates with medical therapy are estimated to occur in 50% of patients at 6 to 36 months.[6]

Whether or not restoration of sinus rhythm should be a goal of therapy is a matter of debate in the literature. Several trials, including the Atrial Fibrillation Follow-Up Investigation of Rhythm Management (AFFIRM) trial, report no benefit of rhythm control over rate control in the treatment of atrial fibrillation.[7,8] These trials, however, examined pharmacologic rhythm control strategies. Further analysis of the AFFIRM data showed that the presence of atrial fibrillation was associated with a 47% increased mortality compared with sinus rhythm. Use of an antiarrhythmic medication was associated with a 49% increased mortality, suggesting that any mortality benefit from maintenance of sinus rhythm was offset by increased mortality from currently available antiarrhythmics.[9] Catheter ablation for atrial fibrillation offers a nonpharmacologic means of restoring sinus rhythm and improves mortality and quality of life compared with antiarrhythmic drugs.[10,11]

FUNDAMENTALS OF RADIOFREQUENCY CATHETER ABLATION

In 1979, Vedel and coauthors[12] reported complete heart block after multiple attempts at direct current

---

A version of this article originally appeared in the *Medical Clinics of North America*, volume 92, issue 1.
[a] Cardiac Pacing and Electrophysiology, Cleveland Clinic Cleveland, OH, USA
[b] Department of Cardiology, University of Foggia, Foggia, Italy
[c] Texas Cardiac Arrhythmia Institute at St. David's Medical Center, Austin, TX; USA
[d] Case Western Reserve University, Cleveland, OH, USA
[e] Division of Cardiology, Stanford University, Stanford, CA, USA
[f] California Pacific Medical Center Atrial Fibrillation and Arrhythmia Program, San Francisco, CA, USA
* Corresponding author. 1015 East 32 Street, Suite 516, Austin, TX 78705, USA.
E-mail address: dr.natale@gmail.com (A. Natale).

cardioversion while a recording catheter was positioned at the bundle of His. The investigators hypothesized that current shunting through the recording catheter injured the conduction system, leading to heart block. Subsequently, percutaneous catheter ablation for treatment of cardiac arrhythmias was developed and, in the infancy of this technique, atrial fibrillation was among the first arrhythmias treated. Patients who had atrial fibrillation and rapid ventricular rates refractory to medical therapy were offered ablation of the atrioventricular (AV) node using high-energy direct current delivered to the region of the AV junction.[13,14] Although effective, this technique was associated with a high rate of life-threatening complications.[15]

Use of radiofrequency energy in catheter ablation was found to improve efficacy of ablation and the safety profile, and quickly supplanted direct current catheter ablation.[16–18] Radiofrequency catheter ablation delivers an alternating current, typically at frequencies of approximately 500 kHz, which generates myocardial lesions through thermal injury. Current disperses radially from the delivery electrode to a dispersive electrode placed on the skin, with impedance, voltage drop, and power dissipation greatest at the interface of the electrode and tissue. Heating of the tissue in close contact to the delivery electrode is caused by resistance as current passes through, and is referred to as direct heating. Thermal energy from this area is transferred back to the delivery electrode and the surrounding tissue through conduction. Conductive or indirect heating accounts for a larger volume of thermal injury in the radiofrequency ablation lesion than does resistive or direct heating. Temperature rise is rapid in the zone of resistive heating and immediately adjacent areas; however, temperature rise is slower as the distance from this area increases, and can continue to rise at remote sites even after delivery of current has ceased.[19]

Lesion size is influenced by several factors. Increasing the length or diameter of the delivery electrode, the contact area, and the source power all result in a larger radius of direct heating and, thus larger lesion size. Circulating blood results in convective cooling. Although convective cooling within the tissue limits lesion size, cooling of the catheter tip through convection allows improved power delivery, which increases lesion size and allows for more rapid lesion formation. Although lesion size is proportional to the peak temperature achieved, at temperatures of 100°C and above, char and coagulum form and can increase impedance dramatically.[19] Within the tissue, temperatures in excess of 100°C cause the sudden

production of steam, which can lead to an explosive venting to the endocardial or epicardial surface, called a *pop*.

Convective cooling of the tissue–catheter interfaces caused by circulating blood and, when used, with irrigation of the catheter tip may cause temperatures at this interface to be lower than peak tissue temperatures achieved within the tissue. As a result, thermal sensors in the catheter tip often underestimate peak in-lesion temperatures. The authors have found that with nonirrigated catheter tips, measured temperature is not reliable and instead microbubble monitoring with intracardiac echocardiography is a more effective strategy for regulation of energy delivery.[20] Because microbubble monitoring is not feasible with open-tip irrigated catheters, tissue disruption is minimized with careful limitation of the maximum temperature and power and monitoring of the impedance.

ATRIOVENTRICULAR NODE ABLATION
Overview

Like medical therapy for atrial fibrillation, catheter ablation for atrial fibrillation can be divided into two general strategies: rate control and rhythm control. Within the field of catheter ablation, rate can be controlled through modifying the AV node or ablating the node and implanting a permanent pacemaker. Curative catheter ablation achieves rhythm control through targeting the triggers of atrial fibrillation, restoring sinus rhythm, and preventing future recurrences.

The technique of AV node ablation predated the development of curative ablation techniques for atrial fibrillation. AV node modification targets the slow pathway, resulting in increased AV node refractoriness and slower ventricular rates without causing AV block. This technique is used rarely, because complete heart block is common and malignant ventricular arrhythmias can be seen after the procedure. AV node ablation does not cure atrial fibrillation and requires placement of a permanent pacemaker to ensure adequate ventricular rates. Ideally, the most proximal portion of the AV node is targeted, leaving the distal portion intact, resulting in complete heart block. Although this is the desired result of the procedure it maximizes the likelihood of leaving patients with an escape rhythm, which is desirable if a pacemaker malfunction occurs. Because of its many limitations, including the requirement of a permanent pacemaker and the failure to address the long-term risk for stroke, and given the possible benefits of restoring sinus rhythm, AV node ablation is restricted primarily to patients refractory to medical therapy and who have contraindications to curative atrial fibrillation ablation, such as significant comorbidities and poor life expectancy.

Techniques

Before AV node ablation, pacing of the ventricle should be ensured. This function can be achieved through implanting a permanent pacemaker before AV node ablation or placing a temporary transvenous pacemaker before ablation and then implanting a permanent pacemaker immediately after the procedure. The first strategy has the advantage of allowing any possible postimplantation device malfunctions to be addressed before AV node ablation. Placing a dual-chamber pacemaker with mode switching capabilities allows for AV synchrony during sinus rhythm or atrial pacing.

Ablation of the AV node usually is performed through the right side of the heart, with radiofrequency ablation most often used. However, in approximately 5% to 10% of cases, the AV node can be ablated only through the left side of the heart, necessitating arterial access and a retrograde approach to apply lesions below to the aortic valve.[21] Use of cryoablation is described but does not seem to offer benefit over radiofrequency ablation.[22] Typically, the His bundle is identified, and the ablation catheter is then withdrawn toward the right atrium to a site that shows an atrial-to-ventricular electrogram ratio of 1:1 to 1:2 and a small His signal (**Fig. 1**). Care should be taken to map adequately and ensure catheter stability, because ineffective lesions may result in edema without successful ablation. This complication may make successful ablation more difficult through obscuring electrograms and increasing the distance to the target tissue. Effective lesions at an appropriate target site often induce an accelerated junctional rhythm early in the radiofrequency application, which subsequently resolves to a slower junctional or ventricular escape as radiofrequency application continues.

Outcomes and Limitations

Success rates for AV node ablation are near 100%.[23–27] The procedure improves quality of life and may improve left ventricular ejection fraction modestly, probably from improved rate control.[23,24,28–30] In addition to these benefits, AV node ablation usually can be performed quickly, which may be advantageous for patients unable to endure more protracted ablation procedures. Additionally, the procedure typically can be performed entirely from the right side of the heart, and thus does not require systemic intraoperative anticoagulation and essentially eliminates the risk for thromboembolic complications. After AV node ablation, a high risk for malignant ventricular arrhythmias is present. This risk is eliminated by programming a lower rate of at least 80 to 90 beats per minute for the first 4 to 8 weeks postprocedure.[29,31]

AV node ablation for the treatment of atrial fibrillation has several key limitations. Patients who do not have contraindications must continue on anticoagulation therapy to minimize risk for the cardioembolic complications of atrial fibrillation. Furthermore, patients may continue to have symptoms from atrial fibrillation, such as shortness of breath, despite regularization of the ventricular rhythm with pacing. In addition, patients are

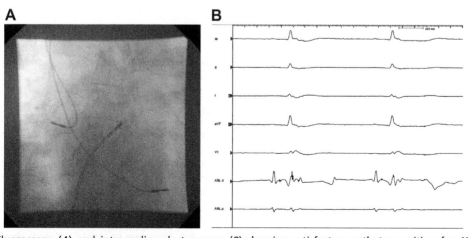

A   **B**

Fig. 1. Fluoroscopy (A) and intracardiac electrograms (B) showing satisfactory catheter position for AV node ablation. The ablation catheter (ABL) is positioned in the region of the slow pathway with approximately equal A and V amplitudes on the distal ablation channel (ABLd) of the intracardiac electrogram. Pacemaker leads are seen in the right atrium (RA) and right ventricle (RV).

exposed to the associated risks for an indwelling cardiac device, including the risk for infection and chronic right ventricular pacing.[32] Patients who have a history of congestive heart failure benefit from biventricular pacing after AV node ablation. No evidence, however, suggests that chronic biventricular pacing in the general population is equivalent to native conduction through the His–Purkinje system.[33] In fact, preliminary results from a randomized study[34] showed better improvement in symptoms, quality of life, and ejection fraction among patients who had congestive heart failure who underwent atrial fibrillation ablation than in those treated with AV node ablation and cardiac resynchronization therapy devices.

CURATIVE CATHETER ABLATION
FOR ATRIAL FIBRILLATION
Background and Overview

Catheter ablation techniques aimed at curing atrial fibrillation rather than simply controlling the ventricular response target the triggers and substrate of atrial fibrillation. Curative catheter ablation techniques initially attempted to mimic the lesions created by the surgical Maze procedure.[35–37] In 1998, Haissaguerre and colleagues[38] described focal firing as an important source of ectopic beats, which could lead to atrial fibrillation, and reported that these foci respond to ablation. Experts believe that as many as 94% of these triggers originate from the pulmonary veins.[39] This finding led to focal ablation within the pulmonary veins to eliminate these triggers.

Further studies propelled the evolution of the technique to the circumferential isolation of the pulmonary veins, which has since become the cornerstone of curative atrial fibrillation ablation. Patients who have paroxysmal atrial fibrillation and a structurally normal heart may expect a high rate of cure from isolation of the pulmonary veins alone. This outcome represents, however, a small number of patients who have atrial fibrillation presenting for ablation. Most patients, especially those who have dilated or scarred atria and chronic atrial fibrillation, do not have the same rate of cure with simple isolation of the pulmonary veins.[40]

Areas of focal firing outside the pulmonary veins in the left and right atria also initiate atrial fibrillation.[41] Ablation of additional triggers outside the pulmonary veins and addition of lesions to interrupt the maintenance of atrial fibrillation may be required to improve long-term success in these substrate modification populations. These adjunctive lesion sets have become an integral component of curative atrial fibrillation ablation for most patients.

More recently, ablation targeting complex fragmented atrial electrograms (CFAEs) has been shown to result in sinus rhythm maintenance in approximately 80% of patients who had paroxysmal and persistent atrial fibrillation. However, these results originated from a single center and have not been replicated by other investigators.[42]

Current techniques for curative atrial fibrillation ablation can be categorized broadly as anatomic ablation or electrogram-guided isolation. Anatomic ablation currently relies on electroanatomic mapping systems to create a three-dimensional representation of the left atrium and pulmonary veins. The position of the ablation catheter can be visualized within this representation, and the location of ablation points marked with respect to the anatomy. Ablation lesions are placed circumferentially around the pulmonary veins, individually or often encircling two ipsilateral pulmonary veins simultaneously. Local electrograms can be measured from the ablation catheter and can help determine the duration of each lesion. Careful inspection for gaps allowing persistent conduction between the left atrium and the pulmonary veins is not performed, however. Persistent conduction between the pulmonary veins and left atrium can be shown in up to 60% of the pulmonary veins after anatomic ablation.[43,44]

In contrast to this technique, electrogram-guided isolation relies on a second mapping catheter with a ring-shaped array of electrodes. This array is placed at the ostium of each pulmonary vein during isolation. In the authors' approach, lesions are delivered circumferentially around the antrum of each individual pulmonary vein, and the ring catheter is used to interrogate the circumference of the pulmonary vein antra to find gaps that can be closed (**Fig. 2**). Electrogram guidance of pulmonary vein antrum isolation (PVAI) improves long-term success compared with a purely anatomic approach.[43,45]

Patient Selection

As with any invasive procedure, patient selection is critical to optimizing the safety and success of PVAI. Although some data suggest increased mortality associated with atrial fibrillation and antiarrhythmic medications, much more study is required to elucidate the magnitude of these risks and the impact PVAI might have on them. Therefore, the diagnosis of atrial fibrillation alone is not sufficient to warrant PVAI. Furthermore, PVAI, like all invasive procedures, carries inherent risks that may be increased by patient age and

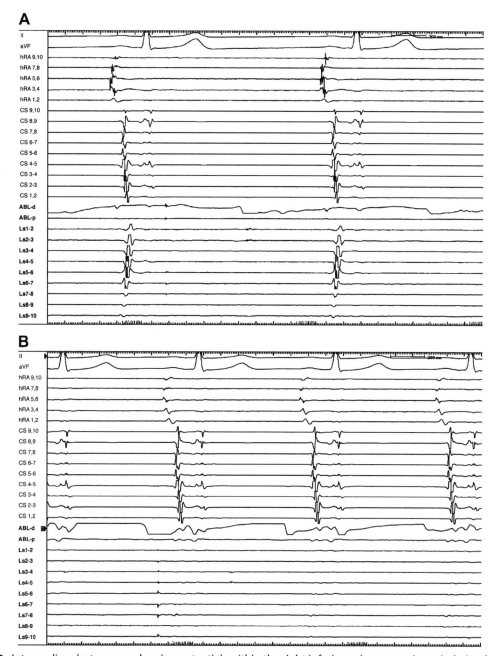

Fig. 2. Intracardiac electrograms showing potentials within the right inferior pulmonary vein preisolation (A) and absence of potentials on the mapping ring catheter (LS 1–10) postisolation (B).

comorbidities. Finally, patient features have been shown to impact the likelihood of success. All of these factors play an important role in determining the appropriateness of PVAI.

Although some data suggest that PVAI may be superior to medical therapy for first-line therapy of atrial fibrillation, current guidelines recommend that, in most patients, treatment with at least one antiarrhythmic drug be tried and fail before atrial fibrillation ablation is considered.[46]

Current indications include symptomatic atrial fibrillation refractory to or intolerant of medical therapy. Additionally, patients in whom anticoagulation is indicated secondary to atrial fibrillation, but who cannot tolerate or whose occupations or activities preclude long-term anticoagulation, may be considered candidates for PVAI regardless of the presence of symptoms. Finally, patients who desire not to take antiarrhythmics or long-term anticoagulation sometimes are considered for PVAI.

PVAI should not be considered for any patients who cannot reasonably be expected to tolerate the procedure. For instance, patients who have severe dementia or decompensated heart failure are unlikely to be able to endure a potentially long procedure that requires their cooperation and for them to remain supine. Because the procedure requires aggressive intraoperative anticoagulation, active bleeding or a history of a severe bleeding diathesis is a contraindication. Patients in persistent or permanent atrial fibrillation should not undergo PVAI if they would not be considered candidates for cardioversion. Adequate anticoagulation of sufficient duration should be ensured just as it would be before cardioversion. If patients have a history of prior ablations or open heart surgery, structural abnormalities such as pulmonary vein stenosis should be ruled out. Congenital heart defects, including repaired atrial septal defects, can add to the technical difficulty but they not absolute contraindications if the procedure is performed in centers where clinicians are experienced in the technique.[47]

Certain patient features are found to be associated with increased or decreased likelihood of success and may help in patient selection and counseling. Patients who have atrial fibrillation that is shorter in duration and paroxysmal and those who have normal-sized atria are more likely to have their atrial fibrillation cured by PVAI. Conversely, patients who have long-standing, permanent atrial fibrillation and those who have dilated atria or known atrial scarring are less likely to experience complete cure after PVAI.[48,49]

The preoperative assessment should include a careful history and physical examination. Patients who have allergies to intravenous contrast dye should be prepared according to standard procedures. Many operators obtain preoperative CT scan or MRI optimized for imaging of the pulmonary veins before PVAI; however, this is not absolutely necessary unless patients have a history of an ablation in the left heart. Antiarrhythmic medications can suppress spontaneous firing and fractionation of the electrograms used to guide ablation.

Therefore, antiarrhythmic medications should be discontinued with approximately a five half-life washout period before the procedure (a longer period around 6 months is required for amiodarone). Continued full anticoagulation with warfarin therapy could decrease the risk for periprocedure thromboembolic events and is not interrupted for PVAI.[50] Patients not previously on chronic anticoagulation are started on warfarin, with a goal international normalized ratio of two to three, at least 3 weeks before PVAI, and this is continued for at least 3 to 6 months after the procedure. Patients must remain in a fasting state before the procedure and should be instructed to expect an overnight hospital admission for observation after the procedure.

Technical Aspects

Pulmonary veins are approached using a transseptal approach, necessitating multiple venous sheaths for the delivery of catheters. Transseptal catheters are delivered through sheaths typically placed in the right femoral vein. Additionally, an intracardiac echocardiogram (ICE) probe may be introduced through the left or right femoral vein. Placement of a coronary sinus catheter provides an additional fluoroscopic landmark to guide catheter positioning and is used as a reference point for certain electroanatomic mapping systems. Additionally, a coronary sinus catheter may help differentiate left- versus right-sided arrhythmogenic triggers.[51] This device typically is placed through the right internal jugular vein or through the right subclavian vein.

Electrogram-guided ablation requires an ablation and a mapping catheter be placed into the left atrium; thus, two transseptal sheaths are needed. Fluoroscopic and ICE visualization of the transseptal needle and the anatomic landmarks should guide transseptal puncture. Care must be taken to ensure that punctures are performed through the inferior interatrial septum, where it is thinner and easier to cross than the more muscular superior septum. Additionally, placing transseptal puncture posteriorly places the catheters close to the posterior left atrium and the pulmonary veins, facilitating reach of the catheters to these targets (**Fig. 3**). Before the transseptal puncture, unfractionated heparin should be bolused and

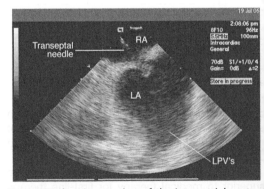

Fig. 3. ICE showing tenting of the intra-atrial septum with the transseptal needle at a satisfactory location on the septum across from the left pulmonary vein (LPVs). The right atrial (RA) and left atrial (LA) are shown.

a drip initiated. A target activated clotting time of 350 to 400 seconds is used at the authors' institution and decreases perioperative thromboembolic events compared with lower targets.[52]

The muscular sleeves of the pulmonary veins are the most common site of triggers of atrial fibrillation.[38,39] Although early approaches used focal lesions within individual pulmonary veins to ablate these foci, they were associated with an increased rate of pulmonary vein stenosis and higher rates of recurrence compared with circumferential isolation.[53,54] Discrete electrical connections between the left atrium and the pulmonary veins often can be identified; however, a segmental approach that targets only these connections has a higher rate of recurrence than circumferential techniques.[39,55–58]

Occasionally, individual pulmonary veins may be identified as the triggers of atrial fibrillation in a given patient. It may be tempting to isolate only the veins identified as harboring triggers in these cases. Failure to isolate all the pulmonary veins, however, yields a lower long-term success rate and, if attempted at all, probably should be reserved for younger patients.[59–61] Purely anatomic ablation is associated with a high incidence of persistent conduction between the pulmonary veins and left atrium and is associated with rates of success inferior to electrogram-guided isolation.[43–45] Thus, the authors believe that electrogram-guided isolation is preferred over anatomic techniques.

Although it is known that most triggers of atrial fibrillation arise from the muscular sleeves of the pulmonary veins, the junction of the pulmonary veins with the left atrium is not a discrete ostium. Instead, these junctions are conically shaped, and the triggers found within the pulmonary veins often exist proximally in this junction. This understanding has shaped the development of catheter ablation for atrial fibrillation from a distal ablation procedure isolating the pulmonary veins at the ostium, what is commonly known as pulmonary vein isolation (PVI), to a more proximal isolation of the entire pulmonary vein antrum, referred to as PVAI (**Figs. 4** and **5**). The pulmonary vein antra isolated with this technique encompass the pulmonary veins, the left atrial roof, the left atrial posterior wall, and a portion of the interatrial septum anterior to the right pulmonary veins (**Fig. 6**).[62,63]

Adjunctive Curative Ablation Techniques

In addition to isolation of the pulmonary veins, adjunctive targets often are ablated in an attempt to prevent short- and long-term recurrences of atrial fibrillation and the development of other atrial arrhythmias. The left atrial posterior wall, interatrial septum, and ligament of Marshall are

identified as sites of ectopic beats initiating atrial fibrillation.[64] Ablation in these areas may improve overall success, especially in patients who have permanent atrial fibrillation. Initiation of atrial flutter, left-sided atrial flutter, atrial tachycardia, and microreentrant atrial flutter may complicate atrial fibrillation ablation.

Ablation lines placed on the posterior wall and roof of the left atrium, typically connecting the left superior pulmonary vein to the right superior pulmonary vein, decrease the risk for developing left atrial arrhythmias, decrease inducibility of atrial fibrillation, and improve long-term success after atrial fibrillation ablation.[65,66] In addition, mitral valve isthmus lines decrease the likelihood of recurrent atrial fibrillation in patients who have permanent atrial fibrillation. This may be secondary to compartmentalization of the left atrium or substrate modification in the region of the ligament of Marshal and around the coronary sinus.[67] In addition to these sites, areas of complex fractionated electrograms are implicated in the development of atrial fibrillation. These areas are found most commonly in the pulmonary veins, on the interatrial septum and left atrial roof, and at the coronary sinus ostium. Limited data suggest that ablation at the sites of complex fractionated electrograms as a stand-alone strategy may be associated with a high rate of success in eliminating atrial fibrillation,[42,68] Finally, some investigators advocate ablation to target autonomic innervation of the left atrium and pulmonary veins. In patients showing autonomic effect while ablation occurs around one or more of the pulmonary veins, denervation of the pulmonary veins, as demonstrated by abolition of the evoked vagal reflex, may improve freedom from atrial fibrillation recurrence.[69,70]

Additional ablation sites within the right atrium may improve the efficacy of PVAI in certain populations. The superior vena cava (SVC) is a common site of atrial fibrillation triggers. Isolation of the SVC through creating a circumferential ablation line at the junction of the right atrium and SVC may improve the success of atrial fibrillation ablation, especially in patients who have permanent atrial fibrillation (**Fig. 7**).[64,71–73] The crista terminalis and the coronary sinus ostium are identified as sites of ectopic beats triggering atrial fibrillation.[64] Empiric ablation of the coronary sinus, however, does not seem to improve the overall success of PVAI.[74]

The authors' opinion is that inclusion of adjunctive lesions has been an important component of the PVAI technique for some time. Early experience prompted experts to incorporate isolation of the SVC, and the antrum approach includes isolation of the posterior wall, left atrial roof, and interatrial

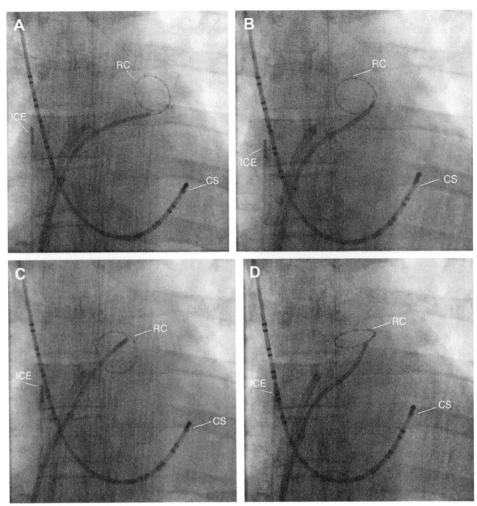

Fig. 4. Fluoroscopic images illustrating movement of the ring mapping catheter (RC) in the antrum of the left superior pulmonary vein, including the os (*A*), superoposterior antrum (*B*), inferoposterior antrum (*C*), and roof (*D*). The coronary sinus catheter (CS) and ICE probe are seen.

septum and extends anterior to the right pulmonary veins. Additionally, in patients who have permanent atrial fibrillation, the left atrium is interrogated routinely for areas of complex fractionated electrograms, and the septal ablation is extended to include the mitral valve annulus. Challenge with high doses of isoproterenol or adenosine is considered to uncover additional triggers, especially in nonparoxysmal atrial fibrillation.

End Points

The procedural end point depends on the strategy used for ablation, including entry block around the ostium or antrum of the pulmonary veins for electrogram-guided atrial fibrillation ablation. A ring or circular mapping catheter with tightly spaced electrodes is used to detect any electrical gaps within the encircling lesions, and confirms block of atrial signal into the pulmonary veins. Confirmation of exit block from the pulmonary veins is documented through pacing within the pulmonary veins, or when independent firing in the pulmonary veins is found.[23] During circumferential anatomic ablation, the end point is abolition of local electrograms detected by the ablation catheter. Electrical isolation of the pulmonary veins is not required or achieved in most pulmonary veins. Limited and contradictory data associate termination of atrial fibrillation during ablation and the inability to induce atrial fibrillation further with improved long-term success.[75–77]

Outcomes and Limitations

Curative catheter ablation for atrial fibrillation has evolved to produce a high overall success rate and low incidence of complications. Studies examining

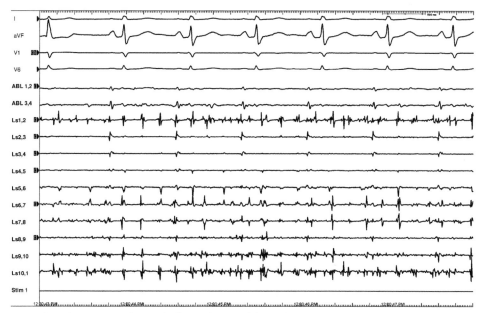

Fig. 5. Intracardiac electrogram obtained after isolation of the right superior pulmonary vein showing fibrillation within the vein recorded by the ring catheter (LS 1–10), whereas the atria remain in sinus rhythm as recorded on the surface leads (I, aVF, V1, and V6).

the cost-effectiveness of atrial fibrillation ablation suggest that cost-equivalency of curative atrial fibrillation ablation to medical management is reached after approximately 5 years.[78]

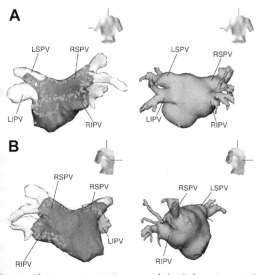

Fig. 6. Electroanatomic images of the left atrium with (A) and without (B) PVAI lesions as seen from PA and RAO perspectives. The antrum included the entire posterior wall and extended anterior to the right PVs along the left septum. Entrance block is the end point of the procedure. Further ablation of the superior vena cava (SVC) along the ostium is also performed if mapping shows PV-like potentials around this region and when high output pacing does not capture the phrenic nerve.

Success rates are highest when treating patients who have paroxysmal atrial fibrillation. In this population, a success rate of 80% to 85% is reasonable.[45,65,79] When recurrences occur, they often are related to focal areas of recovery, leading to conduction gaps across previous ablation lines.[80–83] A second procedure to reisolate the pulmonary veins often provides cure in these patients. Success rates in patients who have permanent atrial fibrillation generally are reported closer to 50% to 60% with a single procedure.[71,75,84,85] Repeat ablation for those experiencing recurrence improves overall success rates to 75% to 90%.[71,85]

As with most technical procedures, experience is an important factor in attaining optimal outcomes, and centers with higher volumes have higher rates of cure.[86] Assessment of recurrences varies in the literature, with some investigators relying solely on symptoms, and others routinely performing ambulatory rhythm monitoring to capture asymptomatic recurrences.

Some data suggest that asymptomatic recurrences after atrial fibrillation ablation are uncommon, occurring only in approximately 2% of the population.[87] Others report higher rates of asymptomatic recurrences. In general, studies with higher reported rates included patients who were continued long term on antiarrhythmic drugs, which may mask symptoms of recurrences. The authors' practice is to discontinue all antiarrhythmic drugs 4 weeks after ablation and not to use

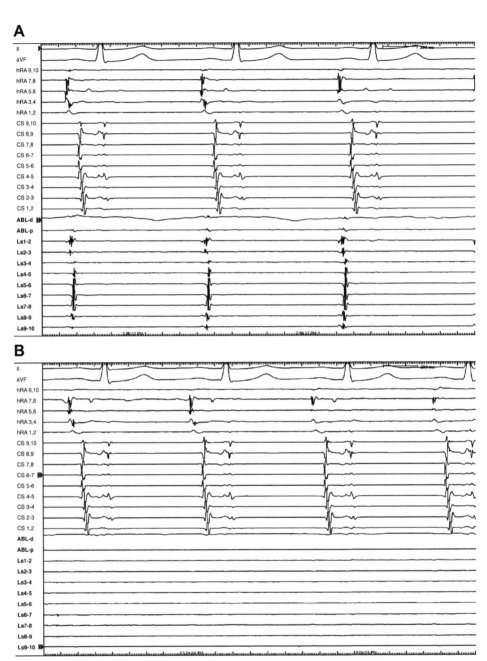

Fig. 7. Intracardiac electrograms showing potentials at the junction of the right atrium and SVC preisolation (A) and absence of potentials on the mapping catheter channels (LS 1–10) post isolation (B).

amiodarone after the procedure. Although success, defined as freedom from atrial fibrillation, may not occur in all patients, those who experience atrial fibrillation recurrence still may benefit from an improvement in symptoms through a reduction in the frequency of episodes or from an improved response to previously ineffective antiarrhythmic medications.

Perhaps the greatest challenge associated with PVAI is the technical difficulty of creating circumferential isolation using multiple discrete ablation points. Electroanatomic mapping systems may help overcome this challenge to some extent, but operator skill and experience are essential for success.

Other challenges associated with PVAI could arise from the transseptal puncture or problems with patient cooperation. Placement of transseptal punctures posteriorly on the interatrial septum is critical to optimizing the reach of the catheters to the veins on the posterior wall of the left atrium. Occasionally, the septum may be thickened or fibrous, making it extremely resistant to puncture. ICE is invaluable to visualizing the septum and left atrial structures, thus improving optimal placement of the transseptal punctures.

Ability of patients to cooperate also may pose important challenges during atrial fibrillation ablation. Deep respirations can diminish catheter stability severely, often drawing catheters from an ostial location into the pulmonary veins. Careful titration of sedation to optimize patient comfort while permitting cooperation, especially during critical stages of the procedure, can minimize this difficulty.

In addition to these challenges, radiation exposure is an important consideration for patients and operators during atrial fibrillation ablation. Duration of fluoroscopy can vary widely depending on patient characteristics, technique used, and operator experience. Fluoroscopy times of 60 to 70 minutes are not uncommon. Electroanatomic mapping systems reduce fluoroscopic times.[88–92] Common practices should be used to reduce radiation dose, including decreasing frame rates, reducing magnification, and reducing the field with shutters. The development of atrial arrhythmias, such as atrial flutter, also may also be a challenge to performing a successful PVI. Depending on the ablation approach, 3% to 30% of patients are reported to develop small-loop atrial reentry, which can be difficult to map.[93,94]

The overall rate of major complications associated with ostial PVI is reported at 4% to 6%.[85,86,95] Perforation leading to tamponade may occur in approximately 1% of cases.[86] This complication often is amenable to treatment with a percutaneous pericardial drain, but may rarely require thoracotomy and pericardial window. Posterior perforation and formation of a left atrial-esophageal fistula are reported. Power titration using detection of microbubbles on ICE is reported to prevent this complication. In addition, use of a radio-opaque esophageal temperature probe allows visualization of the esophageal course and monitoring of esophageal temperatures during ablation.

Radiofrequency current delivery should be terminated when the esophageal temperature increases, and not resumed in that location until temperatures return to baseline. No cases of left atrial-esophageal fistula formation have been reported when this technique is used. Other experts use ingested barium paste to localize the esophagus and help avoid this complication.

Phrenic nerve injury leading to diaphragmatic paralysis or gastric emptying syndrome is reported at a rate of 0.1% to 0.48%. This complication commonly is associated with ablation in the regions of the right superior pulmonary vein, left atrial appendage, and SVC. Recovery is seen in approximately 66% of cases.[86,96,97] Fluoroscopic visualization of the diaphragm while ablating in these areas may show diaphragmatic stimulation during radiofrequency ablation and allow energy delivery to be terminated before permanent injury to the phrenic nerve occurs. Before radiofrequency current is delivered over the lateral aspects of the SVC–right atrial junction, pacing at high output may reveal phrenic nerve stimulation, evidenced by diaphragmatic stimulation, indicating that ablation in that region is unsafe.

Cerebrovascular accidents and transient ischemic attacks are feared complications of any left-sided ablation procedure, including PVAI. Rates are reported at approximately 0.5% to 2.5%.[86,98,99] Targeting an activated clotting time of 350 to 400 seconds compared with lower activated clotting time targets significantly reduces the risk for thromboembolic events during PVAI, with a reported event rate of less than 0.5%.[52]

Severe symptomatic pulmonary vein stenosis may complicate PVI but has become rare, because the technique has moved from ablating distally within the pulmonary veins to a more proximal approach of isolating the pulmonary vein antra. Mild to moderate pulmonary stenosis does not limit flow significantly and is not associated with symptoms. Severe stenosis is reported in 15% to 20% of patients undergoing ablation within the pulmonary veins.[100] Isolation at the pulmonary vein ostium rather than focal ablation within the pulmonary veins is associated with pulmonary vein stenosis rates of 1% to 2%.[54,86,100–102] Using ICE to visualize the pulmonary veins and isolating even more proximally in the pulmonary vein antra further reduces the risk for pulmonary vein stenosis (**Fig. 8**).[20,100] Even when severe, pulmonary

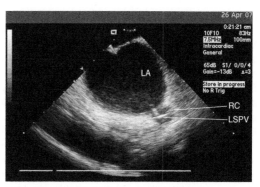

Fig. 8. ICE showing left atrium (LA) and the ring catheter (RC) at the ostium of the left superior pulmonary vein (LSPV).

vein stenosis may be asymptomatic. However, early and repeated angioplasty and stenting have been shown to be an effective treatment option and only a fraction of patients continue to have chronic symptoms.[54,86,103]

Follow-Up

Postablation follow-up should assess the efficacy of the procedure, screen for complications, and address postablation medical therapy for atrial fibrillation. Patients are discharged with a transtelephonic monitor and instructions to transmit rhythm strips whenever they feel symptoms consistent with a recurrence. Additionally, routine transmissions scheduled several times weekly screen for recurrence. Recurrences of atrial fibrillation and episodes of atrial tachycardia or atypical atrial flutter are common within the first few weeks after PVAI. These early recurrences often are related to inflammation from the ablation and resolve completely as inflammation subsides. As a result, recurrences within the first 6 to 8 weeks are not considered an indication that the procedure failed. For this same reason, antiarrhythmic medications typically are restarted immediately after PVAI and discontinued after 8 weeks. To further screen for asymptomatic recurrences, 24-hour holter monitoring is performed at 3 months' follow-up and every 3 months thereafter. Outpatient follow-up is routinely scheduled at 3 months after PVAI to evaluate for symptomatic recurrence and have a CT scan performed to assess for pulmonary vein stenosis/occlusion.[54] If even mild stenosis is detected, the CT scan is repeated at the next follow-up visit. Warfarin is continued perioperatively and at least until the 3- to 6-month follow-up visit. Discontinuation of warfarin after PVAI is under investigation. The decision to terminate anticoagulation after PVAI must be made on an individual basis after risk for recurrence is carefully assessed and discussed with the patient.

Future Advances

Much of the effort in advancing curative atrial fibrillation ablation is directed toward meeting the technical demands of isolating the pulmonary veins. Balloon catheters, alternative ablative energy sources, and remote catheter manipulation all strive to diminish these technical demands. Balloon catheters theoretically could assist operators in stabilizing a catheter in a pulmonary vein and allow circumferential delivery of ablative energy. These catheters, however, must be able to accommodate the widely variable anatomy found in the pulmonary veins. Additionally, they must ensure ablation energy is not delivered too

distally in to the pulmonary veins. High-intensity ultrasound, cryotherapy, and diode laser are potential alternatives to radiofrequency ablation, and could be combined with balloon catheter technology to create circumferential lesions with a few applications, further reducing the technical challenge of circumferential isolation and potentially reducing the time required for ablation. To be viable alternatives, these sources must be able to reliably produce lesions at a consistent depth and have a safety profile at least equal to that of radiofrequency energy.[104]

Large magnets may be used to steer a soft-tipped catheter, allowing remote guidance of lesion delivery. Robotic catheter navigation systems also allow remote manipulation of catheters. Both strategies have the potential to dramatically reduce operators' radiation exposure and improve catheter stability and fine manipulation. When combined with electroanatomic mapping, these systems conceivably could automate much of the ablation procedure. To gain widespread use, however, these systems must meet demands of time-saving, ease of use, and cost-effectiveness.[105–107]

In addition, investigators have been focusing recently on two additional parameters that could be monitored when performing mapping and ablations in the cardiac chambers. New sensors have been introduced in catheter and long sheath that measure the force (in grams) applied by the catheter to the tissue and the phase angle the catheter forms on the cardiac surface when delivering energy. When better developed, this information will help improve the effectiveness of the lesions, and hence the success rate and safety of catheter ablation.[108,109] The field of catheter ablation for atrial fibrillation has grown and evolved rapidly over recent years and is expected to continue.

REFERENCES

1. Lloyd-Jones DM, Wang TJ, Leip EP, et al. Lifetime risk for development of atrial fibrillation: the Framingham heart study. Circulation 2004;110(9) 1042–6.
2. Risk factors for stroke and efficacy of antithrombotic therapy in atrial fibrillation. Analysis of pooled data from five randomized controlled trials. Arch Intern Med 1994;154(13):1449–57.
3. Wolf PA, Abbott RD, Kannel WB. Atrial fibrillation as an independent risk factor for stroke: the Framingham Study. Stroke 1991;22(8):983–8.
4. Benjamin EJ, Wolf PA, D'Agostino RB, et al. Impact of atrial fibrillation on the risk of death: the Framingham heart study. Circulation 1998;98(10):946–52.

5. Kannel WB, Wolf PA, Benjamin EJ, et al. Prevalence, incidence, prognosis, and predisposing conditions for atrial fibrillation: population-based estimates. Am J Cardiol 1998;82(8A):2N–9N.

6. Chung MK. Atrial fibrillation: rate control is as good as rhythm control for some, but not all. Cleve Clin J Med 2003;70(6):567–73.

7. Van Gelder IC, Hagens VE, Bosker HA, et al. A comparison of rate control and rhythm control in patients with recurrent persistent atrial fibrillation. N Engl J Med 2002;347(23):1834–40.

8. Wyse DG, Waldo AL, DiMarco JP, et al. A comparison of rate control and rhythm control in patients with atrial fibrillation. N Engl J Med 2002;347(23):1825–33.

9. Corley SD, Epstein AE, DiMarco JP, et al. Relationships between sinus rhythm, treatment, and survival in the atrial fibrillation follow-up investigation of rhythm management (AFFIRM) study. Circulation 2004;109(12):1509–13.

10. Wazni OM, Marrouche NF, Martin DO, et al. Radiofrequency ablation vs antiarrhythmic drugs as first-line treatment of symptomatic atrial fibrillation: a randomized trial. J Am Med Assoc 2005; 293(21):2634–40.

11. Pappone C, Rosanio S, Augello G, et al. Mortality, morbidity, and quality of life after circumferential pulmonary vein ablation for atrial fibrillation: outcomes from a controlled nonrandomized long-term study. J Am Coll Cardiol 2003;42(2):185–97.

12. Vedel J, Frank R, Fontaine G, et al. [Permanent intra-hisian atrioventricular block induced during right intraventricular exploration]. Arch Mal Coeur Vaiss 1979;72(1):107–12 [in French].

13. Gallagher JJ, Svenson RH, Kasell JH, et al. Catheter technique for closed-chest ablation of the atrioventricular conduction system. N Engl J Med 1982; 306(4):194–200.

14. Scheinman MM, Morady F, Hess DS, et al. Catheter-induced ablation of the atrioventricular junction to control refractory supraventricular arrhythmias. J Am Med Assoc 1982;248(7):851–5.

15. Evans GT, Scheinman MM, Scheinman MM, et al. The percutaneous cardiac mapping and ablation registry: final summary of results. Pacing Clin Electrophysiol 1988;11(11 Pt 1):1621–6.

16. Chen SA, Tsang WP, Hsia CP, et al. Catheter ablation of free wall accessory atrioventricular pathways in 89 patients with Wolff-Parkinson-White syndrome—comparison of direct current and radiofrequency ablation. Eur Heart J 1992;13(10): 1329–38.

17. Morady F, Calkins H, Langberg JJ, et al. A prospective randomized comparison of direct current and radiofrequency ablation of the atrioventricular junction. J Am Coll Cardiol 1993;21(1):102–9.

18. Olgin JE, Scheinman MM. Comparison of high energy direct current and radiofrequency catheter ablation of the atrioventricular junction. J Am Coll Cardiol 1993;21(3):557–64.

19. Haines DE. The biophysics of radiofrequency catheter ablation in the heart: the importance of temperature monitoring. Pacing Clin Electrophysiol. 1993; 16(3 Pt 2):586–91.

20. Marrouche NF, Martin DO, Wazni O, et al. Phased-array intracardiac echocardiography monitoring during pulmonary vein isolation in patients with atrial fibrillation: impact on outcome and complications. Circulation 2003;107(21):2710–6.

21. Kalbfleisch SJ, Williamson B, Man KC, et al. A randomized comparison of the right- and left-sided approaches to ablation of the atrioventricular junction. Am J Cardiol 1993;72(18): 1406–10.

22. Dubuc M, Khairy P, Rodriguez-Santiago A, et al. Catheter cryoablation of the atrioventricular node in patients with atrial fibrillation: a novel technology for ablation of cardiac arrhythmias. J Cardiovasc Electrophysiol 2001;12(4):439–44.

23. Weerasooriya R, Davis M, Powell A, et al. The Australian intervention randomized control of rate in atrial fibrillation trial (AIRCRAFT). J Am Coll Cardiol. 2003;41(10):1697–702.

24. Verma A, Newman D, Geist M, et al. Effects of rhythm regularization and rate control in improving left ventricular function in atrial fibrillation patients undergoing atrioventricular nodal ablation. Can J Cardiol 2001;17(4):437–45.

25. Wood MA, Kay GN, Ellenbogen KA. The North American experience with the ablate and pace trial (APT) for medically refractory atrial fibrillation. Europace 1999;1(1):22–5.

26. Brignole M, Menozzi C, Gianfranchi L, et al. Assessment of atrioventricular junction ablation and VVIR pacemaker versus pharmacological treatment in patients with heart failure and chronic atrial fibrillation: a randomized, controlled study. Circulation 1998;98(10):953–60.

27. Fitzpatrick AP, Kourouyan HD, Siu A, et al. Quality of life and outcomes after radiofrequency His-bundle catheter ablation and permanent pacemaker implantation: impact of treatment in paroxysmal and established atrial fibrillation. Am Heart J 1996;131(3):499–507.

28. Natale A, Zimerman L, Tomassoni G, et al. Impact on ventricular function and quality of life of transcatheter ablation of the atrioventricular junction in chronic atrial fibrillation with a normal ventricular response. Am J Cardiol 1996;78(12):1431–3.

29. Wood MA, Brown-Mahoney C, Kay GN, et al. Clinical outcomes after ablation and pacing therapy for atrial fibrillation: a meta-analysis. Circulation 2000; 101(10):1138–44.

30. Natale A, Zimerman L, Tomassoni G, et al. AV node ablation and pacemaker implantation after

withdrawal of effective rate-control medications for chronic atrial fibrillation: effect on quality of life and exercise performance. Pacing Clin Electrophysiol 1999;22(11):1634–9.

31. Geelen P, Brugada J, Andries E, et al. Ventricular fibrillation and sudden death after radiofrequency catheter ablation of the atrioventricular junction. Pacing Clin Electrophysiol 1997;20(2 Pt 1):343–8.

32. Wilkoff BL, Cook JR, Epstein AE, et al. Dual-chamber pacing or ventricular backup pacing in patients with an implantable defibrillator: the dual chamber and VVI implantable defibrillator (DAVID) trial. J Am Med Assoc 2002;288(24):3115–23.

33. Doshi RN, Daoud EG, Fellows C, et al. Left ventricular-based cardiac stimulation post AV nodal ablation evaluation (the PAVE study). J Cardiovasc Electrophysiol 2005;16(11):1160–5.

34. Khan M, Jais P, Cummings J, Di Biase L, et al. Results of randomized controlled trial of pulmonary vein antrum isolation vs. AV node ablation with Biventricular pacing for treatment of atrial fibrillation in patients with congestive heart failure (PABA CHF). N Engl J Med, in press.

35. Cox JL, Canavan TE, Schuessler RB, et al. The surgical treatment of atrial fibrillation. II. Intraoperative electrophysiologic mapping and description of the electrophysiologic basis of atrial flutter and atrial fibrillation. J Thorac Cardiovasc Surg 1991;101(3):406–26.

36. Padanilam BJ, Prystowsky EN. Should atrial fibrillation ablation be considered first-line therapy for some patients? Should ablation be first-line therapy and for whom? The antagonist position. Circulation 2005;112(8):1223–9 [discussion: 1230].

37. Packer DL, Asirvatham S, Munger TM. Progress in non-pharmacologic therapy of atrial fibrillation. J Cardiovasc Electrophysiol 2003;14(Suppl 12):S296–309.

38. Haissaguerre M, Jais P, Shah DC, et al. Spontaneous initiation of atrial fibrillation by ectopic beats originating in the pulmonary veins. N Engl J Med 1998;339(10):659–66.

39. Chen SA, Hsieh MH, Tai CT, et al. Initiation of atrial fibrillation by ectopic beats originating from the pulmonary veins: electrophysiological characteristics, pharmacological responses, and effects of radiofrequency ablation. Circulation 1999;100(18):1879–86.

40. Verma A, Wazni OM, Marrouche NF, et al. Pre-existent left atrial scarring in patients undergoing pulmonary vein antrum isolation: an independent predictor of procedural failure. J Am Coll Cardiol 2005;45(2):285–92.

41. Natale A, Pisano E, Beheiry S, et al. Ablation of right and left atrial premature beats following cardioversion in patients with chronic atrial fibrillation refractory to antiarrhythmic drugs. Am J Cardiol 2000;85(11):1372–5.

42. Nademanee K, McKenzie J, Kosar E, et al. A new approach for catheter ablation of atrial fibrillation: mapping of the electrophysiologic substrate J Am Coll Cardiol 2004;43:2044–53.

43. Kanagaratnam L, Tomassoni G, Schweikert R, et al Empirical pulmonary vein isolation in patients with chronic atrial fibrillation using a three-dimensiona nonfluoroscopic mapping system: long-term follow-up. Pacing Clin Electrophysiol 2001;24(12): 1774–9.

44. Hocini M, Sanders P, Jais P, et al. Prevalence of pulmonary vein disconnection after anatomical ablation for atrial fibrillation: consequences of wide atrial encircling of the pulmonary veins. Eur Heart J 2005;26(7):696–704.

45. Mantovan R, Verlato R, Calzolari V, et al. Comparison between anatomical and integrated approaches to atrial fibrillation ablation: adjunctive role of electrical pulmonary vein disconnection J Cardiovasc Electrophysiol 2005;16(12):1293–7.

46. Fuster V, Reyen LE, Cannom DS, et al. ACC/AHA, ESC 2006 Practice guidelines for the management of patients with atrial fibrillation. J Am Coll Cardio 2006;48(4):e149–246.

47. Lakkireddy D, Rangisetty U, Prasad S, et al. Intracardiac echo guided radiofrequency catheter ablation of atrial fibrillation in patients with atrial septal defec (ASD) or patent foramen ovale (PFO) repair: a feasibility, safety and Efficacy study. J Cardiovasc Electrophysiol, 2008 Jul 25. [Epub ahead of print].

48. Kannel WB, Abbott RD, Savage DD, et al. Epidemiologic features of chronic atrial fibrillation: the Framingham study. N Engl J Med 1982;306(17): 1018–22.

49. Oral H, Knight BP, Tada H, et al. Pulmonary vein isolation for paroxysmal and persistent atrial fibrillation. Circulation 2002;105(9):1077–81.

50. Wazni OM, Beheiry S, Fahmy T, et al. Atrial fibrillation ablation in patients with therapeutic international normalized ratio: comparison of strategies of anticoagulation management in the periprocedural period. Circulation 2007;116:2531–4.

51. Ashar MS, Pennington J, Callans DJ, et al. Localization of arrhythmogenic triggers of atrial fibrillation. J Cardiovasc Electrophysiol 2000;11(12) 1300–5.

52. Wazni OM, Rossillo A, Marrouche NF, et al. Embolic events and char formation during pulmonary vein isolation in patients with atrial fibrillation: impact of different anticoagulation regimens and importance of intracardiac echo imaging. J Cardiovasc Electrophysiol 2005;16(6):576–81.

53. Robbins IM, Colvin EV, Doyle TP, et al. Pulmonary vein stenosis after catheter ablation of atrial fibrillation. Circulation 1998;98(17):1769–75.

54. Di Biase L, Fahmy TS, Wazni OM, et al. Pulmonary vein total occlusion following catheter ablation for atrial fibrillation: clinical implications after long term follow-up. J Am Coll Cardiol 2006;48:2493–9

55. Nilsson B, Chen X, Pehrson S, et al. Recurrence of pulmonary vein conduction and atrial fibrillation after pulmonary vein isolation for atrial fibrillation: a randomized trial of the ostial versus the extraostial ablation strategy. Am Heart J 2006; 152(3):e531–8.

56. Oral H, Scharf C, Chugh A, et al. Catheter ablation for paroxysmal atrial fibrillation: segmental pulmonary vein ostial ablation versus left atrial ablation. Circulation 2003;108(19):2355–60.

57. Hocini M, Haissaguerre M, Shah D, et al. Multiple sources initiating atrial fibrillation from a single pulmonary vein identified by a circumferential catheter. Pacing Clin Electrophysiol 2000;23(11 Pt 2):1828–31.

58. Haissaguerre M, Shah DC, Jais P, et al. Electrophysiological breakthroughs from the left atrium to the pulmonary veins. Circulation 2000;102(20):2463–5.

59. Oral H, Chugh A, Good E, et al. A tailored approach to catheter ablation of paroxysmal atrial fibrillation. Circulation 2006;113(15):1824–31.

60. Katritsis DG, Ellenbogen KA, Panagiotakos DB, et al. Ablation of superior pulmonary veins compared to ablation of all four pulmonary veins. J Cardiovasc Electrophysiol 2004;15(6):641–5.

61. Gerstenfeld EP, Callans DJ, Dixit S, et al. Incidence and location of focal atrial fibrillation triggers in patients undergoing repeat pulmonary vein isolation: implications for ablation strategies. J Cardiovasc Electrophysiol 2003;14(7):685–90.

62. Kanj M, Wazni O, Natale A. Pulmonary vein antrum isolation. Heart Rhythm 2007;4(Suppl 3):S73–9.

63. Kanj MH, Wazni OM, Natale A. How to do circular mapping catheter-guided pulmonary vein antrum isolation: the Cleveland clinic approach. Heart Rhythm 2006;3(7):866–9.

64. Lin WS, Tai CT, Hsieh MH, et al. Catheter ablation of paroxysmal atrial fibrillation initiated by non-pulmonary vein ectopy. Circulation 2003;107(25):3176–83.

65. Hocini M, Jais P, Sanders P, et al. Techniques, evaluation, and consequences of linear block at the left atrial roof in paroxysmal atrial fibrillation: a prospective randomized study. Circulation 2005;112(24):3688–96.

66. Pappone C, Manguso F, Vicedomini G, et al. Prevention of iatrogenic atrial tachycardia after ablation of atrial fibrillation: a prospective randomized study comparing circumferential pulmonary vein ablation with a modified approach. Circulation 2004;110(19):3036–42.

67. Fassini G, Riva S, Chiodelli R, et al. Left mitral isthmus ablation associated with PV Isolation: long-term results of a prospective randomized study. J Cardiovasc Electrophysiol 2005;16(11):1150–6.

68. Rostock T, Rotter M, Sanders P, et al. High-density activation mapping of fractionated electrograms in the atria of patients with paroxysmal atrial fibrillation. Heart Rhythm 2006;3(1):27–34.

69. Bauer A, Deisenhofer I, Schneider R, et al. Effects of circumferential or segmental pulmonary vein ablation for paroxysmal atrial fibrillation on cardiac autonomic function. Heart Rhythm 2006;3(12): 1428–35.

70. Pappone C, Santinelli V, Manguso F, et al. Pulmonary vein denervation enhances long-term benefit after circumferential ablation for paroxysmal atrial fibrillation. Circulation 2004;109(3):327–34.

71. Calo L, Lamberti F, Loricchio ML, et al. Left atrial ablation versus biatrial ablation for persistent and permanent atrial fibrillation: a prospective and randomized study. J Am Coll Cardiol 2006;47(12): 2504–12.

72. Goya M, Ouyang F, Ernst S, et al. Electroanatomic mapping and catheter ablation of breakthroughs from the right atrium to the superior vena cava in patients with atrial fibrillation. Circulation 2002; 106(11):1317–20.

73. Tsai CF, Tai CT, Hsieh MH, et al. Initiation of atrial fibrillation by ectopic beats originating from the superior vena cava: electrophysiological characteristics and results of radiofrequency ablation. Circulation 2000;102(1):67–74.

74. Kanj M, Muelet J, Phillips K, Barrett C, et al. Empiric coronary sinus ablation during pulmonary venous isolation does not improve the success of AF ablation. Heart Rhythm 2007;4(Suppl):5–22.

75. Richter B, Gwechenberger M, Filzmoser P, et al. Is inducibility of atrial fibrillation after radio frequency ablation really a relevant prognostic factor? Eur Heart J 2006;27(21):2553–9.

76. Oral H, Chugh A, Lemola K, et al. Noninducibility of atrial fibrillation as an end point of left atrial circumferential ablation for paroxysmal atrial fibrillation: a randomized study. Circulation 2004;110(18):2797–801.

77. Haissaguerre M, Sanders P, Hocini M, et al. Changes in atrial fibrillation cycle length and inducibility during catheter ablation and their relation to outcome. Circulation 2004;109(24):3007–13.

78. Khaykin Y. Cost-effectiveness of catheter ablation for atrial fibrillation. Curr Opin Cardiol 2007;22(1):11–7.

79. Liu X, Long D, Dong J, et al. Is circumferential pulmonary vein isolation preferable to stepwise segmental pulmonary vein isolation for patients with paroxysmal atrial fibrillation? Circ J 2006;70(11):1392–7.

80. Mesas CE, Augello G, Lang CC, et al. Electroanatomic remodeling of the left atrium in patients undergoing repeat pulmonary vein ablation: mechanistic insights and implications for ablation. J Cardiovasc Electrophysiol 2006;17(12):1279–85.

81. Rostock T, O'Neill MD, Sanders P, et al. Characterization of conduction recovery across left atrial linear lesions in patients with paroxysmal and persistent atrial fibrillation. J Cardiovasc Electrophysiol 2006;17(10):1106–11.

82. Ouyang F, Antz M, Ernst S, et al. Recovered pulmonary vein conduction as a dominant factor for recurrent atrial tachyarrhythmias after complete

circular isolation of the pulmonary veins: lessons from double Lasso technique. Circulation 2005; 111(2):127–35.

83. Cappato R, Negroni S, Pecora D, et al. Prospective assessment of late conduction recurrence across radiofrequency lesions producing electrical disconnection at the pulmonary vein ostium in patients with atrial fibrillation. Circulation 2003;108(13):1599–604.

84. Oral H, Pappone C, Chugh A, et al. Circumferential pulmonary-vein ablation for chronic atrial fibrillation. N Engl J Med 2006;354(9):934–41.

85. Cheema A, Dong J, Dalal D, et al. Long-term safety and efficacy of circumferential ablation with pulmonary vein isolation. J Cardiovasc Electrophysiol 2006;17(10):1080–5.

86. Cappato R, Calkins H, Chen SA, et al. Worldwide survey on the methods, efficacy, and safety of catheter ablation for human atrial fibrillation. Circulation 2005;111(9):1100–5.

87. Oral H, Veerareddy S, Good E, et al. Prevalence of asymptomatic recurrences of atrial fibrillation after successful radiofrequency catheter ablation. J Cardiovasc Electrophysiol 2004;15(8):920–4.

88. Estner HL, Deisenhofer I, Luik A, et al. Electrical isolation of pulmonary veins in patients with atrial fibrillation: reduction of fluoroscopy exposure and procedure duration by the use of a non-fluoroscopic navigation system (NavX). Europace 2006;8(8):583–7.

89. Tondo C, Mantica M, Russo G, et al. A new nonfluoroscopic navigation system to guide pulmonary vein isolation. Pacing Clin Electrophysiol 2005;28(Supp 1):S102–5.

90. Karch MR, Zrenner B, Deisenhofer I, et al. Freedom from atrial tachyarrhythmias after catheter ablation of atrial fibrillation: a randomized comparison between 2 current ablation strategies. Circulation 2005;111(22):2875–80.

91. Wood MA, Christman PJ, Shepard RK, et al. Use of a non-fluoroscopic catheter navigation system for pulmonary vein isolation. J Interv Card Electrophysiol 2004;10(2):165–70.

92. Macle L, Jais P, Scavee C, et al. Pulmonary vein disconnection using the LocaLisa three-dimensional nonfluoroscopic catheter imaging system. J Cardiovasc Electrophysiol 2003;14(7):693–7.

93. Cummings JE, Schweikert R, Saliba W, et al. Left atrial flutter following pulmonary vein antrum isolation with radiofrequency energy: linear lesions or repeat isolation. J Cardiovasc Electrophysiol 2005;16(3):293–7.

94. Deisenhofer I, Estner H, Zrenner B, et al. Left atrial tachycardia after circumferential pulmonary vein ablation for atrial fibrillation: incidence, electrophysiological characteristics, and results of radiofrequency ablation. Europace 2006;8(8):573–82.

95. Stabile G, Bertaglia E, Senatore G, et al. Feasibility of pulmonary vein ostia radiofrequency ablation in patients with atrial fibrillation: a multicenter study (CACAF pilot study). Pacing Clin Electrophysiol 2003;26(1 Pt 2):284–7.

96. Sacher F, Monahan KH, Thomas SP, et al. Phrenic nerve injury after atrial fibrillation catheter ablation characterization and outcome in a multicenter study. J Am Coll Cardiol 2006;47(12):2498–503.

97. Bai R, Patel MD, Di Biase L, et al. Phrenic nerve injury after catheter ablation: should we worry about this complication? J Cardiovasc Electrophysiol 2006;17:944–8.

98. Mansour M, Ruskin J, Keane D. Efficacy and safety of segmental ostial versus circumferential extra-ostial pulmonary vein isolation for atrial fibrillation. J Cardiovasc Electrophysiol 2004;15(5):532–7.

99. Zhou L, Keane D, Reed G, et al. Thromboembolic complications of cardiac radiofrequency catheter ablation: a review of the reported incidence, pathogenesis and current research directions. J Cardiovasc Electrophysiol 1999;10(4):611–20.

100. Saad EB, Rossillo A, Saad CP, et al. Pulmonary vein stenosis after radiofrequency ablation of atrial fibrillation: functional characterization, evolution, and influence of the ablation strategy. Circulation 2003;108(25):3102–7.

101. Purerfellner H, Cihal R, Aichinger J, et al. Pulmonary vein stenosis by ostial irrigated-tip ablation: incidence, time course, and prediction. J Cardiovasc Electrophysiol 2003;14(2):158–64.

102. Kato R, Lickfett L, Meininger G, et al. Pulmonary vein anatomy in patients undergoing catheter ablation of atrial fibrillation: lessons learned by use of magnetic resonance imaging. Circulation 2003;107(15):2004–10.

103. Saad EB, Marrouche NF, Saad CP, et al. Pulmonary vein stenosis after catheter ablation of atrial fibrillation: emergence of a new clinical syndrome. Ann Intern Med 2003;138(8):634–8.

104. Barrett C, Natale A. Towards balloon based technologies—all that glitters is not gold. J Cardiovasc Electrophysiol 2008 Jun 12 [Epub ahead of print].

105. Di Biase L, Fahmy TS, Patel D, et al. Remote magnetic navigation: human experience in pulmonary vein ablation. J Am Coll Cardiol 2007;50:868–74.

106. Pappone C, Vicedomini G, Manguso F, et al. Robotic magnetic navigation for atrial fibrillation ablation. J Am Coll Cardiol 2006;47(7):1390–400.

107. Saliba WI, Reddy VK, Oussama W, et al. Atrial fibrillation ablation using a robotic catheter remote control system: initial human experience and long-term follow-up results. J Am Coll Cardiol 2008;51:2407–11.

108. Di Biase L, Arruda M, Armaganijan L, et al. Real Time Monitoring of Tip Electrode-Tissue Orientation and Contact Force: Optimizing Accuracy and Safety of Mapping and Ablation Procedures. J Am Coll Cardiol 2008;51(10 Suppl. 1):811–3 [A 26, abstract oral presentation].

109. Di Biase L, Cummings JE, Barrett C, et al. Relationship between Catheter force, popping and char formation: experience with robotic navigation. J Am Coll Cardiol 2008;51(10 Suppl. 1):1036–302 [A 376, ABSTRACTS - Best Poster Award Competition]

Surgical Approaches for Atrial Fibrillation

Adam E. Saltman, MD, PhD[a],*, A. Marc Gillinov, MD[b]

KEYWORDS

- Atrial fibrillation • Ablation • Left atrial appendage
- Mitral valve disease • Maze procedure

Although it long has been recognized that atrial fibrillation (AF) is common in patients presenting for mitral valve surgery and other forms of cardiac surgery, ablation of AF in such patients has recently become more popular. This change in surgical practice is attributable to new data clarifying the pathogenesis and dangers of untreated AF along with the development of new ablation technologies that facilitate ablation. For cardiac surgery patients presenting with AF, surgeons now offer a more complete operation that corrects the structural heart disease and the AF simultaneously. In addition, surgeons are rapidly developing easier and more sophisticated, minimally invasive, epicardial, beating-heart approaches for stand-alone AF ablation. The purposes of this review are to (1) review the rationale for surgical ablation of AF in cardiac surgery patients, (2) describe the classic maze procedure and its results, (3) detail new approaches to surgical ablation of AF, (4) emphasize the importance of management of the left atrial (LA) appendage, and (5) consider challenges and future directions in the ablation of AF in cardiac surgery patients.

RATIONALE FOR SURGICAL ABLATION
Atrial Fibrillation Prevalence

Because AF is particularly common in patients who have mitral valve dysfunction, most studies examining concomitant ablation—and surgical ablation in general—focus on this group. AF is present in up to 50% of patients undergoing mitral valve surgery and in 1% to 6% of patients presenting for coronary artery bypass grafting or aortic valve surgery.[1–4] As in the general population, the prevalence of AF in patients who have mitral valve disease increases with increasing patient age. In patients who have mitral valve dysfunction, AF is a marker of advanced cardiovascular disease and often is associated with the onset or exacerbation of heart failure.[5] Compared with patients who have mitral valve dysfunction who do not have AF, those who have AF have higher New York Heart Association functional class, more severe left ventricular dysfunction, and greater left atrial size.[4,6–9]

Risks of Atrial Fibrillation

AF is associated with increased mortality and morbidity in patients who have mitral valve dysfunction and coronary artery bypass graft. In patients who have degenerative mitral valve disease, AF is an independent risk factor for cardiac mortality and morbidity.[1–4] In patients undergoing mitral valve surgery, persistence of postoperative AF is a marker and a risk factor for increased mortality;[10,11] in addition, AF is associated with morbidity that includes stroke, other thromboembolism, and anticoagulant-related hemorrhage. In some patients, AF causes symptomatic tachycardia, reduced cardiac output, and tachycardia-induced cardiomyopathy. This is deleterious particularly in patients who have structural heart disease and reduced cardiac output. For these reasons, the presence of AF should be included in planning the operative strategy for cardiac surgery patients,

A version of this article originally appeared in *Medical Clinics of North America*, volume 92, issue 1.
This work was supported by the Atrial Fibrillation Innovation Center, a Third Frontier Project Funded by the State of Ohio.
[a] Cardiothoracic Surgery Research, Maimonides Medical Center, 4802 10th Avenue, Brooklyn, NY 11219, USA
[b] Atrial Fibrillation Center, Cleveland Clinic Foundation, 9500 Euclid Avenue, Cleveland, OH, USA
* Corresponding author. Division of Cardiothoracic Surgery, Maimonides Medical Center, 4802 10th Avenue, Brooklyn, NY 11219.
E-mail address: USAadamsaltman@mac.com (A.E. Saltman).

Cardiol Clin 27 (2009) 179–188
doi:10.1016/j.ccl.2008.09.012
0733-8651/08/$ – see front matter © 2009 Elsevier Inc. All rights reserved.

noting that the risk associated with the added rhythm treatment is low.[12,13]

The onset of AF is a relative indication for mitral valve surgery in those who have known mitral valve dysfunction.[2] And once AF appears, it is uncommon for mitral valve surgery alone to restore sinus rhythm.[6–8] When AF has been present for 3 months or less, particularly if it is paroxysmal, lone mitral valve surgery may convert as many as 80% of patients,[6,7] but when the duration of preoperative AF exceeds 6 months, 70% to 80% of patients remain in AF if they do not undergo rhythm correction.[6,7] Therefore, ablation should be added to a mitral valve procedure in any patient who has had AF for more than 6 months or in whom AF is persistent or permanent. Such procedures, performed on this patient group, uniformly have enjoyed high success in restoring sinus rhythm and improving cardiac function.[14,15]

Atrial Fibrillation Mechanisms and the Implications for Surgical Ablation

The clinical presentation of AF varies widely among individuals. The current treatment guidelines account for this somewhat by classifying AF as paroxysmal, persistent, or permanent.[16] Even though the pathogenesis of all types remains incompletely understood, there is agreement that patients who have persistent and permanent AF most likely have a more complex pathophysiology. Unfortunately, among those who have coexistent mitral valve disease, permanent AF is the most common form.[17,18] It is, therefore, not surprising that there is little consensus concerning which ablation strategy to use at the time of surgery, so procedural details and techniques vary widely.

Endocardial electrophysiologic mapping has demonstrated that the pulmonary veins and posterior left atrium are critical anatomic sites in humans who have isolated AF.[19,20] Mapping studies performed during concomitant heart surgery also support the importance of the left atrium as the driving chamber in patients who have mitral valve disease.[21–26] Often, regular and repetitive rapid activation can be identified in the posterior left atrium in the regions of the pulmonary vein orifices and LA appendage;[21–25] however, some patients manifest dominant right atrial focal or re-entrant activation.[21]

These findings emphasize the need for an individualized approach to each patient. But until real-time, intraoperative mapping becomes routine,[26] a more-or-less constant, all-encompassing anatomic approach based on empiric results is reasonable. Over the past 5 to 10 years, this line of attack has become the foundation for catheter-based AF ablation; tracking down and destroying individual AF triggers has given way to the complete encirclement of the pulmonary veins and posterior left atrial wall.[27–31] A left atrial procedure that includes a box-like lesion around all four pulmonary veins and a lesion to the mitral annulus seems to eliminate AF in 70% to 90% of patients who have mitral valve regurgitation.[25,32–35] The addition of right atrial lesions in these patients likely confers some benefit with little additional risk.[36,37] Specific omission of a right atrial isthmus lesion, however, leaves some patients at risk for typical atrial flutter and others at risk for continued AF.[38] Therefore, because right-sided lesions can be created quickly and safely, AF ablation in cardiac surgery patients almost always should include a biatrial lesion set.

THE MAZE PROCEDURE

The Cox maze III operation, or maze procedure, is the gold standard for surgical treatment of AF. It is the most effective curative therapy for AF yet devised for any type of AF and for patients who have or who do not have concomitant cardiac disease.[39–41] In the maze procedure, multiple left and right atrial incisions and cryolesions are placed to isolate triggers and interrupt multiple re-entrant circuits (**Fig. 1**). The maze procedure includes en bloc isolation of the pulmonary veins and posterior left atrium along with excision of the LA appendage; these maneuvers are critical to the efficacy of the procedure in the restoration

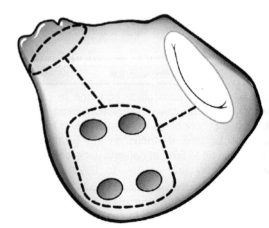

Fig. 1. Left atrial lesion set of the maze procedure. Small circles represent pulmonary vein orifices and white oval represents the mitral valve. Dashed lines represent surgical incisions. (*Reprinted from* The Cleveland Clinic Center for Medical Art & Photography © Copyright 2007. All rights reserved; with permission.)

of sinus rhythm and in the reduction of thrombo-embolic risk.

Although the maze procedure is a complex operation that adds cardiopulmonary bypass and cardiac arrest time, experienced surgeons have performed the classic operation in large numbers of patients having concomitant cardiac surgery.[1–3,6,41] The addition of a maze procedure does not increase operative mortality or morbidity;[42–44] however, it carries with it a 5% to 10% risk for implantation of a permanent pacemaker.[45] This happens most commonly in patients who have pre-existing sinus node dysfunction or in those undergoing multivalve surgery. Recent data demonstrate that the maze procedure has equivalent long-term efficacy at establishing sinus rhythm in patients undergoing lone operations and concomitant procedures; successful restoration of sinus rhythm has been achieved in 70% to 96% of patients.[42–44]

Early postoperative AF is common after a maze procedure, usually abating by 3 months.[42–44] This also is true of catheter-based procedures and should not be confused with a relapse of the presenting disease, although it may be a predictor of long-term outcomes.[46] Although the pathogenesis of failure over the long term is unclear, several risk factors have been identified: increasing left atrial diameter, longer duration of preoperative AF, and advanced patient age all increase the late prevalence of AF.[47–50] Thus, 5 years after a concomitant maze procedure, the predicted prevalence of AF is only 5% in patients who have mitral valve regurgitation who have a 4-cm left atrium; in contrast, the predicted prevalence is 15% in similar patients who have a 6-cm left atrium.[51] Others have identified similar risk factors for AF after the maze procedure, suggesting the possibility that earlier operation and left atrial size reduction in those who have left atrial enlargement (>6 cm) might improve results.[51–53]

The temporal pattern of AF (paroxysmal, persistent, or permanent) does not seem to have an impact on the results of the maze procedure.[44] Similarly, in patients who have mitral valve dysfunction, the cause does not influence results, and there is general agreement that the maze procedure is effective in patients who have rheumatic or degenerative disease.[54,55] Even in patients who have rheumatic disease, biatrial contraction usually is restored.[54]

Beyond restoring sinus rhythm, the maze procedure is associated with additional important clinical benefits in patients who have mitral valve disease. Recent data suggest that restoration of sinus rhythm improves survival in this group,[10] and the risks for stroke, other thromboembolism,

and anticoagulant-related hemorrhage likewise are reduced.[10,11,56,57] The reduced risk for late stroke after a maze procedure deserves particular emphasis. In the largest series focusing on this outcome, Cox and colleagues[57] noted a single late stroke at a mean follow-up of 5 years in 300 patients who had a classic maze procedure. This remarkable late freedom from late stroke likely is attributable to restoration of sinus rhythm in the majority of patients and to excision of the LA appendage, an integral component of the maze procedure.

These results confirm the safety of the maze procedure, its efficacy at restoring sinus rhythm, and the resulting clinical benefits, most notably the virtual elimination of late strokes. Despite these excellent results, the maze procedure has been underused, and today it is almost obsolete. Most surgeons are reluctant to add a maze procedure to the operative course of patients who are having mitral valve surgery or other cardiac surgery. With recent advances in the understanding of the pathogenesis of AF and development of new ablation technologies, however, surgeons increasingly are likely to ablate AF using simpler techniques that require only a few minutes of operative time.

NEW APPROACHES TO SURGICAL ABLATION OF ATRIAL FIBRILLATION
Lesion Sets

Like recent approaches to catheter-based ablation, newer surgical techniques for AF ablation create lines of conduction block in the left atrium.[58–60] Because the left atrium is open during mitral valve procedures, precise creation of lesions is possible. A variety of lesion sets have been used to ablate AF in patients who have mitral valve disease. Most include pulmonary vein isolation, excision or exclusion of the LA appendage, and linear left atrial connecting lesions.[58–62] The pulmonary veins may be isolated with a box-like lesion, as in the maze procedure, or with separate right- and left-sided ovals around the pulmonary veins. With the advantage of direct vision, surgeons easily can create a lesion from the left pulmonary veins to the mitral annulus; this lesion improves results, particularly in patients who have permanent AF and mitral valve disease.[63] In patients who have left atrial enlargement (>6 cm), the authors recommend left atrial reduction, as this may increase restoration of sinus rhythm.

The issue concerning the creation of biatrial lesions (more closely mimicking the Cox maze III set) versus creating left atrial lesions alone remains contentious. It is easier and faster to create a more limited lesion set; yet recent data indicate that patients undergoing right and left atrial treatment have a better long-term result at maintaining sinus rhythm.[37] Through the judicious selection of a technology or multiple technologies, it is becoming possible to create right-sided lesions without opening the right atrium or prolonging cardiopulmonary bypass time or aortic cross-clamp time. In this manner, the largest number of patients can be treated in the most efficacious and safest fashion.

Surgical Ablation for Lone Atrial Fibrillation

When considering the number of patients presenting to operating rooms with AF in combination with coronary or valvular disease, even if all undergo concomitant ablation, it is unlikely that more than 40,000 patients would be treated annually. This is a small fraction of the total number of people suffering from this disease. A much larger patient population, therefore, could benefit from stand-alone AF ablation. It is difficult, however, to justify using cardiopulmonary bypass and cardioplegic arrest, especially through a sternotomy, to open the heart for the surgical treatment of lone AF: witness the relatively poor adoption of the maze procedure over the past 20 years despite its established safety and efficacy.

To bring an effective therapy to the largest number of patients, therefore, there has been recent activity directed toward developing an epicardial approach to ablation that can be performed on a beating heart, preferably through small access incisions or ports. Such an approach should be able to overcome the disadvantages associated with the traditional Cox maze operation (significant morbidity, lengthy operative time, and extended recuperation) and the endocardial, catheter-based techniques (indirect visualization, ablation within a flowing blood pool, and inability to manage the LA appendage).

The first report of such a minimally invasive, epicardial ablation performed on a beating heart appeared in 2003.[64] Since then, three main, less invasive surgical technologies have been developed and used for the ablation of lone AF: robotics,[65] thoracoscopics (endoscopy),[66–68] and minithoracotomies.[69,70] Each has its own advantages and disadvantages but all provide physicians with access to the entire atrial epicardium of a beating heart, whereupon lesions can be placed with precision and immediate visual feedback. Pulmonary vein isolation, for example, is easily accomplished in this manner, and LA appendage management is straightforward.

It is not possible to state conclusively which approach or which ablative technology used in a minimally invasive setting provides superior results. The numbers of patients treated are small and there are technologic hurdles to be overcome (mitral annular and tricuspid isthmus lesion creation, for example). Refinements in approach and technology are progressing rapidly and new tools and methods are becoming available.

A Review of the Available Energy Sources

The classic lesion creation method is cutting and sewing tissue. Once the healing process is complete, there remains a scar composed mostly of collagen and little cellular material. It is not electrically conductive and the lesion is, by definition, transmural. The goal of any energy source, therefore, is to create a similar scar by exposing tissue to extremes of temperature, inducing thermal injury, coagulation necrosis, and healing.

To produce such an irreversible injury, the tissue must be heated to 50°C or frozen to −60°C.[71,72] The quantity of tissue injured usually is directly proportional to the duration of time for which it is held at either temperature. The various energy sources differ mainly in the method by which they transfer energy to the tissue and how deeply that energy is conducted into the tissue. Heat-based energy sources include radiofrequency, laser, microwave, and high-intensity focused ultrasound. Cold-based sources include argon and nitrous oxide gases. As of 2008, all these devices are Food and Drug Administration–labeled for the ablation of soft tissues or cardiac tissue but not for treatment of AF. The specific treatment of AF is considered, therefore, off-label use.

Despite clearly different energy forms and application methods, when applied to the left-atrial endocardium of the arrested heart there seems to be little difference in safety or efficacy among the devices.[73] For example, surveying the use of the dry, unipolar radiofrequency probe (Cobra ESTECH, San Ramon, California) in more than 1100 patients, Khargi and colleagues[73] found that it was effective at freeing patients from AF between 42% and 92% of the time. But there are several complications attributed to the use of the probe, the most worrisome being esophageal injuries, resulting in death 60% of the time.[74,75] Adverse events can occur with any technology when applied incorrectly,[76] but as more experience is gained and safer methods of ablation developed (eg, placing a cold, wet sponge between the posterior wall of the left atrium and the esophagus or shielding the probe in nonconducting sheaths), these injuries have become a rarity.

THE LEFT ATRIAL APPENDAGE

Between 60% and 90% of stroke-causing emboli in patients who have AF originate in the LA appendage,[77–79] giving it the moniker, "our most lethal human attachment."[80,81] Therefore, excision or exclusion of the LA appendage is a critical component of operations to treat AF; as discussed previously, this may explain in part the exceedingly low risk for stroke after the maze procedure. Ligation of the LA appendage in patients who have mitral valve regurgitation and who have AF reduces the late risk for thromboembolic events even if patients do not have intraoperative ablation.[73]

Surgical technique has an impact on results of LA appendage ligation, with incomplete ligation increasing the risk for thromboembolism.[82,83] Currently used techniques include exclusion by suture ligation or noncutting stapler and excision with suture closure or stapling.[83] The authors currently favor surgical excision of the appendage with standard cut-and-sew techniques as complete elimination with minimal cul-de-sac formation is most likely. Development of devices designed specifically for management of the LA appendage will facilitate this procedure. Published preclinical experience with several new LA appendage management devices is promising, and clinical trials are anticipated in the near future (**Figs. 2** and **3**).[84–87]

CHALLENGES AND FUTURE DIRECTIONS

One of the most significant obstacles facing the widespread adoption of surgical AF ablation is lack of data. Large, controlled studies describing well-defined patient populations, detailed techniques, and outcomes are missing from the literature. Electrophysiology colleagues are addressing this need and studies are underway. The advances necessary to improve AF ablation in cardiac surgery patients, therefore, must include (1) uniform definitions and methodology for reporting results, (2) improved technology to facilitate the ablation procedure and its intraoperative assessment, and (3) refinement of minimally invasive procedures.

Reporting Results

Standard terminology and methodology for reporting results has been absent from the cardiac surgery literature, and current reporting is haphazard and rightly subject to criticism.[88–90] Although there are guidelines for categorizing the clinical pattern of AF, these are applied inconsistently. Techniques for postablation rhythm assessment vary, with no generally accepted standard. Technologies for long-term and continuous rhythm monitoring are becoming available but they are costly and not yet convenient. Data obtained with such systems could be analyzed in uniform fashions to determine (1) absolute freedom from AF, (2) changes in the AF burden for individual patients, and (3) prevalence of AF in treated populations.[88–90]

Ablation Technology and Intraoperative Assessment

Current surgical ablation technology has several limitations. No single ablation device can create all of the maze lesions from the epicardial aspect.[91,92] When working from the endocardium, collateral tissue injury is possible. In addition, because real-time mapping is not yet available, the exact ablation procedure cannot yet be tailored to each patient's particular electrophysiologic

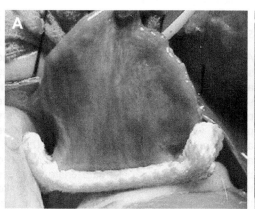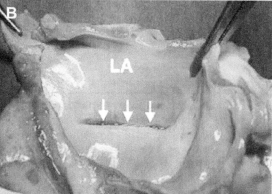

Fig. 2. LA appendage exclusion with a specially designed, cloth-covered clip. (A) Epicardial view of the clip placed on the canine LA appendage. (B) Endocardial view of the excluded appendage orifice 90 days after clip application. Arrows indicate residual LA appendage ostium.

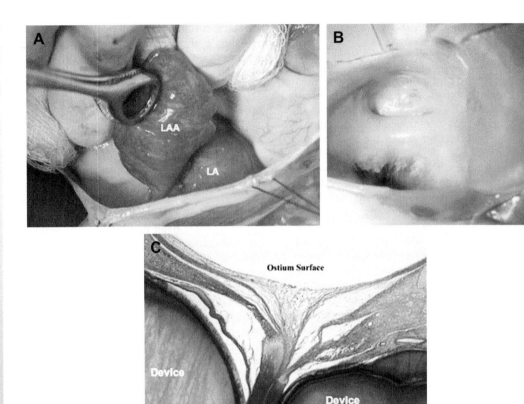

Fig. 3. LA appendage exclusion with a specially designed transmural fixation device. (*A*) Epicardial view of the clip placed on the canine LA appendage (LAA). (*B*) Endocardial view of the excluded appendage orifice 30 days after clip application. (*C*) Photomicrograph of a section taken transversely across the appendage orifice, showing complete endothelialization of the orifice without thrombus.

characteristics. Many of these problems are not unique to surgeons and their instruments but are shared by the electrophysiologists and are among the foremost challenges facing the device industry today. It is safe to say, however, that the next generation of ablation tools, capable of measuring impulse conduction and lesion effectiveness in real time, will greatly improve results and permit for the first time a tailored and more effective approach.

Minimally Invasive Approaches

Although most valve surgeries are performed via the median sternotomy, it is now possible to perform minimally invasive procedures and achieve excellent results with less morbidity and mortality.[93–96] Ablative procedures—stand alone and concomitant—also are being done through these small right thoracotomies or partial upper sternotomies with a variety of technologies.[97–107] They are technically challenging, however, as minimally invasive or keyhole approaches remain hampered by difficult access to the posterior left atrium and LA appendage. Additional refinements in exposure, manipulation, ablation technology, and lesion assessment are necessary to facilitate the widespread application of minimally invasive cardiac surgery with ablation.

SUMMARY

AF is common in patients presenting for cardiac surgery. Left untreated, AF increases morbidity and jeopardizes survival. Recent data demonstrate that AF ablation improves outcomes in these patients. Therefore, virtually all cardiac surgery patients who present with AF should receive a concomitant AF ablation procedure. The cut-and-sew maze procedure is obsolete, replaced by operations that use alternate energy sources to create lines of conduction block rapidly with little risk for bleeding. Minimally invasive cardiac surgery for AF ablation now is possible. Continued progress will facilitate tailored ablation approaches for individual patients and improve results. Development of new devices to facilitate minimally invasive exclusion of the LA appendage may offer a new alternative to patients who have AF and are at risk for stroke.

REFERENCES

1. Cox JL. Intraoperative options for treating atrial fibrillation associated with mitral valve disease. J Thorac Cardiovasc Surg 2001;122:212–5.
2. Ad N, Cox JL. Combined mitral valve surgery and the Maze III procedure. Semin Thorac Cardiovasc Surg 2002;14:206–9.
3. Grigioni F, Avierinos JF, Ling LH. Atrial fibrillation complicating the course of degenerative mitral regurgitation: determinants and long-term outcome. J Am Coll Cardiol 2002;40:84–92.
4. Quader MA, McCarthy PM, Gillinov AM, et al. Does preoperative atrial fibrillation reduce survival after coronary artery bypass grafting? Ann Thorac Surg 2004;77:1514–22.
5. Kareti KR, Chiong JR, Hsu SS, et al. Congestive heart failure and atrial fibrillation: rhythm versus rate control. J Card Fail 2005;11(3):164–72.
6. Obadia JF, el Farra M, Bastien OH. Outcome of atrial fibrillation after mitral valve repair. J Thorac Cardiovasc Surg 1997;114:179–85.
7. Chua YL, Schaff HV, Orsulak TA. Outcome of mitral valve repair in patients with preoperative atrial fibrillation. Should the maze procedure be combined with mitral valvuloplasty? J Thorac Cardiovasc Surg 1994;107:408–15.
8. Lim E, Barlow CW, Hosseinpour AR, et al. Influence of atrial fibrillation on outcome following mitral valve repair. Circulation 2001;104-I-59–I63.
9. Jessurun ER, van Hemel NM, Kelder JC. Mitral valve surgery and atrial fibrillation: is atrial fibrillation surgery also needed? Eur J Cardiothorac Surg 2000;17:530–7.
10. Bando K, Kasegawa H, Okada Y. The impact of pre- and postoperative atrial fibrillation on outcome after mitral valvuloplasty for nonischemic mitral regurgitation. J Thorac Cardiovasc Surg 2005;129: 1032–40.
11. Bando K, Kobayashi J, Kosakai Y. Impact of Cox maze procedure on outcome in patients with atrial fibrillation and mitral valve disease. J Thorac Cardiovasc Surg 2002;124:575–83.
12. Molloy TA. Midterm clinical experience with microwave surgical ablation of atrial fibrillation. Ann Thorac Surg 2005;79(6):2115–8.
13. Ngaage DL, Schaff HV, Mullany CJ, et al. Influence of preoperative atrial fibrillation on late results of mitral repair: is concomitant ablation justified? Ann Thorac Surg 2007;84(2):434–42 [discussion 442–33].

14. Hematpour K, Steinberg JS. Treatment of atrial fibrillation in hypertrophic cardiomyopathy. Anadolu Kardiyol Derg 2006;(6 Suppl 2):44–8.
15. Stulak JM, Schaff HV, Dearani JA, et al. Restoration of sinus rhythm by the Maze procedure halts progression of tricuspid regurgitation after mitral surgery. Ann Thorac Surg 2008;86(1):40–4 [discussion 44–5].
16. Fuster V, Ryden LE, Cannom DS, et al. ACC/AHA/ ESC 2006 Guidelines for the Management of Patients with Atrial Fibrillation: a report of the American College of Cardiology/American Heart Association Task Force on Practice Guidelines and the European Society of Cardiology Committee for Practice Guidelines (Writing Committee to Revise the 2001 guidelines for the management of patients with atrial fibrillation): developed in collaboration with the European Heart Rhythm Association and the Heart Rhythm Society. Circulation 2006; 114(7):e257–354.
17. Wu T-J, Kerwin WF, Hwang C. Atrial fibrillation: focal activity, re-entry, or both? Heart Rhythm 2004;1: 117–20.
18. Savelieva I, Camm J. Update on atrial fibrillation: part I. Clin Cardiol 2008;31(2):55–62.
19. Haissaguerre M, Jais P, Shah DC, et al. Spontaneous initiation of atrial fibrillation by ectopic beats originating in the pulmonary veins. N Engl J Med 1998;339(10):659–66.
20. Todd DM, Skanes AC, Guiraudon G, et al. Role of the posterior left atrium and pulmonary veins in human lone atrial fibrillation: electrophysiological and pathological data from patients undergoing atrial fibrillation surgery. Circulation 2003;108(25):3108–14.
21. Nitta T, Ishii Y, Miyagi Y. Concurrent multiple left atrial focal activations with fibrillatory conduction and right atrial focal or reentrant activation as the mechanism in atrial fibrillation. J Thorac Cardiovasc Surg 2004;127:770–8.
22. Yamauchi S, Ogasawara H, Saji Y. Efficacy of intraoperative mapping to optimize the surgical ablation of atrial fibrillation in cardiac surgery. Ann Thorac Surg 2002;74:450–7.
23. Harada A, Konishi T, Fukata M. Intraoperative map guided operation for atrial fibrillation due to mitral valve disease. Ann Thorac Surg 2000;69:446–50.
24. Harada A, Sasake K, Fukushima T, et al. Atrial activation during chronic atrial fibrillation in patients with isolated mitral valve disease. Ann Thorac Surg 1996;61:104–12.
25. Sueda T, Imai K, Ishii O. Efficacy of pulmonary vein isolation for the elimination of chronic atrial fibrillation in cardiac valvular surgery. Ann Thorac Surg 2001;71:1189–93.
26. Schuessler RB. Do we need a map to get through the maze? J Thorac Cardiovasc Surg 2004;127: 627–8.

27. Pappone C, Santinelli V, Manguso F, et al. Pulmonary vein denervation enhances long-term benefit after circumferential ablation for paroxysmal atrial fibrillation. Circulation 2004;109(3):327–34.

28. Oral H, Scharf C, Chugh A, et al. Catheter ablation for paroxysmal atrial fibrillation: segmental pulmonary vein ostial ablation versus left atrial ablation. Circulation 2003;108(19):2355–60.

29. Marrouche NF, Dresing T, Cole C, et al. Circular mapping and ablation of the pulmonary vein for treatment of atrial fibrillation: impact of different catheter technologies. J Am Coll Cardiol. 2002; 40(3):464–74.

30. Markowitz SM. Ablation of atrial fibrillation: patient selection, technique, and outcome. Curr Cardiol Rep 2008;10(5):360–6.

31. Yamada T, McElderry HT, Doppalapudi H, et al. Catheter ablation of focal triggers and drivers of atrial fibrillation. J Electrocardiol 2008;41(2): 138–43.

32. Kondo N, Takahashi K, Minakawa M. Left atrial maze procedure: a useful addition to other corrective operations. Ann Thorac Surg 2003;75:1490–4.

33. Gaita F, Gallotti R, Calo L. Limited posterior left atrial cryoablation in patients with chronic atrial fibrillation undergoing valvular heart sugery. J Am Coll Cardiol 2000;36:159–66.

34. Tuinenburg AE, van Gelder IC, Tieleman R. Minimaze suffices as adjunct to mitral valve surgery in patients with preoperative atrial fibrillation. J Cardiovasc Electrophysiol 2000;11:960–7.

35. Kalil RAK, Lima GG, Leiria TLL, et al. Simple surgical isolation of pulmonary veins for treating secondary atrial fibrillation in mitral valve disease. Ann Thorac Surg 2002;73(4):1169–73.

36. Deneke T, Khargi K, Grewe PH, et al. Left atrial versus bi-atrial Maze operation using intraoperatively cooled-tip radiofrequency ablation in patients undergoing open-heart surgery: safety and efficacy. J Am Coll Cardiol 2002;39(10):1644–50.

37. Barnett SD, Ad N. Surgical ablation as treatment for the elimination of atrial fibrillation: a meta-analysis. J Thorac Cardiovasc Surg 2006;131(5):1029–35.

38. Usui A, Inden Y, Mizutani S. Repetitive atrial flutter as a complication of the left-sided simple maze procedure. Ann Thorac Surg 2002;73:1457–9.

39. Cox JL, Schuessler RB, Boineau JP. The development of the Maze procedure for the treatment of atrial fibrillation. Semin Thorac Cardiovasc Surg 2000;12(1):2–14.

40. McCarthy PM, Gillinov AM, Castle L, et al. The Cox-Maze procedure: the Cleveland Clinic experience. Semin Thorac Cardiovasc Surg 2000;12(1):25–9.

41. Schaff HV, Dearani JA, Daly RC, et al. Cox-Maze procedure for atrial fibrillation: Mayo Clinic experience. Semin Thorac Cardiovasc Surg 2000;12(1):30–7.

42. Prasad SM, Maniar HS, Camillo CJ, et al. The Cox maze III procedure for atrial fibrillation: long-term efficacy in patients undergoing lone versus concomitant procedures. J Thorac Cardiovasc Surg 2003;126(6):1822–8.

43. Gillinov AM. Ablation of atrial fibrillation in mitral valve surgery. Curr Opin Cardiol 2005;20:107–14.

44. Gillinov AM, Sirak JH, Blackstone EH. The Cox maze procedure in mitral valve disease: predictors of recurrent atrial fibrillation. J Thorac Cardiovasc Surg 2005;130:1653–60.

45. Reston JT, Shuhaiber JH. Meta-analysis of clinical outcomes of maze-related surgical procedures for medically refractory atrial fibrillation. Eur J Cardiothorac Surg 2005;28(5):724–30.

46. Richter B, Gwechenberger M, Socas A, et al. Frequency of recurrence of atrial fibrillation within 48 hours after ablation and its impact on long-term outcome. Am J Cardiol 2008;101(6):843–7.

47. Scherer M, Dzemali O, Aybek T. Impact of left atrial size reduction on chronic atrial fibrillation in mitral valve surgery. J Heart Valve Dis 2003;12:469–74.

48. Gaynor SL, Schuessler RB, Bailey MS, et al. Surgical treatment of atrial fibrillation: predictors of late recurrence. J Thorac Cardiovasc Surg 2005; 129(1):104–11.

49. Isobe F, Kawashima Y. The outcome and indications of the Cox maze III procedure for chronic atrial fibrillation with mitral valve disease. J Thorac Cardiovasc Surg 1998;116:220–7.

50. Kosakai Y, Kawaguchi AT, Isobe F, et al. Modified maze procedure for patients with atrial fibrillation undergoing simultaneous open heart surgery. Circulation 1995;92(9 Suppl):II359–64.

51. Chen MC, Chang JP, Guo GB, et al. Atrial size reduction as a predictor of the success of radiofrequency maze procedure for chronic atrial fibrillation in patients undergoing concomitant valvular surgery. J Cardiovasc Electrophysiol 2001;12(8): 867–74.

52. Kim YH, Lee SC, Her AY, et al. Preoperative left atrial volume index is a predictor of successful sinus rhythm restoration and maintenance after the maze operation. J Thorac Cardiovasc Surg 2007;134(2):448–53.

53. Marui A, Nishina T, Tambara K, et al. A novel atrial volume reduction technique to enhance the Cox maze procedure: initial results. J Thorac Cardiovasc Surg 2006;132(5):1047–53.

54. Lee JW, Park NH, Choo SJ. Surgical outcome of the maze procedure for atrial fibrillation in mitral valve disease: rheumatic versus degenerative. Ann Thorac Surg 2003;75:57–61.

55. Jatene MB, Marcial MB, Tarasoutchi F. Influence of the maze procedure on the treatment of rheumatic atrial fibrillation - evaluation of rhythm control and

clinical outcome in a comparative study. Eur J Cardiothorac Surg 2000;17:117–24.

56. Handa N, Schaff HV, Morris JJ. Outcome of valve repair and the Cox maze procedure for mitral regurgitation and associated atrial fibrillation. J Thorac Cardiovasc Surg 1999;118:628–35.

57. Cox JL, Ad N, Palazzo T. Impact of the maze procedure on the stroke rate in patients with atrial fibrillation. J Thorac Cardiovasc Surg 1999;118:833–40.

58. Gillinov AM, Blackstone EH, McCarthy PM. Atrial fibrillation: current surgical options and their assessment. Ann Thorac Surg 2002;74(6):2210–7.

59. Gillinov AM, McCarthy PM. Advances in the surgical treatment of atrial fibrillation. Cardiol Clin 2004;22:147–57.

60. Gillinov AM, McCarthy PM, Marrouche N, et al. Contemporary surgical treatment for atrial fibrillation. Pacing Clin Electrophysiol 2003;26(7 Pt 2):1641–4.

61. Raman J, Ishikawa S, Storer MM. Surgical radiofrequency ablation of both atria for atrial fibrillation: results of a multicenter trial. J Thorac Cardiovasc Surg 2003;126:1357–66.

62. Sie HT, Beukema WP, Elvan A. Long-term results of irrigated radiofrequency modified maze procedure in 200 patients with concomitant cardiac surgery: six years experience. Ann Thorac Surg 2004;77:512–6.

63. Luria DM, Nemec J, Etheridge SP. Intra-atrial conduction block along the mitral valve annulus during accessory pathway ablation: evidence for a left atrial "isthmus". J Cardiovasc Electrophysiol 2001;12:744–9.

64. Saltman AE, Rosenthal LS, Francalancia NA, et al. A completely endoscopic approach to microwave ablation for atrial fibrillation. Heart Surg Forum 2003;6(3):E38–41.

65. Reade CC, Johnson JO, Bolotin G, et al. Combining robotic mitral valve repair and microwave atrial fibrillation ablation: techniques and initial results. Ann Thorac Surg 2005;79(2):480–4.

66. Salenger R, Lahey SJ, Saltman AE. The completely endoscopic treatment of atrial fibrillation: report on the first 14 patients with early results. Heart Surg Forum 2004;7(6):E555–8.

67. Pruitt JC, Lazzara RR, Dworkin GH, et al. Totally endoscopic ablation of lone atrial fibrillation: initial clinical experience. Ann Thorac Surg 2006;81(4):1325–30 [discussion 1330–21].

68. Bisleri G, Manzato A, Argenziano M, et al. Thoracoscopic epicardial pulmonary vein ablation for lone paroxysmal atrial fibrillation. Europace 2005;7(2):145–8.

69. Wolf RK, Schneeberger EW, Osterday R, et al. Video-assisted bilateral pulmonary vein isolation and left atrial appendage exclusion for atrial fibrillation. J Thorac Cardiovasc Surg 2005;130(3):797–802.

70. Cox JL, Ad N. The importance of cryoablation of the coronary sinus during the Maze procedure. Semin Thorac Cardiovasc Surg 2000;12:20–4.

71. Nath S, Lynch C 3rd, Whayne JG, et al. Cellular electrophysiological effects of hyperthermia on isolated guinea pig papillary muscle. Implications for catheter ablation. Circulation 1993;88(4):1826–31.

72. Lustgarten DL, Keane D, Ruskin J. Cryothermal ablation: mechanism of tissue injury and current experience in the treatment of tachyarrhythmias. Prog Cardiovasc Dis 1999;41(6):481–98.

73. Khargi K, Hutten BA, Lemke B, et al. Surgical treatment of atrial fibrillation; a systematic review. Eur J Cardiothorac Surg 2005;27(2):258–65.

74. Gillinov AM, Pettersson G, Rice TW. Esophageal injury during radiofrequency ablation for atrial fibrillation. J Thorac Cardiovasc Surg 2001;122(6):1239–40.

75. Doll N, Borger MA, Fabricius A, et al. Esophageal perforation during left atrial radiofrequency ablation: is the risk too high? J Thorac Cardiovasc Surg 2003;125(4):836–42.

76. Manasse E, Medici D, Ghiselli S, et al. Left main coronary arterial lesion after microwave epicardial ablation. Ann Thorac Surg 2003;76(1):276–7.

77. Ohara K, Hirai T, Fukuda N, et al. Relation of left atrial blood stasis to clinical risk factors in atrial fibrillation. Int J Cardiol 2008.

78. Mobius-Winkler S, Schuler GC, Sick PB. Interventional treatments for stroke prevention in atrial fibrillation with emphasis upon the WATCHMAN device. Curr Opin Neurol 2008;21(1):64–9.

79. Hur J, Kim YJ, Nam JE, et al. Thrombus in the left atrial appendage in stroke patients: detection with cardiac CT angiography–A preliminary report. Radiology 2008;249:81–7.

80. Johnson WD, Ganjoo AK, Stone CD. The left atrial appendage: our most lethal human attachment! Surgical implications. Eur J Cardiothorac Surg 2000;17:718–22.

81. Garcia-Fernandez MA, Perez-David E, Quiles J. Role of left atrial appendage obliteration in stroke reduction in patients with mitral valve prosthesis: a transesophageal echocardiographic study. J Am Coll Cardiol 2003;42:1253–8.

82. Rosenzweig BP, Katz E, Kort S. Thromboembolus from a ligated left atrial appendage. J Am Soc Echocardiogr 2001;14:396–8.

83. Gillinov AM, Pettersson G, Cosgrove DM. Stapled excision of the left atrial appendage. J Thorac Cardiovasc Surg 2004;129:679–80.

84. Kamohara K, Fukamachi K, Ootaki Y. A novel device for left atrial appendage exclusion. J Thorac Cardiovasc Surg 2005;130:1639–44.

85. Kamohara K, Fukamachi K, Ootaki Y, et al. Evaluation of a novel device for left atrial appendage exclusion: the second-generation atrial exclusion device. J Thorac Cardiovasc Surg 2006;132(2): 340–6.

86. Salzberg SP, Gillinov AM, Anyanwu A, et al. Surgical left atrial appendage occlusion: evaluation of a novel device with magnetic resonance imaging. Eur J Cardiothorac Surg 2008;34:766–70.

87. Saltman AE, Virmani R, Mohan A. Development and testing of a novel device for left atrial appendage occlusion. Kos, Greece: International Society for Cardiothoracic Surgery; 2008.

88. Pacifico A, Henry PD. Ablation for atrial fibrillation: are cures really achieved? J Am Coll Cardiol 2004;43:1940–2.

89. Gillinov AM, McCarthy PM, Blackstone EH. Surgical ablation of atrial fibrillation with bipolar radiofrequency. J Thorac Cardiovasc Surg 2004;129: 1322–9.

90. Shemin RJ, Cox JL, Gillinov AM, et al. Guidelines for reporting data and outcomes for the surgical treatment of atrial fibrillation. Ann Thorac Surg 2007;83(3):1225–30.

91. Gillinov AM, Saltman AE. Ablation of atrial fibrillation with concomitant cardiac surgery. Semin Thorac Cardiovasc Surg 2007;19(1):25–32.

92. Gillinov AM. Advances in surgical treatment of atrial fibrillation. Stroke 2007;38(Suppl 2):618–23.

93. Loulmet DF, Patel NC, Jennings JM, et al. Less invasive intracardiac surgery performed without aortic clamping. Ann Thorac Surg 2008;85(5):1551–5.

94. Umakanthan R, Leacche M, Petracek MR, et al. Safety of minimally invasive mitral valve surgery without aortic cross-clamp. Ann Thorac Surg 2008;85(5):1544–9 [discussion 1549–50].

95. Greco E, Zaballos JM, Alvarez L, et al. Video-assisted mitral surgery through a micro-access: a safe and reliable reality in the current era. J Heart Valve Dis 2008;17(1):48–53.

96. Mohamed KS. Minimally invasive right posterior minithoracotomy for open-heart procedures. Asian Cardiovasc Thorac Ann 2007;15(6):468–71.

97. Doll N, Kiaii BB, Fabricius AM, et al. Intraoperative left atrial ablation (for atrial fibrillation) using a new argon cryocatheter: early clinical experience. Ann Thorac Surg 2003;76(5):1711–5.

98. Mohr FW, Fabricius AM, Falk V, et al. Curative treatment of atrial fibrillation with intraoperative radiofrequency ablation: Short-term and midterm results. J Thorac Cardiovasc Surg 2002;123(5):919–27.

99. Edgerton JR, Edgerton ZJ, Weaver T, et al. Minimally invasive pulmonary vein isolation and partial autonomic denervation for surgical treatment of atrial fibrillation. Ann Thorac Surg 2008;86(1):35–8 [discussion 39].

100. Wolf RK. Minimally invasive surgical treatment of atrial fibrillation. Semin Thorac Cardiovasc Surg 2007;19(4):311–8.

101. Matsutani N, Takase B, Ozeki Y, et al. Minimally invasive cardiothoracic surgery for atrial fibrillation: a combined Japan-US experience. Circ J 2008; 72(3):434–6.

102. Pruitt JC, Lazzara RR, Ebra G. Minimally invasive surgical ablation of atrial fibrillation: the thoracoscopic box lesion approach. J Interv Card Electrophysiol 2007;20(3):83–7.

103. Gillinov AM, Saltman AE. Surgical approaches for atrial fibrillation. Med Clin North Am 2008;92(1): 203–15, xii.

104. Gillinov AM, Svensson LG. Ablation of atrial fibrillation with minimally invasive mitral surgery. Ann Thorac Surg 2007;84(3):1041–2.

105. Moten SC, Rodriguez E, Cook RC, et al. New ablation techniques for atrial fibrillation and the minimally invasive cryo-maze procedure in patients with lone atrial fibrillation. Heart Lung Circ 2007;(16 Suppl 3):S88–93.

106. Suwalski P, Suwalski G, Wilimski R, et al. Minimally invasive off-pump video-assisted endoscopic surgical pulmonary vein isolation using bipolar radiofrequency ablation—preliminary report. Kardiol Pol 2007;65(4):370–4 [discussion 375–6].

107. Saltman AE. Minimally invasive surgery for atrial fibrillation. Semin Thorac Cardiovasc Surg 2007; 19(1):33–8.

Atrial Fibrillation: Goals of Therapy and Management Strategies to Achieve the Goals

Benzy J. Padanilam, MD, Eric N. Prystowsky, MD*

KEYWORDS

- Atrial fibrillation • Management • Rate control
- Rhythm control • Anticoagulation

Atrial fibrillation (AF) may be associated with disabling symptoms and complications, such as stroke and tachycardia-induced cardiomyopathy. Although AF, per se, is rarely a life-threatening arrhythmia, it was associated with decreased overall survival in the Framingham Heart Study.[1] The three major therapeutic strategies in managing AF include prevention of stroke, rate control, and rhythm control. Anticoagulation with warfarin reduces the risk for stroke. Therapies to achieve symptom control and prevention of tachycardia-mediated cardiomyopathy are often similar. For example, ventricular rate control during AF or maintenance of sinus rhythm may improve symptoms and prevent tachycardia-induced cardiomyopathy. When clinical goals are not met using one strategy, the alternate strategy can be pursued in the same patient. Current therapies of AF have not demonstrated survival benefits, and future research needs to focus on the goals of improving the survival of patients who have AF. Development of strategies for the primary prevention of AF is another area of great significance for research considering the high prevalence of the disease. Until such therapeutic options become available, prevention of the disease-related complications and control of symptoms may be considered the primary goals of AF management (**Box 1**).

GOALS OF THERAPY
Prevention of Thromboembolism

AF, with its accompanying loss of organized atrial contraction, can lead to stagnation of blood, especially in the left atrial appendage, with resultant thrombus formation and embolism. There is also some evidence that AF is associated with a hypercoagulable state, further promoting thromboembolism.[2,3] Stroke, the most common thromboembolic event in AF, occurs at a higher frequency in individuals who have AF, and approximately 36% of all strokes in individuals aged 80 to 89 years are attributed to AF.[4] Furthermore, strokes occurring in patients who have AF tend to have a higher degree of severity.[5] Individuals who have AF are not at equal risk for thromboembolic events, and several predisposing clinical factors can identify those patients at high risk. Anticoagulation with warfarin is the current standard of therapy for preventing thromboembolism in patients at high risk for stroke. The goal of anticoagulation is to prevent AF-related thromboembolic complications without increasing the risks for bleeding significantly. There is evidence that suggests warfarin therapy is underused in patients who have AF;[6,7] more widespread use of warfarin therapy in appropriate patients is another goal to be achieved. An important lesson learned from recent clinical trials of AF management is that

A version of this article originally appeared in *Medical Clinics of North America*, volume 92, issue 1.
The Care Group, LLC, 8333 Naab Road, Suite 400, Indianapolis, IN 46260–1919, USA
* Corresponding author.
E-mail address: eprystow@thecaregroup.com (E.N. Prystowsky).

Cardiol Clin 27 (2009) 189–200
doi:10.1016/j.ccl.2008.09.006

> **Box 1**
> **Goals of atrial fibrillation therapy**
>
> Prevention of stroke (thromboembolism)
>
> Prevention of tachycardia-induced cardiomyopathy
>
> Symptom relief
>
> Improved survival
>
> Primary prevention

patients at high risk for stroke who seem to be maintaining sinus rhythm while receiving antiarrhythmic medications still require warfarin therapy.[8,9] These patients have a continued risk for stroke, possibly from clinically unrecognized episodes of AF.

Prevention of Tachycardia-Induced Cardiomyopathy

Untreated AF often is associated with rapid ventricular rates. In experimental models, ventricular dysfunction can occur as soon as 24 hours and continue to deteriorate for 3 to 5 weeks with rapid pacing rates. Recovery of ventricular function with cessation of pacing could start within 48 hours, and normalization can occur within 1 to 2 weeks.[10] Patients who have AF and prolonged periods of rapid ventricular rates may develop left ventricular (LV) dysfunction, although the severity and temporal course of its onset vary significantly among individuals. In a study of AV node ablation and permanent pacemaker placement for AF refractory to medical therapy, 37% (105 of 282) of patients had an LV ejection fraction of 40% or less,[11] indicating a high prevalence of cardiomyopathy in such patients. Control of ventricular rates, by rate or rhythm control strategies, when undertaken early after AF onset, can prevent subsequent development of cardiomyopathy. If patients already have developed tachycardia-induced ventricular dysfunction at presentation, the immediate goal is to reverse this process with aggressive rate control or cardioversion to sinus rhythm. In such patients, particular attention should be paid to avoid recurrent AF with prolonged periods of rapid ventricular rates, because rather quick development of LV failure and incidents of sudden death are reported in the literature with recurrent tachycardia-induced cardiomyopathy.[12]

Control of Symptoms

Patients who have AF exhibit a panoply of clinical presentations, ranging from none to disabling symptoms. Common symptoms include anxiety, palpitations, dyspnea, dizziness, chest pain, and fatigue. Several hemodynamic derangements, including rapid ventricular rates, loss of organized atrial contraction, irregularity of cardiac rhythm, and bradycardia (resulting particularly from sinus pauses when AF episodes terminate), may be the underlying cause of the symptoms related to AF. Although the Atrial Fibrillation Follow-up Investigation of Rhythm Management (AFFIRM) trial[8] demonstrated that symptoms can be controlled equally well with a rate control or rhythm control strategy, clinicians encounter many patients who have AF who need sinus rhythm to feel better. This may be particularly relevant in younger patients and those who have paroxysmal AF. The loss of regularity and fine autonomic control of cardiac rhythm and the loss of atrial contribution to ventricular filling may be postulated as playing a bigger role in the hemodynamics of these patients, accounting for the lack of success of rate control. When a rate control strategy is selected, it is important to allow adequate time for symptoms to improve, because in many patients, it can take several months for good symptom relief after achieving rate control. Control of symptoms rather than elimination of all symptoms may be an acceptable goal in many patients based on a risks/benefits analysis of the available therapeutic options.

Future Goals

Improvement in survival should be a goal of AF therapy. Elucidation of basic mechanisms of the disease and targeted therapy that does not have significant adverse effects (eg, atrial-specific antiarrhythmic drugs),[13] continued anticoagulation in patients taking antiarrhythmic drugs for rhythm control,[14] and catheter ablation strategies to cure AF could potentially improve patient survival. Preliminary data comparing ablation with antiarrhythmic medications show favorable outcomes for the ablation strategy.[15,16]

Primary prevention of AF is an important public health goal because it affects an estimated 2.2 million people in the United States[17] and its prevalence is rising.[18] Preliminary data suggest that the use of medications, such as angiotensin-converting enzyme inhibitors, angiotensin receptor blockers, and 3-hydroxy-3-methylglutaryl coenzyme A (HMG-CoA) reductase inhibitors in addition to dietary intake of fish and n-3 polyunsaturated fatty acids may reduce AF incidence.[13] Whether or not treatment of disease states, such as hypertension and heart failure, that have a known association with AF could lead to a decreased incidence of AF also needs evaluation.

THERAPEUTIC OPTIONS
Anticoagulation

Risk stratification

Because anticoagulation therapy is inherently associated with an increased risk for bleeding complications, such therapy is limited to patients who have AF and are deemed to be at high risk for thromboembolism. Collective information from various clinical trials of anticoagulation therapy has identified several risk factors that predispose persons who have AF to thromboembolism.[19] Gage and colleagues[20] developed a scoring system for stroke risk prediction called CHADS2 using these risk factors. Each of the letters in this acronym represents a risk factor—congestive heart failure, hypertension, age, diabetes, and stroke. Previous stroke or transient ischemic attack (TIA) is the strongest predictor of stroke, and therefore carries two points, whereas the other risk factors carry one point each. The American College of Cardiology (ACC)/American Heart Association (AHA)/European Society of Cardiology (ESC) guidelines on AF management use the CHADS2 scoring for risk classification.[21] **Box 2** summarizes the ACC/AHA/ESC system of dividing predisposing factors into less validated or weaker risk factors, moderate risk factors, and high risk factors. Patients who have any high risk factor or more than one moderate risk factor are considered at high risk (>4% annual risk) for stroke, and warfarin is recommended. Those who have no risk factors are considered at low risk (<2% annual risk) for stroke and are generally prescribed aspirin

---

Box 2
Risk factors for thromboembolism

Less validated risk

Female gender

Age 65 to 74 years

Coronary artery disease

Thyrotoxicosis

Moderate risk

Age 75 years or older

Hypertension

LV ejection fraction 35% or less

Heart failure

Diabetes mellitus

High risk

Previous stroke, TIA, embolism

Mitral stenosis

Prosthetic heart valve

Box 3
Risk category and recommended therapy

No risk factors: aspirin (81 mg/d or 325 mg/d)

One moderate risk factor: aspirin or warfarin

Any high risk factor or more than one moderate risk factor: warfarin

---

(**Box 3**). Patients who have one moderate risk factor have an intermediate risk (2.8% annual risk) for stroke.[20,21] Treatment decisions are individualized in these latter patients, and warfarin or aspirin may be used.[21]

Warfarin

Warfarin therapy is highly effective, compared with placebo, in reducing (by 61%) the stroke risk in patients who have AF.[22] Strokes occurring in patients who have AF while they are taking warfarin therapy also are less severe.[23] In clinical studies, an international normalized ratio (INR) between 2.0 and 3.0 correlates to maximum protection against strokes with minimum bleeding risks.[24] Warfarin has several drawbacks, including a 1% to 1.5% risk for major bleeding complications.[19] The risk for bleeding may be higher in women and in the elderly, who also are at the highest risk for embolic stroke from AF.[25,26] The risk for bleeding seems higher at initiation of warfarin, and a recent study has noted a threefold increase in bleeding risk during the first 3 months of therapy.[27]

Alternatives to warfarin

Aspirin is significantly less effective than warfarin, with a stroke reduction of only 19%.[22] Aspirin, however, is recommended in lower risk patients because of its favorable side-effect profile and ease of use. In a clinical study of high-risk patients, a combination of aspirin and clopidogrel was inferior to warfarin for stroke prevention.[28] Ximelagatran (an oral direct thrombin inhibitor) did not meet US Food and Drug Administration approval because of concerns regarding its hepatotoxicity and clinical trial design.[29] Nonpharmacologic stroke prevention, a consideration only in high-risk patients who are not candidates for warfarin, has not been well studied. Approaches include surgical left atrial appendage removal and catheter-based left atrial appendage occlusion.[30,31]

Anticoagulation management before cardioversion

The use of anticoagulation before and after cardioversion (electrical or pharmacologic) requires special consideration because of increased risk for stroke noted in retrospective studies after cardioversion.[32] According to the current guidelines,[21] patients may be cardioverted without anticoagulation if the duration of AF is less than 48 hours. When the duration of AF is unknown or greater than 48 hours, anticoagulation with warfarin should be instituted with a therapeutic INR for at least 3 weeks before and 4 weeks after the cardioversion.[21] An alternative approach is a transesophageal echocardiogram to exclude the presence of left atrial thrombus,[33] followed by cardioversion. In this approach, it is not necessary to have 3 weeks of therapeutic INR before the cardioversion and patients who do not have a therapeutic INR may be given intravenous unfractionated heparin or subcutaneous low-molecular-weight heparin to achieve immediate anticoagulation.[33,34] Cardioversion, however, should be followed by continued unfractionated or low-molecular-weight heparin therapy until the INR is therapeutic, and warfarin should be continued for at least 4 weeks.

Rate Control and Rhythm Control

The two basic therapeutic options to control symptoms in AF are rhythm control, in which sinus rhythm is re-established, and rate control, in which patients remain in AF with control of ventricular rates. Pharmacologic and nonpharmacologic options are available for both of these strategies.

Although re-establishing the normal rhythm (the rhythm control strategy) may seem to be intuitively superior, clinical studies show no significant difference in major clinical outcomes between this strategy and that of rate control. Five randomized clinical trials looked at total mortality, thromboembolic events, hemorrhage, and symptomatic improvement and found no statistically significant differences in outcomes between the pharmacologic rate control and rhythm control strategies.[8,9,35–37] The mean age of participants in the largest of these trials (AFFIRM) was 69.7 years, leading many clinicians to choose rate control as a preferred strategy in older less symptomatic patients.

The reasons for the lack of advantage of sinus rhythm maintenance in clinical trials are not clear but could relate to the toxicity associated with antiarrhythmic medications, negating the advantages of sinus rhythm. Another important factor may be the discontinuation of anticoagulation in patients, seemingly maintaining sinus rhythm in such trials. In fact, one of the important messages from rate control versus rhythm control trials is the need for continued anticoagulation therapy in high-risk patients while they are clinically maintaining sinus rhythm on antiarrhythmic medications. Preliminary evidence suggesting that the toxicity of current antiarrhythmic medications may negate the advantages of sinus rhythm is as follows. A retrospective subanalysis of the on-treatment outcomes in the AFFIRM study suggests that a strategy to maintain sinus rhythm without the adverse effects of antiarrhythmic medications may confer a survival advantage.[14] Radiofrequency ablation trials also shed some light on this debate. In a nonrandomized study, Pappone and colleagues[15] compared the outcomes in a selected group of 589 patients who underwent circumferential pulmonary vein ablation with those in 582 age- and gender-matched cohort patients who received antiarrhythmic medications to maintain sinus rhythm. After a median follow-up of 900 days, the observed survival was longer and the quality of life was better for patients who underwent ablation. Radiofrequency pulmonary vein isolation was a superior first-line therapy compared with antiarrhythmic drug therapy in a small randomized trial of 70 patients.[16] Finally, in patients who had heart failure, ablation resulted in improved heart function even when heart rates were well controlled before ablation.[38,39] Thus, future use of antiarrhythmic medications with a better side-effect profile and advancements in ablation techniques could lead to better outcomes with rhythm control strategy.

Choice of strategy

The choice of a particular strategy should be dictated by the clinical scenario, with a preference toward rate control in less symptomatic elderly patients. Rate control also may be preferred in patients who are noncompliant or decline hospitalization and cardioversion, because the rhythm control strategy may require a higher number of hospitalizations.[8] Patients in whom the only antiarrhythmic choice is amiodarone also are potential candidates for an initial rate control strategy. An initial rhythm control strategy may be appropriate in younger symptomatic patients, newly diagnosed patients who have lone AF, and those who have AF believed to be secondary to a precipitating event. Although a retrospective analysis suggested improved survival by maintaining sinus rhythm in patients who had heart failure,[8,40,41] results of the recent randomized prospective trial of 1376 patients who had heart failure and a left ventricular ejection fraction (LVEF) less than 35% showed no significant differences in outcomes between a rhythm control and rate control strategy.[42]

Definition of rate control

The best parameters for rate control in AF are not well defined, but the AFFIRM study criteria generally are recommended[8,21] (ventricular rate ≤80 beats per minute at rest and a maximum of <110 beats per minute during a 6-minute walk or an average heart rate <100 beats per minute during 24-hour ambulatory monitoring with no heart rate >110% of the maximal age-predicted exercise heart rate). It is unclear whether or not strict heart rate control is essential for good outcomes, especially in patients who do not have LV dysfunction and significant symptoms. Cooper and colleagues[43] analyzed the outcomes in different quartiles of heart rate control in the AFFIRM study (heart rate quartiles at rest: 44–69, 70–78, 79–87, and 88–148 beats per minute and heart rate quartiles with a 6-minute walk: 53–82, 83–92, 93–106 and 107–220 beats per minute) and found no differences in overall survival or quality of life. These data may indicate that strict heart rate control may not be essential for good outcomes in some patients. At the authors' institution, physicians prefer to regulate the heart rate for AF in each patient's normal daily activity profile. To accomplish this, the daily heart rate trend graphs from 24-hour electrocardiographic (ECG) recordings are used and medications are adjusted to maintain average rates for each hour of less than 100 beats per minute and for a 24-hour period of approximately 70 to 80 beats per minute.[44]

Therapeutic options for rate control

Beta-blockers, nondihydropyridine calcium channel blockers, and digoxin are the usual pharmacologic agents used for rate control. Digoxin is less effective than beta-blockers and calcium channel blockers, particularly during exercise, but has a synergistic effect when added to them.[45] Beta-blockers are preferred as an initial AV blocking agent when there is LV dysfunction associated with AF.[46,47] Calcium channel blockers, verapamil and diltiazem in a sustained released form, often are well tolerated by patients who have bronchospastic disease. At times, it is useful to give smaller doses of two classes of drugs to minimize adverse effects. Amiodarone and clonidine also have been used for rate control purposes in limited situations.[21,48] AV junction ablation with permanent pacemaker implantation (ablate and pace strategy) is a highly effective method for rate control but is usually reserved for situations in which pharmacologic options are ineffective. Clinical studies have demonstrated improvement in quality of life and LV function with such an approach.[49,50] Concerns with this approach include patients becoming pacemaker dependent, provocation of fatal ventricular arrhythmias, and the more recently described deleterious effects of permanent right ventricular pacing.[51] Consideration may be given to biventricular pacing for patients who have

significant LV dysfunction undergoing AV junction ablation for AF rate control to address the potential deleterious effects of right ventricular pacing in that situation.[52–54]

Rhythm control with antiarrhythmic medications

Antiarrhythmic medications, by changing the electrophysiologic properties of atrial tissue, can terminate AF or prevent its recurrence. The Vaughan-Williams classification divides these agents into class IA, IB, and IC (sodium channel blockers); class II (beta-blockers); class III (potassium channel blockers); and class IV (calcium channel blockers). Only class I and class III agents are referred to as antiarrhythmic medications in this article because beta-blockers and calcium channel blockers do not have the ability to cardiovert AF or maintain sinus rhythm after cardioversion of AF.

Choice of antiarrhythmic medication

Selection of antiarrhythmic agents should be directed by a safety-based approach (**Fig. 1**). The class IC agent flecainide increased mortality in the setting of previous myocardial infarction and ventricular ectopy in the Cardiac Arrhythmia Suppression Trial.[55] Based on this information, the class IC agents flecainide and propafenone are considered to be contraindicated in patients who have AF with ischemic heart disease.[21] Class IC agents do not increase mortality in patients who have structurally normal hearts,[56] however, making them one of the initial agents of choice for treatment of AF. Class III (sotalol and dofetilide) and class IA (quinidine, procainamide, and disopyramide) agents prolong cardiac repolarization, and therefore can be associated with the torsades de pointes form of ventricular tachycardia. Although many patients at risk can be identified by monitoring for early proarrhythmia and QT prolongation on ECG, late episodes of torsades de pointes can occur, particularly in the setting of hypokalemia, bradycardia, or renal dysfunction.[57] Amiodarone is a multi-ion channel-blocking agent (included in class III) and prolongs QT interval but has a low risk for causing torsades de pointes. Amiodarone is the most effective antiarrhythmic drug available, and in the Canadian Trial of Atrial Fibrillation, only 35% of patients taking amiodarone had recurrent AF compared with 63% of those taking propafenone or sotalol during a mean follow-up of 468 (±150) days.[58] Amiodarone, however, has many organ toxicities—thyroid, pulmonary, neurologic, hepatic, optic neuropathy (rare), and dermatologic effects[59]—that limit its usefulness. In a meta-analysis of 44 antiarrhythmic

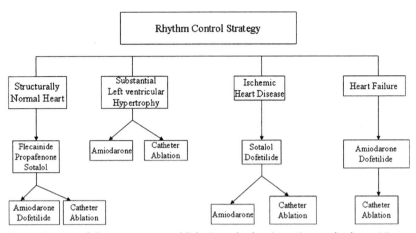

Fig. 1. Approach to selection of therapy to re-establish sinus rhythm in patients who have AF.

medication trials (11,322 patients), sotalol, dofetilide, or amiodarone did not show any significant change in mortality compared with placebo, and the same review showed increased mortality associated with the use of class IA drugs compared with placebo.[56]

When selecting an antiarrhythmic medication for AF treatment, first determine if the heart structurally is normal. The initial choice of an antiarrhythmic medication in patients who have structurally normal hearts and normal 12-lead ECGs is flecainide, propafenone, or sotalol. In the presence of LV hypertrophy (>1.4 cm), amiodarone is the preferred initial therapy because of the perceived potential for proarrhythmia with other agents.[21] Only amiodarone and dofetilide are demonstrated not to decrease survival in the setting of heart failure, making them the preferred agents for these patients. Patients who have ischemic heart disease usually are given sotalol or dofetilide as an initial agent. Sotalol and dofetilide are excreted through the kidneys and should be avoided in patients who have significant renal dysfunction. Bradycardia accentuates QT prolonging effects of sotalol and dofetilide, and patients may require permanent pacing to facilitate the use of these agents in this scenario. Finally, consider avoiding these latter medications in patients who have complex medical regimens, particularly if significant variations in serum electrolytes could occur.

Outpatient initiation of antiarrhythmic medications

Dofetilide therapy always is initiated in a hospital with daily 12-lead ECGs and telemetry monitoring for at least 3 days. All other antiarrhythmic medications can be initiated in an outpatient setting in patients who have no or minimal heart disease per current guidelines.[21] In the presence of heart disease, the authors recommend starting sotalol during constant heart rhythm monitoring in a hospital. Patients who are in AF at the time of therapy initiation also are candidates for inpatient treatment because they may have unidentified sinus node dysfunction, leading to significant bradycardia with conversion of AF to sinus rhythm. One exception is amiodarone initiation at low doses of 200 to 600 mg/d. Here, drug loading takes several weeks, and it is impractical to monitor patients in the hospital. When drugs are initiated on an outpatient basis, the authors recommend 12-lead ECGs 2 to 3 days after each dose change. ECGs are analyzed for excessive prolongation of the QT interval (corrected QT interval [QT$_c$] >500 milliseconds) with sotalol and for prolongation of the PR interval and QRS duration with flecainide or propafenone.

Cardioversion

Conversion of AF to sinus rhythm can be done using synchronized external shocks or antiarrhythmic medications at loading doses. Anticoagulation issues must be addressed before pharmacologic or electrical cardioversions. AF, unlike atrial flutter, is not a rhythm that can be terminated with overdrive pacing. A "pill-in-the-pocket" strategy of outpatient cardioversion may be attempted using loading doses of propafenone or flecainide in some patients.[60] The first such attempt, however, should be done in a hospital setting[21] to establish safety. Administration of beta-blockers or calcium channel blockers is recommended at least 30 minutes before administration of high-dose propafenone or flecainide to prevent development of atrial flutter with 1:1 atrioventricular conduction leading to potentially life-threatening ventricular rates.[21]

Nonpharmacologic rhythm control

When rhythm maintenance is needed and antiarrhythmic medications are ineffective, radiofrequency catheter ablation approaches may be considered. Recent observations from Haissaguerre and colleagues[61,62] have demonstrated that the initiators of AF typically originate in the pulmonary veins and that electrical isolation of these veins often prevents AF. Many different ablation techniques subsequently have been described, and the best AF ablation technique to eliminate AF in individual patients has yet to be defined.[63] The surgical maze procedure to cure AF is highly effective, but this is typically reserved for patients who have failed the catheter ablation approach or for patients undergoing another open-heart procedure, when it is added onto the primary procedure.[64]

MANAGEMENT STRATEGIES BASED ON CLINICAL PRESENTATIONS

Initial Approach to any Patients who Have Atrial Fibrillation

History, physical examination, and laboratory tests

Initial evaluation of AF should include a clinical history regarding the time of onset and the nature of patient's symptoms (**Fig. 2**). Attention should be directed to identifying a possible precipitating event that led to AF. Symptoms suggestive of complications, such as heart failure and stroke, also should be part of the history. Physical examination is directed to vital signs and cardiovascular and other system examinations, especially to increase the information obtained from the history. Initial laboratory testing should include a complete blood cell count, a metabolic panel, and renal and thyroid function evaluations. A two-dimensional echocardiogram is indicated in most patients to identify causative factors for AF and to evaluate for LV dysfunction.

Hemodynamics

Initial attention is directed to the hemodynamic stability of patients. AF, particularly with rapid ventricular rates, can result in severe hemodynamic compromise, especially in patients who have heart disease in which cardiac output is heavily dependent on the atrial contribution and diastolic filling time of the ventricle. Examples include hypertrophic cardiomyopathy with its associated noncompliant ventricles, diastolic dysfunction, and severe mitral stenosis. Significant hemodynamic instability also can occur in scenarios in which there is preexisting hemodynamic compromise, such as sepsis, myocardial infarction, or pulmonary

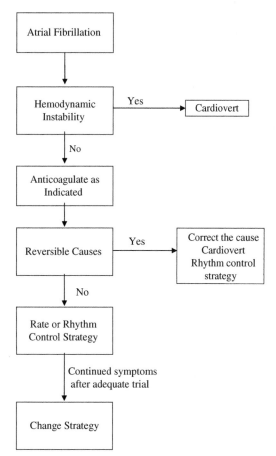

Fig. 2. General approach to patients presenting with AF.

embolism. Patients who have life-threatening hemodynamic compromise need emergent cardioversion without consideration of anticoagulation status. These patients also are at risk for recurrent AF after the cardioversion and may need treatment with intravenous antiarrhythmic drugs, such as amiodarone, to maintain sinus rhythm or to control ventricular rates during AF. Digoxin is another agent that can provide rate control without causing hypotension; however, its effectiveness is minimized in these states of high sympathetic tone.

Precipitating factors

Once the hemodynamic status is addressed, potential precipitating events that caused AF are evaluated. Examples of cardiac disorders that may underlie AF include pericarditis, heart failure, thoracic surgery, Wolff-Parkinson-White syndrome, and mitral stenosis. Several noncardiac conditions also can precipitate AF, for example, pneumonia, pulmonary embolism, acute hypoxia, thyrotoxicosis, and alcohol binge drinking. Although AF may not recur when precipitating factors are eliminated, there is a distinct possibility that AF episodes may continue to occur and that the correlation was coincidental or the precipitating event simply brought out the underlying causative AF pathophysiology. Therefore, AF in patients who have possible precipitating events is initially managed the same way as is AF in other patients with regard to anticoagulation. Anticoagulation should be considered in all high-risk patients with the understanding that it can be discontinued if there are no clinical AF recurrences during follow-up. For moderate-risk patients in whom warfarin anticoagulation is optional, waiting to see if AF recurs in the absence of the initial precipitating event before initiating anticoagulation treatment is reasonable. A rhythm control rather than a rate control approach is preferred because of the distinct possibility of long-term sinus rhythm maintenance without antiarrhythmic medications. Short-term antiarrhythmic therapy may be considered if the initial AF episode is persistent.

Newly Diagnosed Atrial Fibrillation

Persistent atrial fibrillation

In patients presenting with new-onset symptoms, it may be worth waiting at least 24 hours to determine if the AF self-terminates. At least one attempt at establishing sinus rhythm is reasonable in most patients who have a new diagnosis of AF, because some patients may maintain sinus rhythm for prolonged periods after an initial cardioversion. Older asymptomatic patients who have no precipitating events for AF may be managed with rate control from the beginning. When AF is diagnosed for the first time in a patient, the time of onset of the arrhythmia may or may not be clear based on clinical history. Because it has an impact on anticoagulation decisions for cardioversion, meticulous attention should be paid to establish the time at which AF started. A history of palpitations and dyspnea is unreliable, particularly in elderly patients, and these may signify AF-related heart failure symptoms rather than the onset of the arrhythmia itself. It may be wise to err on the side of indeterminate time of onset in elderly patients and patients who have multiple stroke risk factors and have the patients undergo 3 weeks of anticoagulation or a transesophageal echocardiogram before cardioversion. If the time of onset is clear and less than 48 hours based on the history, particularly in young patients, cardioversion (electrical or pharmacologic) may be considered without anticoagulation.

Paroxysmal atrial fibrillation

Because AF episodes are self-terminating, cardioversion is unnecessary. Antiarrhythmic medications should be avoided until a pattern of recurrent symptomatic episodes is established. Rate control may be needed and should be guided by symptoms. Patients who have minimally symptomatic and infrequent episodes may not need any treatment other than anticoagulation considerations.

Recurrent Atrial Fibrillation

In most patients, persistent or paroxysmal AF recurs after the initial event. Anticoagulation decisions are made based on the risk profile for stroke and are not affected by the persistent or paroxysmal nature of AF. The decision of pursuing a rhythm or rate control strategy depends on individual patient factors. In general, based on general principles (as discussed previously), rate control is favored in older less symptomatic patients. For patients who have infrequent but highly symptomatic persistent AF episodes, a pill-in-the-pocket strategy may be appropriate and can help to reduce the risk for side effects related to long-term antiarrhythmic therapy. Catheter ablation is an option for persistent and paroxysmal AF when antiarrhythmic therapy is ineffective in controlling symptoms.

Permanent Atrial Fibrillation

Permanent atrial fibrillation is a term applied to cases in which patients are allowed to remain in AF without further attempts at rhythm control, because rhythm control is deemed unnecessary or not attainable with a reasonable risk/benefit ratio. Anticoagulation should be administered when indicated based on risk factors. Ventricular rate control must be addressed in all cases.

Tachycardia-Bradycardia Syndrome

Patients who have paroxysmal AF may have high ventricular rates during AF episodes and bradycardia during sinus rhythm. Similarly, patients who have persistent or permanent AF may present with uncontrolled high ventricular rates at times and symptomatic slow ventricular rates at other times. These two situations, in which tachycardia and bradycardia are present in the same patient present a scenario in which rate control and antiarrhythmic medications are difficult to use. Permanent pacemaker implantation usually is necessary to facilitate appropriate therapy. Sinus node dysfunction may resolve after a successful catheter ablation of AF and may be a consideration, particularly in young patients, to avoid the need for permanent pacing.[65]

Atrial Fibrillation with Heart Failure

Patients presenting with heart failure (systolic or diastolic dysfunction) resulting from AF generally have high ventricular rates. Cardioversion to sinus rhythm and initiation of an antiarrhythmic medication (dofetilide or amiodarone) usually are needed, because such patients often do not tolerate beta-blockers or calcium channel blockers for rate control. The need for cardioversion is less clear when ventricular rates are controlled at presentation.

Postoperative Atrial Fibrillation

AF occurs in approximately one third of patients after open heart surgery.[66] It is an important risk factor for postoperative stroke, and anticoagulation should be instituted despite the increased bleeding risk inherent in this setting.[66–68] A meta-analysis of 42 clinical trials showed benefits of beta-blockers, sotalol, and amiodarone in reducing the incidence of postoperative AF.[69] Beta-blockers are recommended routinely for patients undergoing cardiac surgery, and amiodarone may be considered for patients at high risk for postoperative AF.[21]

Atrial Fibrillation and Wolff-Parkinson-White Syndrome

Wolff-Parkinson-White syndrome presents two specific clinical problems with AF. First, an accessory pathway–mediated atrioventricular reentry tachycardia can degenerate into AF. Second, in some patients who have accessory pathways capable of rapid conduction to the ventricle, the AF may degenerate into ventricular fibrillation and cause sudden death.[70] Electrical cardioversion is necessary if patients are hemodynamically unstable. In stable patients, intravenous procainamide or amiodarone can be used to slow conduction over the accessory pathway. Intravenous beta-blockers and calcium channel blockers could result in hypotension and accelerated conduction over the accessory pathway and are contraindicated in this setting. Digoxin also is contraindicated in this setting because of concerns of accelerated conduction over the accessory pathway and the paradoxical effect of increased ventricular rates from AV node blockade.[21] Definitive therapy is radiofrequency ablation of the accessory pathway.

SUMMARY

The primary goals in the management of patients who have AF are the prevention of stroke and cardiomyopathy and the amelioration of symptoms.

Each patient presents to a physician with a specific constellation of symptoms and signs, but, fortunately, most patients can be assigned to broad categories of therapy. For some, anticoagulation and rate control suffice, whereas others require more aggressive attempts to restore and maintain sinus rhythm. Physicians and patients need to be willing to alter therapeutic plans if an initial strategy of rate or rhythm control is unsuccessful.

REFERENCES

1. Benjamin EJ, Wolf PA, D'Agostino RB, et al. Impact of atrial fibrillation on the risk of death: the Framingham heart study. Circulation 1998;98(10):946–52.
2. Heppell RM, Berkin KE, McLenachan JM, et al. Haemostatic and haemodynamic abnormalities associated with left atrial thrombosis in non-rheumatic atrial fibrillation. Heart 1997;77(5):407–11.
3. Conway DS, Pearce LA, Chin BS, et al. Prognostic value of plasma von Willebrand factor and soluble P-selectin as indices of endothelial damage and platelet activation in 994 patients with nonvalvular atrial fibrillation. Circulation 2003;107(25):3141–5.
4. Wolf PA, Abbott RD, Kannel WB. Atrial fibrillation as an independent risk factor for stroke: the Framingham study. Stroke 1991;22(8):983–8.
5. Lin HJ, Wolf PA, Kelly-Hayes M, et al. Stroke severity in atrial fibrillation. The Framingham study. Stroke 1996;27(10):1760–4.
6. Stafford RS, Singer DE. National patterns of warfarin use in atrial fibrillation. Arch Intern Med 1996; 156(22):2537–41.
7. Waldo AL, Becker RC, Tapson VF, et al. NABOR Steering Committee. Hospitalized patients with atrial fibrillation and a high risk of stroke are not being provided with adequate anticoagulation. J Am Coll Cardiol 2005;46(9):1729–36.
8. Wyse DG, Waldo AL, DiMarco JP, et al. Atrial Fibrillation Follow-up Investigation of Rhythm Management (AFFIRM) Investigators. A comparison of rate control and rhythm control in patients with atrial fibrillation. N Engl J Med 2002;347(23):1825–33.
9. Van Gelder IC, Hagens VE, Bosker HA, et al. Rate Control Versus Electrical Cardioversion for Persistent Atrial Fibrillation Study Group. A comparison of rate control and rhythm control in patients with recurrent persistent atrial fibrillation. N Engl J Med 2002; 347(23):1834–40.
10. Shinbane JS, Wood MA, Jensen DN, et al. Tachycardia-induced cardiomyopathy: a review of animal models and clinical studies. J Am Coll Cardiol 1997;29(4):709–15.
11. Ozcan C, Jahangir A, Friedman PA, et al. Significant effects of atrioventricular node ablation and pacemaker implantation on left ventricular function and

long-term survival in patients with atrial fibrillation and left ventricular dysfunction. Am J Cardiol 2003; 92(1):33–7.

12. Nerheim P, Birger-Botkin S, Piracha L, et al. Heart failure and sudden death in patients with tachycardia-induced cardiomyopathy and recurrent tachycardia. Circulation 2004;110(3):247–52.

13. Padanilam BJ, Prystowsky EN. New antiarrhythmic agents for the prevention and treatment of atrial fibrillation. J Cardiovasc Electrophysiol 2006;17: S62–6.

14. Corley SD, Epstein AE, DiMarco JP, et al. AFFIRM Investigators. Relationships between sinus rhythm, treatment, and survival in the Atrial Fibrillation Follow-up Investigation of Rhythm Management (AFFIRM) Study. Circulation 2004; 109(12):1509–13.

15. Pappone C, Rosanio S, Augello G, et al. Mortality, morbidity, and quality of life after circumferential pulmonary vein ablation for atrial fibrillation: outcomes from a controlled nonrandomized long-term study. J Am Coll Cardiol 2003;42(2):185–97.

16. Wazni OM, Marrouche NF, Martin DO, et al. Radiofrequency ablation vs antiarrhythmic drugs as first-line treatment of symptomatic atrial fibrillation: a randomized trial. JAMA 2005;293(21):2634–40.

17. Feinberg WM, Blackshear JL, Laupacis A, et al. Prevalence, age distribution, and gender of patients with atrial fibrillation. Analysis and implications. Arch Intern Med 1995;155(5):469–73.

18. Wolf PA, Benjamin EJ, Belanger AJ, et al. Secular trends in the prevalence of atrial fibrillation: the Framingham study. Am Heart J 1996;131(4):790–5.

19. Anonymous. Risk factors for stroke and efficacy of antithrombotic therapy in atrial fibrillation. Analysis of pooled data from five randomized controlled trials. Arch Intern Med 1994;154(13):1449–57.

20. Gage BF, Waterman AD, Shannon W, et al. Validation of clinical classification schemes for predicting stroke: results from the National Registry of Atrial Fibrillation. JAMA 2001;285(22):2864–70.

21. Fuster V, Ryden LE, Cannom DS, et al. American College of Cardiology/American Heart Association Task Force on Practice Guidelines; European Society of Cardiology Committee for Practice Guidelines; European Heart Rhythm Association; Heart Rhythm Society. ACC/AHA/ESC 2006 guidelines for the management of patients with atrial fibrillation: a report of the American College of Cardiology/American Heart Association Task Force on Practice Guidelines and the European Society of Cardiology Committee for Practice Guidelines (Writing Committee to Revise the 2001 Guidelines for the Management of Patients With Atrial Fibrillation): developed in collaboration with the European Heart Rhythm Association and the Heart Rhythm Society. Circulation 2006;114(7): e257–354.

22. Hart RG, Halperin JL. Atrial fibrillation and thromboembolism: a decade of progress in stroke prevention. Ann Intern Med 1999;131(9):688–95.

23. Singer DE, Albers GW, Dalen JE, et al. Antithrombotic therapy in atrial fibrillation: the seventh ACCP conference on antithrombotic and thrombolytic Therapy. Chest 2004;126(Suppl 3):429S–56S.

24. Hylek EM, Go AS, Chang Y, et al. Effect of intensity of oral anticoagulation on stroke severity and mortality in atrial fibrillation. N Engl J Med 2003; 349(11):1019–26.

25. Hart RG, Halperin JL, Pearce LA, et al. Stroke Prevention in Atrial Fibrillation Investigators. Lessons from the stroke prevention in Atrial Fibrillation Trials. Ann Intern Med 2003;138(10):831–8.

26. Friberg J, Scharling H, Gadsboll N, et al. Copenhagen City Heart Study. Comparison of the impact of atrial fibrillation on the risk of stroke and cardiovascular death in women versus men (The Copenhagen City Heart Study). Am J Cardiol 2004;94(7): 889–94.

27. Hylek EM, Evans-Molina C, Shea C, et al. Major hemorrhage and tolerability of warfarin in the first year of therapy among elderly patients with atrial fibrillation. Circulation 2007;115(21):2689–96.

28. Connolly S, Pogue J, Hart R, et al. ACTIVE Writing Group on behalf of the ACTIVE Investigators. Clopidogrel plus aspirin versus oral anticoagulation for atrial fibrillation in the Atrial Fibrillation Clopidogrel Trial with Irbesartan for Prevention of Vascular Events (ACTIVE W): a randomised controlled trial. Lancet 2006;367(9526):1903–12.

29. Kaul S, Diamond GA, Weintraub WS. Trials and tribulations of non-inferiority: the ximelagatran experience. J Am Coll Cardiol 2005;46(11):1986–95.

30. Blackshear JL, Johnson WD, Odell JA, et al. Thoracoscopic extracardiac obliteration of the left atrial appendage for stroke risk reduction in atrial fibrillation. J Am Coll Cardiol 2003;42(7):1249–52.

31. Ostermayer SH, Reisman M, Kramer PH, et al. Percutaneous left atrial appendage transcatheter occlusion (PLAATO system) to prevent stroke in high-risk patients with non-rheumatic atrial fibrillation: results from the International Multi-Center Feasibility Trials. J Am Coll Cardiol 2005;46(1):9–14

32. Arnold AZ, Mick MJ, Mazurek RP, et al. Role of prophylactic anticoagulation for direct current cardioversion in patients with atrial fibrillation or atrial flutter. J Am Coll Cardiol 1992;19(4):851–5.

33. Klein AL, Grimm RA, Murray RD, et al. Assessment of Cardioversion Using Transesophageal Echocardiography Investigators. Use of transesophageal echocardiography to guide cardioversion in patients with atrial fibrillation. N Engl J Med 2001;344(19) 1411–20.

34. Stellbrink C, Nixdorff U, Hofmann T, et al. ACE (Anticoagulation in Cardioversion Using Enoxaparin

Study Group. Safety and efficacy of enoxaparin compared with unfractionated heparin and oral anti-coagulants for prevention of thromboembolic complications in cardioversion of nonvalvular atrial fibrillation: the Anticoagulation in Cardioversion Using Enoxaparin (ACE) trial. Circulation 2004; 109(8):997–1003.

35. Carlsson J, Miketic S, Windeler J, et al. STAF Investigators. Randomized trial of rate-control versus rhythm-control in persistent atrial fibrillation: the Strategies of Treatment of Atrial Fibrillation (STAF) study. J Am Coll Cardiol 2003;41(10):1690–6.

36. Hohnloser SH, Kuck KH, Lilienthal J. Rhythm or rate control in atrial fibrillation—Pharmacological Intervention in Atrial Fibrillation (PIAF): a randomised trial. Lancet 2000;356(9244):1789–94.

37. Opolski G, Torbicki A, Kosior DA, et al. Investigators of the Polish How to Treat Chronic Atrial Fibrillation Study. Rate control vs rhythm control in patients with nonvalvular persistent atrial fibrillation: the results of the Polish How to Treat Chronic Atrial Fibrillation (HOT CAFE) Study. Chest 2004;126(2): 476–86.

38. Hsu LF, Jais P, Sanders P, et al. Catheter ablation for atrial fibrillation in congestive heart failure. N Engl J Med 2004;351(23):2373–83.

39. Gentlesk PJ, Sauer WH, Gerstenfeld EP, et al. Reversal of left ventricular dysfunction following ablation of atrial fibrillation. J Cardiovasc Electrophysiol 2007; 18(1):9–14.

40. Deedwania PC, Singh BN, Ellenbogen K, et al. Spontaneous conversion and maintenance of sinus rhythm by amiodarone in patients with heart failure and atrial fibrillation: observations from the Veterans Affairs Congestive Heart Failure Survival Trial of Antiarrhythmic Therapy (CHF-STAT). The Department of Veterans Affairs CHF-STAT Investigators. Circulation 1998;98(23):2574–9.

41. Pedersen OD, Bagger H, Keller N, et al. Efficacy of dofetilide in the treatment of atrial fibrillation-flutter in patients with reduced left ventricular function: a Danish Investigations of Arrhythmia and Mortality on Dofetilide (DIAMOND) substudy. Circulation 2001; 104(3):292–6.

42. Roy D, Talajic M, Nattel S, et al. Rhythm control versus rate control for atrial fibrillation and heart failure. N Engl J Med 2008;358:2667.

43. Cooper HA, Bloomfield DA, Bush DE, et al. AFFIRM Study Investigators. Relation between achieved heart rate and outcomes in patients with atrial fibrillation (from the Atrial Fibrillation Follow-up Investigation of Rhythm Management [AFFIRM] Study). Am J Cardiol 2004;93:1247–53.

44. Prystowsky EN. Assessment of rhythm and rate control in patients with atrial fibrillation. J Cardiovasc Electrophysiol 2006;17(2):S7–10.

45. Bjerregaard P, Bailey WB, Robinson SE. Rate control in patients with chronic atrial fibrillation. Am J Cardiol 2004;93(3):329–32.

46. Meng F, Yoshikawa T, Baba A, et al. Beta-blockers are effective in congestive heart failure patients with atrial fibrillation. J Card Fail 2003;9(5):398–403.

47. Khand AU, Rankin AC, Martin W, et al. Carvedilol alone or in combination with digoxin for the management of atrial fibrillation in patients with heart failure? J Am Coll Cardiol 2003;42(11):1944–51.

48. Scardi S, Humar F, Pandullo C, et al. Oral clonidine for heart rate control in chronic atrial fibrillation. Lancet 1993;341(8854):1211–2.

49. Wood MA, Brown-Mahoney C, Kay GN, et al. Clinical outcomes after ablation and pacing therapy for atrial fibrillation: a meta-analysis. Circulation 2000; 101(10):1138–44.

50. Weerasooriya R, Davis M, Powell A, et al. The Australian Intervention Randomized Control of Rate in Atrial Fibrillation Trial (AIRCRAFT). J Am Coll Cardiol 2003;41(10):1697–702.

51. Wilkoff BL, Cook JR, Epstein AE, et al. Dual Chamber and VVI Implantable Defibrillator Trial Investigators. Dual-chamber pacing or ventricular backup pacing in patients with an implantable defibrillator: the Dual Chamber and VVI Implantable Defibrillator (DAVID) trial. JAMA 2002;288(24):3115–23.

52. Simantirakis EN, Vardakis KE, Kochiadakis GE, et al. Left ventricular mechanics during right ventricular apical or left ventricular-based pacing in patients with chronic atrial fibrillation after atrioventricular junction ablation. J Am Coll Cardiol 2004;43(6): 1013–8.

53. Garrigue S, Bordachar P, Reuter S, et al. Comparison of permanent left ventricular and biventricular pacing in patients with heart failure and chronic atrial fibrillation: prospective haemodynamic study. Heart 2002;87(6):529–34.

54. Doshi RN, Daoud EG, Fellows C, et al. PAVE Study Group. Left ventricular-based cardiac stimulation post AV nodal ablation evaluation (the PAVE study). J Cardiovasc Electrophysiol 2005;16(11):1160–5.

55. Preliminary report: effect of encainide and flecainide on mortality in a randomized trial of arrhythmia suppression after myocardial infarction. N Engl J Med 1989;321:406–12.

56. Lafuente-Lafuente C, Mouly S, Longas-Tejero MA, et al. Antiarrhythmic drugs for maintaining sinus rhythm after cardioversion of atrial fibrillation: a systematic review of randomized controlled trials. Arch Intern Med 2006;166(7):719–28 [review] [63 refs].

57. Roden DM, Woosley RL, Primm RK. Incidence and clinical features of the quinidine-associated long QT syndrome: implications for patient care. Am Heart J 1986;111(6):1088–93.

58. Roy D, Talajic M, Dorian P, et al. Amiodarone to prevent recurrence of atrial fibrillation. Canadian Trial of Atrial Fibrillation Investigators. N Engl J Med 2000; 342(13):913–20.

59. Zimetbaum P. Amiodarone for atrial fibrillation. N Engl J Med 2007;356(9):935–41.

60. Alboni P, Botto GL, Baldi N, et al. Outpatient treatment of recent-onset atrial fibrillation with the "pill-in-the-pocket" approach. N Engl J Med 2004; 351(23):2384–91.

61. Haissaguerre M, Jais P, Shah DC, et al. Spontaneous initiation of atrial fibrillation by ectopic beats originating in the pulmonary veins. N Engl J Med 1998;339(10):659–66.

62. Haissaguerre M, Jais P, Shah DC, et al. Electrophysiological end point for catheter ablation of atrial fibrillation initiated from multiple pulmonary venous foci. Circulation 2000;101(12):1409–17.

63. Padanilam BJ, Prystowsky EN. Should ablation be first-line therapy and for whom: the antagonist position. Circulation 2005;112(8):1223–9.

64. Cox J, Schuessler R, Lappas D. An 8½ -year clinical experience with surgery for atrial fibrillation. Ann Surg 1996;224(3):267–75.

65. Hocini M, Sanders P, Deisenhofer I, et al. Reverse remodeling of sinus node function after catheter ablation of atrial fibrillation in patients with prolonged sinus pauses. Circulation 2003;108(10):1172–5.

66. McKeown PP, Gutterman D. Executive summary: American College of Chest Physicians guidelines for the prevention and management of postoperative atrial fibrillation after cardiac surgery. Chest 2005; 128(Suppl 2):1S–5S.

67. Stamou SC, Hill PC, Dangas G, et al. Stroke after coronary artery bypass: incidence, predictors, and clinical outcome. Stroke 2001;32(7): 1508–13.

68. Taylor GJ, Malik SA, Colliver JA, et al. Usefulness of atrial fibrillation as a predictor of stroke after isolated coronary artery bypass grafting. Am J Cardiol 1987; 60(10):905–7.

69. Crystal E, Connolly SJ, Sleik K, et al. Interventions on prevention of postoperative atrial fibrillation in patients undergoing heart surgery: a meta-analysis. Circulation 2002;106(1):75–80.

70. Klein GJ, Bashore TM, Sellers TD, et al. Ventricular fibrillation in the Wolff-Parkinson-White syndrome. N Engl J Med 1979;301(20):1080–5.

Atrial Fibrillation: Unanswered Questions and Future Directions

Vivek Y. Reddy, MD

KEYWORDS

• Atrial fibrillation • Ablation • New technology

Just over a decade ago, Haissaguerre and colleagues[1] provided the seminal demonstration of the role of pulmonary vein (PV) triggers in the pathogenesis of atrial fibrillation (AF) and the potential therapeutic role of catheter ablation to treat patients who have paroxysmal AF. This initial observation ushered in the modern era of catheter ablation to treat patients who have AF, and tremendous progress has been made in understanding its pathogenesis and the catheter approaches to treating this rhythm. Although the current state of AF catheter ablation is well described elsewhere in this issue, this article reflects on some of the major unanswered questions about AF management, and the future technologic and investigational directions being explored in the nonpharmacologic management of AF.

CATHETER ABLATION OF PAROXYSMAL ATRIAL FIBRILLATION

After the initial demonstration that the PVs harbor most of the triggers for paroxysmal AF, the approach to catheter ablation in this patient population evolved considerably. The initial approaches centered on inducing and identifying the specific AF triggering sites within the PVs and targeting these for catheter ablation.[1,2] From a safety and efficacy perspective, empiric isolation of all PVs was clearly a much more suitable strategy.[3–6]

The poor efficacy of ablating AF triggers stems from the difficulty in inducing these initiating foci during any given electrophysiology ablation procedure. During these early procedures, electrophysiologists often spent many hours with multiple catheters positioned in various PVs waiting for AF-initiating premature ectopic depolarizations to occur. Beyond this prolonged case duration, these procedures were often followed by clinical recurrences related to additional initiating foci at sites completely unelicited during the index ablation procedure. By empirically ablating around the PV ostia to isolate all veins electrically, however, one could ensure that no PV triggers would affect the left atrium, proper.

Empiric PV isolation also has one very important safety advantage compared with focal ablation of AF triggers. Briefly, ablation deep within the PVs can result in PV stenosis, a dreaded complication that has a strong tendency to recur as restenosis after balloon venoplasty. If the circumferential isolating ablation lesion set is placed outside the PVs, however, the risk for stenosis is minimized.

Based on the improved efficacy and safety of empiric PV isolation, several approaches have been forwarded to achieve this electrophysiologic end point. These approaches include using contrast angiography to identify and target the PV ostia; targeting the ostia using electroanatomic mapping systems to localize the catheter tip

A version of this article originally appeared in *Medical Clinics of North America*, volume 92, issue 1.

This work was supported in part by the Deane Institute for Integrative Research in Atrial Fibrillation and Stroke. Dr. Reddy has received grant support or served as a consultant to Biosense-Webster, CardioFocus, Cryocath Technologies, GE Medical Systems, Hansen Medical, Philips Medical Systems, ProRhythm, St. Jude Medical, and Stereotaxis.

University of Miami Hospital Cardiovascular Clinic, Electrophysiology, So. Building, 1295 NW 14th Street, Miami, FL 33125, USA

E-mail address: v.reddy@miami.edu

Cardiol Clin 27 (2009) 201–216

doi:10.1016/j.ccl.2008.10.002

0733-8651/08/$ – see front matter © 2009 Elsevier Inc. All rights reserved.

(with or without the incorporation of preacquired three-dimensional CT scans or MRIs); and using intracardiac echocardiography to position a circular mapping catheter at the PV ostia and target the electrograms for ablation. Regardless of the approach used during the index procedure, the mechanism of arrhythmia recurrence is virtually always caused by electrical PV reconnection.[7] That is, point-to-point ablation lesions are placed completely to encircle the PVs during the initial ablation procedure. Because the ablation lesions cannot be directly visualized, however, a surrogate marker for lesion integrity is used: the lack of electrical conduction across the ablation lesions at the end of the procedure. If the tissue at one of these sites is damaged but not fully necrotic from the ablation, however, PV to left atrial conduction can recur several weeks later after tissue healing is complete, leading to clinical AF recurrences. The difference in clinical outcome after ablation of paroxysmal AF is very likely related directly to the ability of the operator to manipulate and stably position the ablation catheter with the requisite force to generate effective ablation lesions.

The most important goal during catheter ablation of paroxysmal AF is to achieve permanent PV isolation. To improve the technical feasibility of the procedure and thereby improve the continuity of the isolating ablation lesion sets, extensive effort has been made to improve the ablation technology. These various technologic advances can be broadly separated into two groups: remote navigation technology to provide for precise navigation with the hope that this translates to improved lesion contiguity, and balloon ablation catheter technology using various ablation energy sources designed to isolate the PVs in a facile manner.

REMOTE NAVIGATION TECHNOLOGY

Currently, two remote navigation systems are available for clinical use: a magnetic navigation system (Niobe II system, Stereotaxis, St. Louis, Missouri) and a robotic navigation system (Sensei system, Hansen Medical, Mountain View, California).

Remote Magnetic Navigation

The magnetic navigation system (**Fig. 1**) uses two large external magnets positioned on either side of the fluoroscopy table to generate a uniform magnetic field (0.08 T) of approximately 15-cm diameter within the patient's chest.[8] Specialized ablation catheters are used with this system; briefly, these catheters are extremely floppy along their distal end, and have magnets embedded at the tip of the catheter. When placed within the patient's heart, the catheter tip aligns with the orientation of the generated magnetic field. The operator uses a software interface to manipulate the magnetic field, and by extension, the tip of the ablation catheter. This ability to manipulate the magnetic field provides the first level of freedom of movement with this system. The other level of freedom

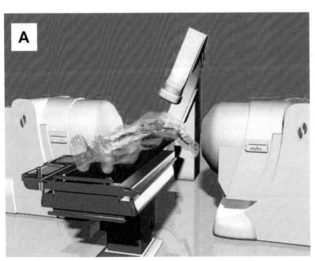
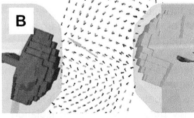
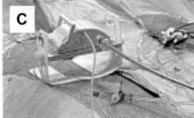

Fig. 1. (*A*) The magnetic navigation system uses two large magnets positioned on either side of the fluoroscopy table. (*B*) These magnets can generate a uniform magnetic field in virtually any direction so that magnetically enabled catheters orient in the same direction as the field. (*C*) A disposable catheter advancement system is positioned at the femoral puncture site to advance or retract the catheter remotely. (*Courtesy of* Stereotaxis, St Louis, Missouri; with permission.)

of movement is the ability remotely to advance or retract the catheter tip. This function is possible using a computer-controlled catheter advancer system consisting of a disposable plastic unit positioned at the femoral catheter insertion site. The catheter shaft is affixed to this unit where it enters the sheath, and can transduce the remote operator instructions to advance or retract the catheter appropriately. This combination of remote catheter advancement-retraction and magnetic field manipulation allows the operator a great deal of flexibility in intracardiac catheter manipulation.

This magnetic navigation system is now integrated with one of the electroanatomic mapping systems (CARTO RMT, Biosense Webster, Diamond Bar, CA). The mapping system can precisely localize the catheter tip in space to a submillimeter resolution (**Fig. 2**A). Through precisely tracking the catheter location, this combination of mapping and navigation systems allows for a novel capability: automated chamber mapping. Briefly, the operator remotely manipulates the catheter within the left atrium to a few defined anatomic locations (eg, the ostia of the various PVs, the mitral valve annulus) and, based on these parameters, the system automatically manipulates the catheter throughout the chamber to facilitate the creation of an electroanatomic map. Future iterations of the software are planned to allow the system automatically to manipulate the catheter tip to create linear ablation lesions with the chamber as per the operator's wishes. The efficiency and

accuracy of these automatic software solutions, however, remain to be determined. The other significant advance is the ability to incorporate preacquired three-dimensional MRIs or CT scans into the system to allow mapping on a realistic model of the heart.

With the current generation software, some clinical data are available on its efficacy for AF ablation. In a consecutive series of 40 patients, Pappone and colleagues[9] used the mapping and navigation systems in tandem to determine the feasibility of circumferential PV ablation in patients undergoing catheter ablation of AF. Using a 4-mm tip ablation catheter (with the requisite embedded magnets), they showed that the left atrium and PVs could be successfully mapped in 38 of 40 patients. Ablation lesions were placed in a circumferential fashion for a maximum of 15 seconds at any endocardial ablation site. They reported that procedure times decreased significantly with increased operator experience. Although this study clearly showed the feasibility of remote mapping of the left atrium and PVs, the procedural end point was not electrical PV isolation in the standard electrophysiologic sense. Instead, the end point was ">90% reduction in the bipolar electrogram amplitude, and/or peak-to-peak bipolar electrogram amplitude <0.1 mV inside the line."[9] The significance of this end point is unclear.

To address some of these uncertainties, DiBiase and colleagues[10] examined the efficacy of PV isolation using this remote navigation system in

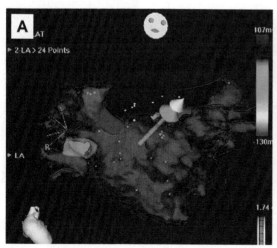
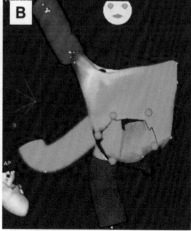

Fig. 2. (*A*) The magnetic navigation system is integrated with an electroanatomic mapping system that also permits integration of three-dimensional CT or MRI models. Once integrated, the magnetic field can be directly controlled with the computer mouse to the desired direction. The yellow arrow represents the current direction of magnetic field and the green arrow represents the desired direction of the field. Note that the catheter is oriented in the same direction as the field. (*B*) Magnetically enabled irrigated ablation catheters are not currently available for clinical use. As shown in this anterior view of the left atrial anatomic map, however, this catheter has been used in experimental protocols to show the ability to map the porcine left atrium and pulmonary veins.

a series of 45 patients using a stepwise approach. First, the ability remotely to map the chamber was again confirmed in this study. Second, these investigators performed circumferential ablation using the same 4-mm tip radiofrequency ablation catheter as described in the initial paper by Pappone and colleagues.[9] When a circular mapping catheter was deployed into the PVs to assess more precisely for vein isolation, no veins in any patient were shown to be electrically isolated. The operators then used the circular mapping catheter to guide the ablation catheter remotely to isolate the vein antra, but electrical disconnection was attained in only four veins in four different patients (8%). In the remaining 41 patients (92%), no evidence was found of disconnection in any of the veins. When the operators then targeted a portion of the veins using a standard manual radiofrequency ablation catheter (ie, not using the remote navigation system), however, they were able to achieve electrical isolation in all attempted veins.

Despite the sharply improved procedural outcome with manual catheter manipulation, concluding that PV isolation is not possible using the magnetic navigation system is inappropriate. Unlike with remote navigation, manual ablation in this study was performed using an irrigated radiofrequency ablation catheter. Unlike with standard radiofrequency ablation, irrigated ablation allows the operator safely to deliver more energy into

the tissue, thereby achieving deeper ablation lesions. Significant charring on the ablation catheter tip was seen in 15 (33%) of 45 procedures when using the standard remote 4-mm tip ablation catheter. The critical information that remains to be determined is whether remote PV isolation can be reproducibly achieved using an irrigated ablation catheter. An irrigated ablation catheter with the requisite embedded magnets to permit remote navigation exists but, at the time of this writing, has not been used clinically. In the experimental animal setting, however, the author has shown that this catheter can be remotely manipulated to map all chambers of the porcine heart (**Fig. 2B**), and can deliver ablation lesions of similar quality to those seen using a manual irrigated ablation catheter (Vivek Y. Reddy, unpublished data, 2006). How this finding translates during clinical use of this remote irrigated catheter will not be known until the ongoing studies are completed.

Remote Robotic Navigation

The remote navigation capability of the robotic system (Sensei) is based on multiple pullwires that control the deflection capability of two steerable sheaths.[11,12] Briefly, this is a "master-slave" electromechanical system that controls an internal steerable guide sheath and an external steerable sheath (**Fig. 3**). The internal sheath contains four

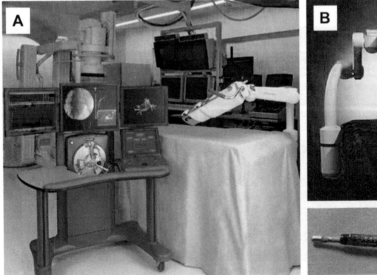
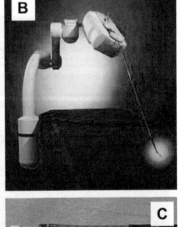
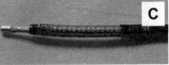

Fig. 3. The primary components of the robotic navigation system are shown (A) including the workstation and the robotic arm (B), which can be mounted at the foot of any standard fluoroscopy table. The two-piece sheath system extends from this robotic arm and is inserted through the femoral venous puncture site. (C) Any standard ablation catheter can be manipulated within the heart by simply placing the catheter within the sheath system so that the tip of the catheter is protruding just beyond the tip of the inner sheath. (*Courtesy of* Hansen Medical Mountain View, California; with permission.)

pullwires located at each quadrant; the range of motion includes deflection in 360 degrees and the ability to insert and withdraw. The external sheath has a single pullwire to permit deflection, and can rotate and insert and withdraw. This combination of movements allows for a broad range of motion in virtually any direction. Unlike the magnetic navigation system, most standard ablation catheters can be used with this system, because the inner steerable sheath can accommodate any catheter up to 8.3-French catheter diameter. By fixing the mapping-ablation catheter so that it is just protruding beyond the tip of the inner system, remotely driving these steerable sheaths translates to remote navigation of the catheter tip. The steerable sheaths are attached to the remote robotic arm unit, which can be mounted to any standard radiography procedure table. Using a software interface, a three-dimensional joystick allows the operator remotely to drive the catheter tip. Movements of the joystick are translated into a complex series of manipulations by the pullwires governing sheath motion.

The author examined the feasibility of synchronizing this robotic navigation system with electroanatomic mapping and three-dimensional CT imaging to perform view-synchronized left atrial ablation (**Fig. 4**).[13] The mapping catheter was remotely manipulated with the robotic navigation system within the registered three-dimensional CT image of the left atrial PVs. The initial porcine experimental phase (N = 9) validated the ability of view-synchronized robotic navigation to guide atrial mapping and ablation. An irrigated radiofrequency ablation catheter was able to be navigated

remotely into all of the PVs, the left atrial appendage, and circumferentially along the mitral valve annulus. In addition, circumferential radiofrequency ablation lesions were applied periosteally to ablate 11 porcine PVs. The consequent clinical phase (N = 9 patients who had AF) established that this paradigm could be successfully applied for all of the major aspects of catheter ablation of paroxysmal or chronic AF: electrical PV isolation in an extraostial fashion, isolation of the superior vena cava, and linear atrial ablation of typical and atypical atrial flutters. The electrophysiologic end point of electrical PV isolation, as verified using a circular mapping catheter, was achieved in all patients. This study showed the safety and feasibility of an emerging paradigm for AF ablation involving the confluence of three technologies: (1) three-dimensional imaging, (2) electroanatomic mapping, and (3) remote navigation. This study involved a minimal number of patients, however, treated by a single center. The long-term safety and efficacy of PV isolation performed by multiple operators in a larger patient cohort using this robotic navigation system remains to be established.

Image Guidance

Three-dimensional imaging is playing an increasingly important role in guiding ablation procedures. It is now standard to integrate patient-specific preacquired three-dimensional models of the left atrium and PVs (generated using either contrast-enhanced CT or MRI) with mapping systems to guide better the ablation procedure (**Fig. 5**).[14–19] This approach is somewhat limited, however, by the variable chamber geometry and size that can

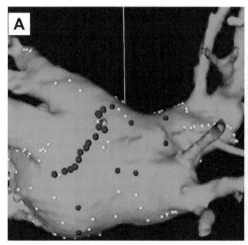
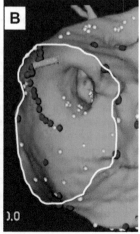

Fig. 4. View-synchronized robotic ablation was performed to treat atrial fibrillation. In this paradigm, the mapping system provided the location of the catheter tip, the CT scan identified where the catheter should be positioned, and the robotic navigation system was used to manipulate the catheter to each location. Shown are an external posterior view (*A*) and a left-sided endoluminal view showing the left pulmonary veins (*B*).

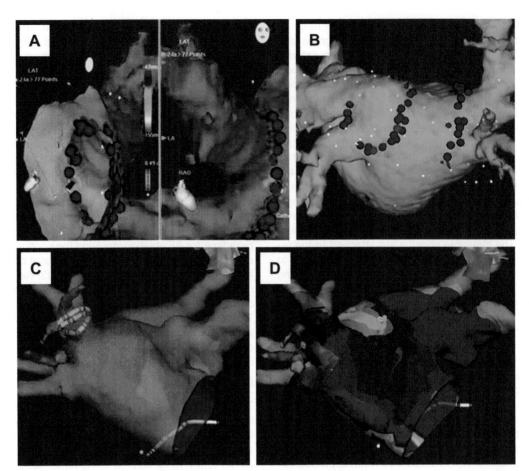

Fig. 5. Three-dimensional CT-MRI integration with electroanatomic mapping systems is now a standard procedure. Once the three-dimensional image is integrated, the ablation catheter can be manipulated to encircle the pulmonary veins with ablation lesions. Shown is integration with either the CARTO RMT (*A, B*) or NavX (*C, D*) systems.

occur as a result of various physiologic factors, such as heart rate, rhythm, and volume state. Accordingly, a significant amount of effort is being devoted to real-time or near real-time imaging of the three-dimensional chamber anatomy during the ablation procedure. The modalities being explored include ultrasound imaging, three-dimensional rotational angiography, and MRI. Although three-dimensional surface transducers are already available for ultrasound imaging, obtaining accurate images of the left atrium and PVs through surface thoracic imaging can be difficult. Three-dimensional intracardiac ultrasound imaging probes do not currently exist; however, localized three-dimensional intracardiac ultrasound probes exist and can be used to generate three-dimensional images. Briefly, this consists of an intracardiac ultrasound catheter with a localization sensor that precisely provides the location and direction of the catheter. Accordingly, a series of high-resolution two-dimensional images can be "stitched" together to generate a near real-time three-dimensional image.

Rotational angiography consists of the injection of contrast followed by rotation of the x-ray fluoroscopy head around the patient to generate a three-dimensional image.[20,21] For example, the contrast can be injected directly into the pulmonary artery, and imaging can be performed during the levo-phase after the contrast traverses the pulmonary vascular bed and flows back through the PVs into the left atrium. As shown in **Fig. 6** a volumetric three-dimensional image of the left atrium and PVs can be generated through properly timing the rotation of the x-ray fluoroscopy unit. The quality of these three-dimensional rotational angiography images was compared with the gold standard, preacquired, three-dimensional CT scans or MRIs in a consecutive series of 42 patients undergoing AF ablation procedures.[2]

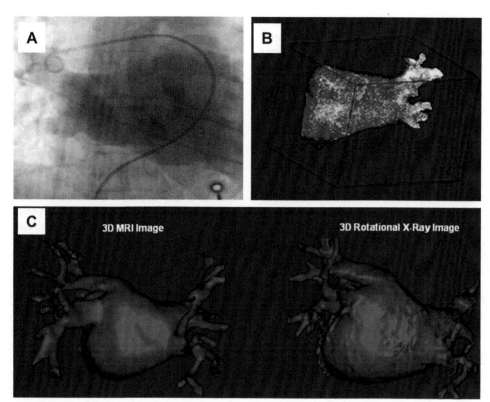

Fig. 6. Rotational angiography imaging can be used to generate volumetric images of the left atrium and pulmonary veins. Contrast is injected from a pigtail catheter positioned in the pulmonary artery, and rotational imaging is performed during the levo phase as the contrast courses back into the left atrium from the pulmonary veins (*A*) to generate a volumetric image of this anatomy (*B*). (*C*) These intraprocedural rotational images are of comparable quality to preacquired three-dimensional MRIs or CT scans.

In this series, most of the three-dimensional rotational angiography acquisitions (71%) were qualitatively sufficient in delineating the left atrial and PV anatomy. A blinded quantitative comparison of PV ostial diameters resulted in an absolute difference of only 2.7 ± 2.3 mm, 2.2 ± 1.8 mm, 2.4 ± 2.2 mm, and 2.2 ± 2.3 mm for the left-superior, left-inferior, right-superior, and right-inferior PVs, respectively. In addition, the feasibility for registering the three-dimensional rotational angiography image with real-time electroanatomic mapping was also shown. More recent reconstruction algorithms that can resolve soft tissue structures are likely further to increase the capability of three-dimensional rotational angiography through improving the image quality of data obtained with the current strategy (of intracardiac contrast injection) and potentially allowing for CT-like imaging of the left atrium and PVs using a peripheral intravenous injection of contrast.

Real-time interventional MRI involves the concept of performing the entire procedure in the MRI environment.[22] In this paradigm, various MRI-compatible catheters are continuously imaged as they are positioned within the patient anatomy. MRI has the advantage of using nonionizing radiation, the ability to resolve soft tissue with high resolution, and the potential for physiologic imaging; for example, during liver tumor ablation, MRI-based thermal imaging has been used directly to image ablation lesion formation. Although this modality is in some respects the most powerful, it is also the one furthest away from clinical practice. A significant amount of research and development is required in the MRI scanning equipment and protocols and MRI-compatible equipment (eg, catheters, patient monitoring equipment). Each of these three-dimensional imaging modalities will likely show a tremendous amount of progress.

BALLOON ABLATION CATHETERS

A significant effort has been put into developing balloon ablation catheter designs quickly, easily, and effectively to isolate the PVs. The first device tested clinically was an ultrasound balloon ablation catheter that delivered energy in a radial fashion at the level of the diameter of the balloon, hence necessitating that the balloon catheter be placed within the PV when delivering energy.[23] This balloon design was suboptimal because the level of electrical isolation typically excluded the proximal portions of the vein, and PV triggers of AF located at this region are not included in the ablation lesion.[24] From a safety perspective, the intravenous location of the energy delivery resulted in PV stenosis. Since this first-generation device, balloon ablation catheters have evolved considerably. Four major balloon-based ablation devices are now used at various stages of clinical evaluation: (1) cryoballoon ablation, (2) endoscopic laser ablation, (3) high-intensity focused ultrasound, and (4) balloon-based radiofrequency ablation (**Fig. 7**). Each of these devices was fashioned to be placed at the PV ostia theoretically to isolate the veins outside their tubular portion.

Balloon Cryoablation

The cryoballoon system is a deflectable catheter (manufactured by Cryocath Technologies, Montreal, Quebec, Canada) with a balloon-within-a-balloon design wherein the cryo refrigerant (N_2O) is delivered within the inner balloon. A constant vacuum is applied between the inner and outer balloons to ensure the absence of refrigerant leakage into the systemic circulation in the event of a breach in the integrity of the inner balloon. The cryoballoon catheter is manufactured in two sizes: 23 mm and 28 mm in diameter. After transseptal puncture, the deflated balloon catheter is deployed through a 12-French catheter deflectable sheath. Once within the left atrium, the inflated balloon is positioned at each respective PV ostium to occlude

blood flow temporarily from the targeted vein. Each balloon-based cryoablation lesion lasts 4 minutes. Because the cyrorefrigerant is delivered to the whole face of the balloon, any tissue in contact with the balloon is ablated. This function can be safely performed because the experimental results have shown that cryothermal ablation is associated with a minimal risk of PV stenosis.[25,26] Similarly, no evidence of stenosis has been seen in the clinical experience, perhaps because at the temperatures achieved with this system, the cryoablative energy is selective toward the cellular elements of the tissue and leaves the connective tissue matrix intact. Accordingly, cryothermy as an energy source seems to have a good safety profile. The long-term efficacy of achieving permanent PV isolation, however, has not been established.

Balloon-Based Visually Guided Laser Ablation

The most unique aspect of this system is the capability for endoscopic visualization using a 2-French catheter endoscope positioned at a proximal location in the balloon. This 12-French catheter laser ablation catheter system (CardioFocus, Marlborough, MA) is delivered using a deflectable sheath. Once in the left atrium, a 20-mm, 25-mm, or 30-mm diameter balloon is inflated and positioned at the PV ostia. The endoscope allows the operator to visualize the internal face of the balloon and identify areas of balloon-tissue contact (blanched white) versus blood (red).[27] An optical fiber that projects a 90-degree to 150-degree arc is advanced and rotated to the desired location for energy delivery. Once the proper location is identified, a diode laser is used to deliver laser energy at 980 nm to isolate electrically the PV. This endoscopic laser balloon catheter provides greater flexibility to the location of energy

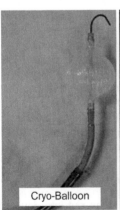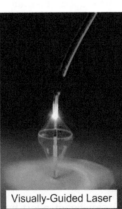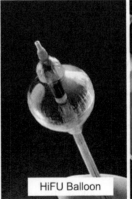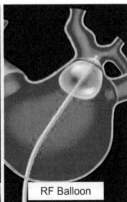

| Cryo-Balloon | Visually-Guided Laser | HiFU Balloon | RF Balloon |

Fig. 7. Four major balloon ablation catheter technologies are currently in clinical trials to assess their safety and efficacy in treating patients who have paroxysmal AF.

deposition and the total amount of energy applied to each site. For example, a greater amount and duration of energy may be applied anteriorly along the ridge between the left-sided PVs and left atrial appendage than that applied along the thinner posterior wall near the course of the esophagus.

Balloon-Based High-Intensity Focused Ultrasound Ablation

The high-intensity focused ultrasound catheter (ProRhythm, Ronkonkoma, NY) is a 14-French catheter system that, once inflated, consists of a fluid-filled balloon in front of a smaller carbon dioxide–filled balloon.[28] The ultrasound transducer delivers energy in a radially directed fashion; this energy reflects off the air-fluid interface to project forward and deposit and concentrate just beyond the face of the balloon. Because of the minimal chance of clot formation when sonicating through blood, contact with the atrial tissue is not necessary for ablation with this catheter. This deflectable catheter is delivered using a nondeflectable 14-French catheter sheath. Lesions are delivered using either a 20-mm or 25-mm diameter balloon catheter for 40 to 60 seconds per lesion. To use this technology to ablate the PVs, a series of partially encircling ablation lesions sometimes must be stitched together as the balloon is precessed about the orifice of each vein.

Balloon-Based Radiofrequency Ablation

This elastic balloon ablation catheter (Toray Industries, Tokyo, Japan) is made of a heat-resistant, antithrombotic resin. Inside the fluid-filled balloon are a coil electrode for the delivery of radiofrequency energy and a thermocouple to monitor the electrode temperature.[29] The radiofrequency generator delivers a high-frequency current (13.56 MHz) to induce capacitive-type heating of the tissue in contact with the balloon. The energy output is modulated to maintain the temperature in the balloon at 60°C to 75°C. During each application of energy, the venous blood is continuously suctioned through the central lumen of the catheter to protect the PV blood from excessive heating, preventing thrombus formation beyond the face of the balloon.

Clinical Overview of Balloon-Based Pulmonary Vein Isolation

Analysis of three-dimensional left atrial–PV surface reconstructions from MRI datasets on patients who had paroxysmal AF showed a marked intrapatient and interpatient variability in PV ostial size and geometry.[30] The challenge to each of the balloon ablation catheters is to negotiate this

venous anatomy so that the lesions are proximal enough to include all of the potentially arrhythmogenic periostial tissue and minimize the risk for PV stenosis. The energy source used also has important implications on the ablation strategy. For example, cryothermal ablation is believed to portend minimal risk for PV stenosis. A balloon cryoablation catheter may be used safely even deep within large common PVs (ie, within the common truck separately to isolate the individual superior and inferior PVs). The adjustable lasing element of the endoscopic balloon catheter, however, allows the operator to vary the circumference and location of the ablative beam. This catheter design may be considerably useful in patients who have veins with marked variability in size and shape. Alternatively, because high-intensity focused ultrasound energy can be delivered through blood with minimal risk, this energy modality might be efficacious in isolating large PV ostial or antral regions through delivering a series of sequential lesions as it is precessed about the long axis of the targeted vein.

Although the clinical experience is still very early, the results from nonrandomized feasibility studies suggest that most patients who have paroxysmal AF can be treated successfully with these balloon devices. Several balloon ablation catheters have received regulatory approval for clinical use in Europe, but none have been approved for general clinical use in the United States. Most of these devices are being studied in a randomized fashion versus antiarrhythmic medications in the United States. These investigations should determine conclusively whether all or any of these catheters can provide facile, safe, and reproducibly effective PV isolation.

CATHETER ABLATION OF NONPAROXYSMAL ATRIAL FIBRILLATION

Unlike catheter ablation of paroxysmal AF, considerably less consensus exists as to the proper approach to catheter ablation of chronic AF. There is a growing understanding that as the pathophysiology of AF progresses from the paroxysmal to the persistent and eventual permanent state, significant electrophysiologic and structural changes occur. These changes in ion channel physiology and increased extracellular fibrosis are believed to potentiate atrial myocardial substrate-driven reentry. When progressing on the continuum from paroxysmal to permanent AF, the pathophysiologic importance of focal triggers diminishes and the importance of substrate-driven reentry increases. Furthermore, because the latter perpetuating sources of AF are typically located outside the PVs in the atrial tissue itself, the efficacy of PV isolation alone is believed to decline in nonparoxysmal AF. This hypothesis has never been addressed conclusively, however, because of the clinical difficulty in achieving permanent PV isolation. That is, because permanent vein isolation is difficult to achieve reproducibly, whether the cause of clinical arrhythmia recurrence is resumption of PV conduction or from the extravenous perpetuators of AF cannot be determined. If one or more of the balloon ablation catheters can consistently achieve permanent PV isolation, this cause can be determined. Because of the limitations of current technology, however, a PV isolation-alone strategy is ineffective in many patients who have nonparoxysmal AF.

Intraoperative mapping studies of AF suggested the role of perpetuators of AF. These studies showed that complex fractionated atrial electrograms (CFAEs) were observed mostly in areas of slow conduction or at pivot points where the wavelets turn around at the end of the arcs of functional blocks (**Fig. 8**).[31] These areas of fractionated electrograms during AF represent either continuous reentry of the fibrillation waves into the same area, or overlap of different wavelets entering the same area at different times. This complex electrical activity was characterized by a short cycle length and heterogeneous temporal and spatial distribution in humans. This observation led Nademanee and colleagues[32] to hypothesize that, if the areas of CFAEs could be identified through catheter mapping during AF, locating the areas where the wavelets reenter would be possible. They showed that they could terminate AF in 95% of patients, and reported that most patients were free of arrhythmia symptoms after these CFAE sites were ablated. These investigators concluded from this experience that CFAE sites represent the electrophysiologic substrate for AF and can be effectively targeted for ablation to achieve normal sinus rhythm.

Despite these encouraging clinical results, one of the difficulties other investigators have encountered in attempting to reproduce these results is the relative subjectivity inherent in defining whether a particular electrogram is complex enough to warrant ablation. To standardize the definition of a CFAE site, signal processing software to analyze atrial electrograms during AF is being developed. Several mapping systems now contain signal processing software to quantify the degree of electrogram complexity. Further clinical work is necessary, however, to determine whether catheter ablation of the sites identified by these software algorithms can truly convert AF into sinus rhythm.

Given the current clinical data, catheter ablation of chronic AF has evolved into an approach that incorporates strategies to address the AF triggers and perpetuators (ie, electrical isolation of the PVs to isolate the former, and ablation within the atria to eliminate the latter). Specifically, this stepwise approach initially involves electrical PV isolation and then targeting of CFAE sites within the left atrium, particularly the interatrial septum, the base of the left atrial appendage, and the inferior left atrium along the coronary sinus.[33] During this progressive ablation strategy, the rhythm often converts from AF to organized macroreentrant or microreentrant atrial tachycardias. These organized atrial tachycardias are then targeted for ablation to terminate the rhythm to sinus. Although feasible, this approach is limited by the long procedural duration and the extremely high rate of atrial tachycardia recurrence mandating second, and even third, ablation procedures.[34]

Further technical and scientific advances are required to refine the ablation approach to overcome these limitations. One promising approach to these reentrant atrial tachycardias is to use multielectrode mapping catheters in conjunction with advanced mapping systems rapidly to map these complex tachycardias (**Fig. 9**). In conclusion, although many questions are unanswered regarding ablation of nonparoxysmal AF, many patients at this end of the disease spectrum clearly require a more extensive procedure that is still being defined.

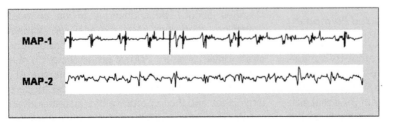

Fig. 8. Shown are two electrograms during AF. MAP-1 is a site with the usual degree of complexity (likely a passive site that would not be targeted for ablation) whereas MAP-2 is a site of complex fractionated activity (this site would be targeted for ablation) Note the continuous nature of electrogram activity in the latter

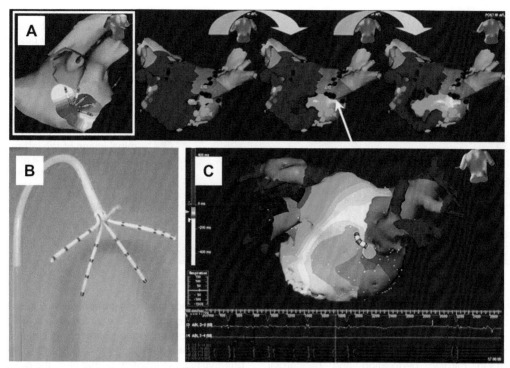

Fig. 9. (A) One paradigm for rapid mapping of an atypical atrial flutter seen during an ablation procedure for nonparoxysmal AF. After isolating the pulmonary veins and placing additional lesions at sites of CFAEs, the rhythm had organized to the atypical flutter. (B) Using a penta-array catheter in conjunction with an electroanatomic mapping system (NavX), the atrium was rapidly mapped. Activation mapping showed an area of percolation of activity (A, arrow) between the previously placed ablation lesions isolating the right inferior pulmonary vein and the inferior left atrium region below the right inferior pulmonary vein. Entrainment of the flutter from this site showed a postpacing interval–tachycardia cycle length. (C) As shown on the activation map projected onto a three-dimensional CT image, an ablation lesion placed at this location terminated and eliminated the flutter.

THE SAFETY OF ATRIAL FIBRILLATION ABLATION

When performed by experienced operators, catheter ablation of AF is not a very high-risk procedure. As with all procedures, however, several potential complications are associated with ablation. Accordingly, improving the safety of the procedure has been and continues to be an important area of investigation. Several complications are associated with AF ablation, but the most important are PV stenosis, thromboembolism and stroke, perforation with cardiac tamponade, phrenic nerve injury, and atrioesophageal fistula.

It is now well established that if too much radiofrequency energy is applied within a PV, stenosis can occur.[35,36] Although this complication was common early in the ablation experience, symptomatic PV stenosis is now uncommon, with a frequency of approximately 1%. This decreased incidence is partly a result of the more careful use of various imaging modalities (eg, intracardiac ultrasound, three-dimensional CT and MRI) to prevent inadvertent ablation deep within a PV (**Fig. 10**). Future developments include continued refinements in real-time imaging, such as three-dimensional ultrasound imaging or direct visual guidance (eg, endoscopic visualization using the laser balloon catheter), and the use of alternative energy modalities, such as cryothermal energy, that seem to have minimal risk for PV stenosis.[37]

During radiofrequency energy delivery, the temperature of the catheter tip increases when in contact with the tissue being ablated. When this temperature exceeds approximately 50°C, however, coagulum can accumulate and embolize to cause a stroke. The simple solution has been to irrigate the tip of the ablation catheter with saline to prevent overheating. Future approaches include the use of other ablation technologies that either work by generating more volumetric heating (eg, focused ultrasound, laser energy) or have an inherently low thrombogenic potential (eg, cryothermal energy).

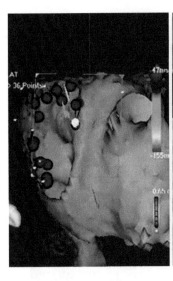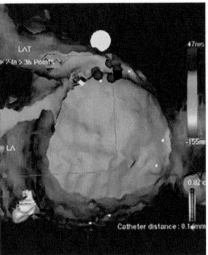

Fig. 10. Using a properly registered CT image, the ablation catheter is precisely positioned at the ridge, separating the left pulmonary veins and left atrial appendage. In avoiding placing the catheter deep inside the pulmonary vein, the risk for pulmonary vein stenosis can be minimized. An endoluminal image of the left pulmonary veins (*left*) and a posterior view with the posterior atrial wall clipped away to show the relative incursion of the ablation catheter into the pulmonary vein (*right*).

When too much radiofrequency energy is delivered into the tissue, steam formation can rapidly occur, culminating in a "pop." Although some of these pops are clinically insignificant, others can result in cardiac perforation and pericardial effusion with tamponade physiology. The amount of power that qualifies as too much varies significantly, however, according to the catheter tip–tissue contact force. That is, mild contact may require 35 W of energy to generate an adequate lesion, but forceful contact with the tissue may require only 15 W, with 35 W causing a pop. One of the important areas of active investigation is the development of a force-sensing mechanism on the catheter tip to optimize energy delivery.

The right phrenic nerve is typically located just lateral to the superior vena cava in proximity to the right superior PV but several centimeters distal to the vein ostium. Phrenic nerve injury can occur if radiofrequency energy is delivered at this location.[38] From a practical perspective, this complication is now uncommon during radiofrequency ablation, because ablation is now typically delivered at the vein ostium and not within the vein. Because of the typical funnel-shaped morphology of the right superior PV, however, balloon ablation catheters tend to lodge further inside the vein. Accordingly, phrenic nerve injury has been a more common issue associated with these devices. One of the important goals in the further development of these balloon catheters is either to minimize the impact of this complication or to avoid this complication altogether.

Although certainly one of the most infrequent complications associated with AF ablation (estimated at less than 1:10,000), atrioesophageal fistula formation remains the most feared because

of its high mortality. This complication occurs from inadvertent damage to the esophagus as ablation energy is applied to the posterior left atrium.[39–41] Although the exact pathophysiology of atrioesophageal fistula formation is unknown, the outcome is dismal.[42] Recent experience suggests that early recognition and treatment may prevent a fatal outcome. With an esophageal ulcer, mild interventions may be required, such as treatment with proton-pump inhibiting medications and not giving patients anything by mouth. Esophageal stent placement has been used successfully, however, in a patient who had a transmural esophageal ulcer, without a frank fistula to the atrium.[43] Furthermore, with prompt recognition that an atrioesophageal fistula has already formed, cardiac surgery can correct the defect.

Although the best strategy is prevention, further work is needed to define best the most appropriate means to avoid esophageal injury. The strategies that are currently being used include minimizing the overall amount of energy delivered to the posterior wall, visualizing the real-time position of the esophagus during catheter ablation with either intracardiac ultrasound or fluoroscopy, and esophageal temperature monitoring to help titrate the magnitude and duration of energy delivery. Two other concepts being explored are the use of a cooling balloon catheter placed inside the esophagus to counteract the thermal effect of the ablation energy and deflecting an endoscope positioned within the esophagus to deviate it away from the ablation catheter.[44,45] Further work is required to determine fully the usefulness of these various maneuvers. This investigation is particularly important as the ablation energy sources become progressively more powerful (eg, balloon ablation catheters).

STROKE PROPHYLAXIS IN PATIENTS WHO HAVE ATRIAL FIBRILLATION

Little doubt exists that warfarin treatment should be instituted in patients who have AF and additional risk factors (eg, advanced age, hypertension, congestive heart failure, diabetes, prior personal history of thromboembolism). Less well-understood, however, is whether successful catheter ablation can substantially and favorably modify this risk to obviate the need for oral anticoagulation treatment. Some data suggest that catheter ablation can favorably modify the risk to a level safe without warfarin.[46] One very important observation from the Atrial Fibrillation Follow-up Investigation of Rhythm Management study, however, was that patients who were believed to be treated successfully with antiarrhythmic medications still developed strokes as a result of asymptomatic AF.[47] Although catheter ablation can treat symptoms of AF, further studies are required to assess fully the effect of ablation on the long-term risk for thromboembolism and stroke.

Several other oral anticoagulant medications are being investigated as alternatives to warfarin (discussed elsewhere in this issue), but none has gained clinical approval. One nonpharmacologic approach is currently being investigated, however, as an alternative to warfarin: the Watchman device. This device consists of a nitinol spline and is covered by a 120-μm pore filter made of polytetrafluoroethylene. When delivered through a long transseptal sheath, it can be placed at the ostium of the left atrial appendage to cause permanent occlusion (**Fig. 11**). After undergoing significant evolution in a preliminary safety study, the device is now being studied in the pivotal phase in the United States.[48] In this US Food and Drug Administration study, patients who have AF and at least one other risk factor for stroke are randomized to treatment with either the Watchman device or continued usual therapy (warfarin), with stroke as the primary end point.[49] This noninferiority study is designed to determine whether the Watchman device can replace warfarin for treating patients who have AF. In addition to assessing the safety of the Watchman device, this study directly assesses the true import of the left atrial appendage in the pathogenesis of stroke in patients who have AF. If positive, the Watchman device may be relevant in managing patients who have asymptomatic AF who do not want to

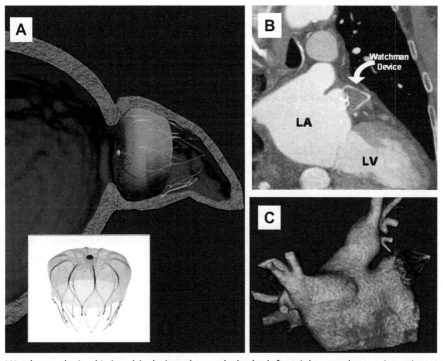

Fig. 11. The Watchman device (A, inset) is designed to occlude the left atrial appendage at its ostium. In a patient treated with this device, two-dimensional (B) and three-dimensional (C) CT images of the left atrium were obtained 1 year after implantation. Note the location of the Watchman device and the absence of contrast in the left atrial appendage, indicating its successful exclusion from the systemic circulation. (Part A Courtesy of Atritech, Plymouth, Minnesota; with permission.)

take warfarin and those who undergo catheter ablation (as concomitant therapy).

SUMMARY

Considerable progress has been made in understanding the pathogenesis of and approaches to the treatment of AF. More unanswered questions than answered questions remain, however, including the following:

What is the best approach to achieve permanent PV isolation?

Which patients who have nonparoxysmal AF can be treated with PV isolation alone?

What is the proper follow-up for patients who have undergone AF ablation?

How much ablation should be performed during catheter-based substrate modification of nonparoxysmal AF?

Which energy sources are the best for achieving long-term safety while maintaining an acceptable level of efficacy?

What are the precise electrogram characteristics during AF that best identify an active source of AF as opposed to irrelevant areas of passive activation?

In which patients can warfarin treatment be stopped after catheter ablation?

Further studies are required to answer these questions.

REFERENCES

1. Haissaguerre M, Jais P, Shah DC, et al. Spontaneous initiation of atrial fibrillation by ectopic beats originating in the pulmonary veins. N Engl J Med 1998;339:659–66.
2. Chen SA, Hsie MH, Tai CT, et al. Initiation of atrial fibrillation by ectopic beats originating from the pulmonary veins: electrophysiological characteristics, pharmacological responses, and effects of radiofrequency ablation. Circulation 1999;100:1879–86.
3. Jais P, Weerasooriya R, Shah DC, et al. Ablation therapy for atrial fibrillation (AF): past, present and future. Cardiovasc Res 2002;54:337–46.
4. Marrouche NF, Dresing T, Cole C, et al. Circular mapping and ablation of the pulmonary vein for treatment of atrial fibrillation: impact of different catheter technologies. J Am Coll Cardiol 2002;40:464–74.
5. Oral H, Scharf C, Chugh A, et al. Catheter ablation for paroxysmal atrial fibrillation: segmental pulmonary vein ostial ablation versus left atrial ablation. Circulation 2003;108:2355–60.
6. Ouyang F, Bansch D, Ernst S, et al. Complete isolation of left atrium surrounding the pulmonary veins:

7. new insights from the double-lasso technique in paroxysmal atrial fibrillation. Circulation 2004;110 2090–6.
7. Callans DJ, Gerstenfeld EP, Dixit S, et al. Efficacy o repeat pulmonary vein isolation procedures in patients with recurrent atrial fibrillation. J Cardiovasc Electrophysiol 2004;15:1050–6.
8. Faddis MN, Chen J, Osborn J, et al. Magnetic guidance system for cardiac electrophysiology: a prospective trial of safety and efficacy in humans J Am Coll Cardiol 2003;42:1952–8.
9. Pappone C, Vicedomini G, Manguso F, et al. Robotic magnetic navigation for atrial fibrillation ablation J Am Coll Cardiol 2006;47:1390–400.
10. DiBiase L, Tahmy TS, Patel D, et al. Remote Magnetic Navigation: human experience in pulmonar vein ablation. J Am Coll Cardiol 2007;50:868–74.
11. Al-Ahmad A, Grossman JD, Wang PJ. Early experience with a computerized robotically controlled catheter system. J Interv Card Electrophysiol 2005 12:199–202.
12. Saliba W, Cummings JE, Oh S, et al. Novel robotic catheter remote control system: feasibility and safety of transseptal puncture and endocardial catheter navigation. J Cardiovasc Electrophysiol 2006;17 1–4.
13. Reddy VY, Neuzil P, Malchano ZJ, et al. View-synchronized robotic image-guided therapy for atrial fibrillation ablation: experimental validation and clinical feasibility. Circulation 2007;115:2705–14.
14. Mikaelian BJ, Malchano ZJ, Neuzil P, et al. Integration of 3-dimensional cardiac computed tomography images with real-time electroanatomic mapping to guide catheter ablation of atrial fibrillation. Circulation 2005;112:E35–6.
15. Noseworthy PA, Malchano ZJ, Ahmed J, et al. The impact of respiration on left atrial and pulmonary venous anatomy: implications for image-guided intervention. Heart Rhythm 2005;2:1173–8.
16. Tops LF, Bax JJ, Zeppenfeld K, et al. Fusion of multi-slice computed tomography imaging with three dimensional electroanatomic mapping to guide radiofrequency catheter ablation procedures. Heart Rhythm 2005;7:1076–81.
17. Kistler PM, Eaerley MJ, Harris S, et al. Validation of three-dimensional cardiac image integration: use of integrated CT image into electroanatomic mapping system to perform catheter ablation of atrial fibrillation. J Cardiovasc Electrophysiol 2006 17:341–8.
18. Dong J, Dickfeld T, Dalal D, et al. Initial experience i the use of integrated electroanatomical mapping with three-dimensional MR/CT images to guide catheter ablation of atrial fibrillation. J Cardiovasc Electrophysiol 2006;17:459–66.
19. Malchano ZJ, Neuzil P, Cury R, et al. Integration of cardiac CT/MR imaging with 3-dimensional

electroanatomical mapping to guide catheter manipulation in the left atrium: implications for catheter ablation of atrial fibrillation. J Cardiovasc Electrophysiol 2006;17:251–5.

20. Orlov MV, Hoffmeister P, Chaudhry GM, et al. Three-dimensional rotational angiography of the left atrium and esophagus—a virtual computed tomography scan in the electrophysiology lab? Heart Rhythm 2007;4:37–43.

21. Thiagalingam A, Manzke R, d'Avila A, et al. Intra-procedural volume imaging of the left atrium and pulmonary veins with rotational x-ray angiography. J Cardiovasc Electrophysiol 2008;19(3):293–300.

22. Thiagalingam A, D'Avila A, Schmidt EJ, et al. Feasibility of MRI-guided mapping and pulmonary vein ablation in a swine model. Heart Rhythm 4(5S):S13.

23. Natale A, Pisano E, Shewchik J, et al. First human experience with pulmonary vein isolation using a through-the-balloon circumferential ultrasound ablation system for recurrent atrial fibrillation. Circulation 2000;102:1879–82.

24. Saliba W, Wilber D, Packer D, et al. Circumferential ultrasound ablation for pulmonary vein isolation: analysis of acute and chronic failures. J Cardiovasc Electrophysiol 2002;13:957–61.

25. Sarabanda AV, Bunch TJ, Johnson SB. Efficacy and safety of circumferential pulmonary vein isolation using a novel cryothermal balloon ablation system. J Am Coll Cardiol 2005;46:1902–12.

26. Reddy VY, Neuzil P, Pitschner HF, et al. Clinical experience with a balloon cryoablation catheter for pulmonary vein isolation in patients with atrial fibrillation: one-year results. Circulation 2005;112:II491–2.

27. Reddy VY, Neuzil P, Themisotoclakis S, et al. Long-term single-procedure clinical results with an endoscopic balloon ablation catheter for pulmonary vein isolation in patients with atrial fibrillation. Circulation 2006;114:II747.

28. Nakagawa H, Antz M, Wong T, et al. Initial experience using a forward directed, high-intensity focused ultrasound balloon catheter for pulmonary vein antrum isolation in patients with atrial fibrillation. J Cardiovasc Electrophysiol 2007;18:1–9.

29. Satake S, Tanaka K, Saito S, et al. Usefulness of a new radiofrequency thermal balloon catheter for pulmonary vein isolation: a new device for treatment of atrial fibrillation. J Cardiovasc Electrophysiol 2003;14:609–15.

30. Ahmed J, Sohal S, Malchano ZJ, et al. Three-dimensional analysis of pulmonary venous ostial and antral anatomy: implications for balloon catheter-based pulmonary vein isolation. J Cardiovasc Electrophysiol 2006;17:251–5.

31. Konings KT, Smeets JL, Penn OC, et al. Configuration of unipolar atrial electrograms during electrically induced atrial fibrillation in humans. Circulation 1997;95:1231–41.

32. Nademanee K, McKenzie J, Kosar E, et al. A new approach for catheter ablation of atrial fibrillation: mapping of the electrophysiologic substrate. J Am Coll Cardiol 2004;43:2044–53.

33. Haïssaguerre M, Sanders P, Hocini M, et al. Catheter ablation of long-lasting persistent atrial fibrillation: critical structures for termination. J Cardiovasc Electrophysiol 2005;16:1125–37.

34. Haïssaguerre M, Hocini M, Sanders P, et al. Catheter ablation of long-lasting persistent atrial fibrillation: clinical outcome and mechanisms of subsequent arrhythmias. J Cardiovasc Electrophysiol 2005;16:1138–47.

35. Robbins IM, Colvin EV, Doyle TP, et al. Pulmonary vein stenosis after catheter ablation of atrial fibrillation. Circulation 1998;98:1769–75.

36. Packer DL, Keelan P, Munger TM, et al. Clinical presentation, investigation, and management of pulmonary vein stenosis complicating ablation for atrial fibrillation. Circulation 2005;111:546–54.

37. Tse HF, Reek S, Timmermans C, et al. Pulmonary vein isolation using transvenous catheter cryoablation for treatment of atrial fibrillation without risk of pulmonary vein stenosis. J Am Coll Cardiol 2003;42:752–8.

38. Bai R, Patel D, Biase LD, et al. Phrenic nerve injury after catheter ablation: should we worry about this complication? J Cardiovasc Electrophysiol 2006;17:944–8.

39. Doll N, Borger MA, Fabricius A, et al. Esophageal perforation during left atrial radiofrequency ablation: is the risk too high? J Thorac Cardiovasc Surg 2003;125:836–42.

40. Sosa E, Scanavacca M. Left atrial-esophageal fistula complicating radiofrequency catheter ablation of atrial fibrillation. J Cardiovasc Electrophysiol 2005;16:249–50.

41. Pappone C, Oral H, Santinelli V, et al. Atrio-esophageal fistula as a complication of percutaneous transcatheter ablation of atrial fibrillation. Circulation 2004;109:2724–6.

42. Cummings JE, Schweikert RA, Saliba WI, et al. Brief communication: atrial-esophageal fistulas after radiofrequency ablation. Ann Intern Med 2006;144:572–4.

43. Bunch TJ, Nelson J, Foley T, et al. Temporary esophageal stenting allows healing of esophageal perforations following atrial fibrillation ablation procedures. J Cardiovasc Electrophysiol 2006;17:435–9.

44. Tsuchiya T, Ashikaga K, Nakagawa S, et al. Atrial fibrillation ablation with esophageal cooling with a cooled water-irrigated intraesophageal balloon: a pilot study. J Cardiovasc Electrophysiol 2007;18:145–50.

45. Yokoyama K, Nakagawa H, Reddy VY, et-al. Esophageal cooling balloon prevents esophageal injury during pulmonary vein ablation in a canine model. Heart Rhythm 4(5S):S12–3.

46. Oral H, Chugh A, Ozaydin M, et al. Risk of thrombo-embolic events after percutaneous left atrial radio-frequency ablation of atrial fibrillation. Circulation 2006;114:759–65.

47. The Atrial Fibrillation Follow-up Investigation of Rhythm Management (AFFIRM) Investigators. A comparison of rate control and rhythm control in patients with atrial fibrillation. N Engl J Med 2002; 347:1825–33.

48. Sick PB, Schuler G, Hauptmann KE, et al. Initial worldwide experience with the WATCHMAN left atrial appendage system for stroke prevention in atrial fibrillation. J Am Coll Cardiol 2007;49:1490–5.

49. Fountain RB, Holmes DR, Chandrasekaran K, et al. The PROTECT AF (WATCHMAN Left Atrial Append-age System for Embolic PROTECTion in Patients with Atrial Fibrillation) trial. Am Heart J 2006;151: 956–61.

Index

Note: Page numbers of article titles are in **boldface** type.

A

A Trial of Dronedarone For Prevention Of
  Hospitalization in Patients with AF trial, 83
Ablation
  atrioventricular junction, in atrial fibrillation
    management, pacing in, 142–143
  atrioventricular node, 162–164. See also
    Atrioventricular node ablation.
  catheter. See *Catheter ablation.*
  in atrial fibrillation management
    historical perspective on, 6
    safety of, 209–210
  laser, balloon-based visually guided, 206–207
  radiofrequency
    balloon-based, in atrial fibrillation
      management, 207
    in stroke prevention in patients with atrial
      fibrillation
      long-term anticoagulation after, 127
      overview after, 131–132
  surgical, in atrial fibrillation management,
    179–188. See also *Atrial fibrillation,
    management of, surgical approaches to.*
  ultrasound, balloon-based high-intensity focused,
    in atrial fibrillation management, 207
ACC/AHA/ESC. See *American College of Cardiology/
  American Heart Association/European Society of
  Cardiology (ACC/AHA/ESC).*
ACC/AHA/HRS. See *American College of Cardiology/
  American Heart Association/Heart Rhythm Society
  (ACC/AHA/HRS).*
ACE-I. See *Angiotensin-converting enzyme inhibitors
  (ACE-I).*
Acid(s), fatty, omega-3, in atrial fibrillation
  management, 117
β-Adrenergic receptor antagonists, in postoperative
  atrial fibrillation prevention, 70
AF-CHF trial. See *Atrial Fibrillation and Congestive
  Heart Failure (AF-CHF) trial.*
AFFIRM trial. See *Atrial Fibrillation Follow-Up
  Investigation of Rhythm Management (AFFIRM)
  trial.*
Age, as factor in atrial fibrillation, 149–150
Aging, in animal models of atrial fibrillation, 51–52
Aldosterone antagonists, in atrial fibrillation
  management, 116
American College of Cardiology/American Heart
  Association/European Society of Cardiology

(ACC/AHA/ESC), 2006 revised Guidelines for the
  Management of Patients with Atrial Fibrillation,
  109, 123, 189
  risk factors for stroke in, 128
American College of Cardiology/American Heart
  Association/Heart Rhythm Society (ACC/AHA/
  HRS), guidelines for atrial fibrillation of, 135–136
American College of Chest Physicians guidelines, 81
American-Australian-African Trial with Dronedarone
  in Atrial Fibrillation or Flutter Patients for the
  Maintenance of Sinus Rhythm, 112
Amiodarone
  after failed electrical cardioversion in atrial
    fibrillation management, 101
  for rhythm control, in atrial fibrillation
    management, 192
  in atrial fibrillation management, 109
    historical perspective on, 4, 5
  in postoperative atrial fibrillation prevention, 71
  in sinus rhythm maintenance, in atrial fibrillation
    management, 109
Amiodarone analogues, in atrial fibrillation
  management, 111–113
ANDROMEDA trial. See *Antiarrhythmic Trial with
  Dronedarone in Moderate to Severe Congestive
  Heart Failure Evaluating Morbidity Decrease
  (ANDROMEDA).*
Anesthesia/anesthetics, for electrical cardioversion in
  atrial fibrillation management, 98–99
Angiotensin receptor blockers, in atrial fibrillation
  management, 115–116
Angiotensin-converting enzyme inhibitors (ACE-I), in
  atrial fibrillation management, 115
Antiarrhythmic drugs
  for rhythm control, in atrial fibrillation
    management, 191–192
  in patients with atrial fibrillation and implantable
    defibrillators
    defibrillation threshold and, 155
    shocks related to, 155
Antiarrhythmic Trial with Dronedarone in Moderate to
  Severe Congestive Heart Failure Evaluating
  Morbidity Decrease (ANDROMEDA), 113
Anticoagulant(s)
  after radiofrequency ablation in stroke prevention
    in patients with atrial fibrillation, long-term use,
    127
  oral, in stroke prevention in patients with atrial
    fibrillation, long-term use issues, 129–131

Cardiol Clin 27 (2009) 217–225
doi:10.1016/S0733-8651(08)00117-3
0733-8651/08/$ – see front matter © 2009 Elsevier Inc. All rights reserved

cardiology.theclinics.com

Anticoagulation
   in atrial fibrillation management, 188–190
      before cardioversion in, 189–190
      in CHF patients, 80–82
      postoperative, 73–74
      risk stratification for, 188–189
      warfarin in, 189
   in patients with implantable defibrillators, 155–156
   pericardioversion, in atrial fibrillation
      management, 94–96
Anti-inflammatory agents, in atrial fibrillation
   management, 116
Apixaban, in stroke prevention in patients with atrial
   fibrillation, 128
ASPECT. See *Atrial Septal Pacing Efficacy Clinical
   Trial (ASPECT)*.
Aspirin, in stroke prevention in patients with atrial
   fibrillation, 125–128
Assessment of Cardioversion using Transesophageal
   Echocardiography trial, 82–83
Association studies, in genetics of atrial fibrillation,
   28, 30
ATI-2001, in atrial fibrillation management, 113
Atorvastatin for Reduction of Myocardial Dysrhythmia
   After Cardiac Surgery study, 116
Atorvastatin Therapy for the Prevention of Atrial
   Fibrillation trial, 116
Atrial Arrhythmia Conversion Trial I and III, 114
Atrial autonomic nerves, structural anatomy of,
   38–39
Atrial burst pacing, in animal models of atrial
   fibrillation, 49–50
Atrial fibrillation
   ACC/AHA/HRS guidelines for, 135–136
   anatomic and neural substrates in pulmonary
      veins during, 37
   animal models of
      aging in, 51–52
      atrial burst pacing in, 49–50
      autonomic stimulation in, 49
      clinical paradigms in, 46–47
      heart failure in, 50–51
      information learned from, **45–54**
      spiral wave model, 45–46
      sterile pericarditis in, 51
   autonomic nervous system and, 39
   "calcium-transient triggering" hypothesis in, 38
   cardiac autonomic innervation during, 37
   cardiovascular conditions associated with, 16
   catheter ablation of, **163–178**
   causes of, historical perspective on, 3
   chronic, classification of, 45
   classification of, 107
   clinical implications of, 69–70
   clinical manifestations of, 17
   complications of, 187
   described, 35, 161

echocardiographic abnormalities associated
   with, 16
epidemiology of
   current perceptions of, **13–24**
   overlapping, 149–152
future directions in, **201–216**
genetics of, **25–33**
   described, 25–26
   genes and loci implicated in, 27
   historical perspective on, 3–4
   studies of, 26–30
      association studies, 28, 30
      candidate gene studies, 28
      linkage analysis, 26–28
      refining of, 30
heart failure with, management of, 195
historical perspective on, **1–12**
   causes, 3
   described, 1
   earliest clinical sightings, 1–2
   ECG, 2–3
   genetics, 3–4
   localizing origin, 4
   management, 4–8. See also *Atrial fibrillation,
      management of, historical perspective on.*
   pathophysiology, 3
   thromboembolism, 6–7
in CHF, **79–93**. See also *Congestive heart failure
   (CHF), atrial fibrillation in.*
in patients with implantable defibrillators,
   151–161. See also *Implantable defibrillators,
   atrial fibrillation in patients with.*
incidence of, 13–14, 25, 69
lone, management of, surgical ablation in, 180
management of, **109–123**. See also specific types
   and agents.
   ablation in, safety of, 209–210
   ACE-I in, 115
   aldosterone antagonists in, 116
   amiodarone analogues in, 111–113
   angiotensin receptor blockers in, 115–116
   anticoagulation in, 188–190
   anti-inflammatory agents in, 116
   ATI-2001 in, 113
   atrial repolarization delaying agents in,
      114–115
   AVE0118 in, 114
   AZD7009 in, 114–115
   azimilide in, 113–114
   balloon ablation catheters in, 205–207
   cardiac resynchronization therapy in, 144–145
   cardioversion in, **95–107**. See also
      *Cardioversion, in atrial fibrillation
      management.*
   celicarone in, 113
   clinical presentations as factor in, 193–195
   costs related to, 18, 25

device-related applications for, 136
dronedarone in, 111–112
future directions in, 8
goals in, **189–200**
    future, 188
    symptom control, 188
    tachycardia-induced cardiomyopathy
       prevention, 188
    thromboembolism prevention, 187–188
heart failure–related, 195
historical perspective on, 4–6
    ablation procedures, 6
    cardioversion, 5–6
    drugs, 4–5
    surgical approaches, 7–8
initial approach in, 193–194
neural modulation in, 40–41
newly diagnosed cases, 194
omega-3 fatty acids in, 117
outpatient vs. inpatient initiation of, 110–111
pacemakers in, **137–150.** See also
    Pacemaker(s), in atrial fibrillation
    management.
paroxysmal atrial fibrillation, 194
permanent atrial fibrillation, 194
persistent atrial fibrillation, 194
pharmacologic, future directions in, 111–115
postoperative atrial fibrillation, 195
rate control in, 107–108, 190–193. See also
    Rate control, in atrial fibrillation
    management.
recurrent atrial fibrillation, 194
remote navigation technology in, 200–205
rhythm control in, 109, 190–193. See also
    Rhythm control, in atrial fibrillation
    management.
serotonin antagonists in, 115
sinus rhythm maintenance in, 109–110
statins in, 116
steroids in, 116
surgical approaches to, **179–188**
    challenges facing, 181–182
    energy sources for, 180
    for lone atrial fibrillation, 180
    future directions in, 181–182
    left atrial appendage, 181
    lesion sets in, 179–180
    maze procedure, 178–179
    minimally invasive, 182
    new approaches, 179–180
    rationale for, 177–178
tachycardia-bradycardia syndrome, 194
tedisamil in, 114
traditional class III agents in, 113–114
vernakalant in, 114
mapping of, historical perspective on, 4
mechanisms of, surgical ablation and, 178

new concepts in, **35–43**
newly diagnosed, management of, 194
nonparoxysmal, management of, catheter
    ablation in, 207–208
origin of, localization of, 4
paroxysmal
    animal models of, sympathetic nerve
       recordings in, 39–40
    management of, 194
       catheter ablation in, 199–200
    vs. persistent, management of, pacing in,
       143–144
pathogenesis of, 69
pathophysiology of, 45–49
    historical perspective on, 3
patterns of, 93
permanent, management of, 194
persistent, management of, 194
    pacing in, 143–144
polymorphisms associated with, 29
postoperative, **69–78.** See also *Postoperative*
    atrial fibrillation.
prevalence of, 13–14, 25, 107, 149
prevention of, adjuvant therapy in, 115–116
prognosis of, 17–18
public health burden of, 18
recurrent, management of, 194
risk factors for, 149–152
    age, 149–150
    Brugada syndrome, 150–152
    cardiovascular, 14–16
    channelopathies, 150–152
    cigarette smoking, 14
    diabetes mellitus, 14–15
    gender, 150
    genetics, 20
    heart failure, 150
    hypertension, 15–16
    long Q syndrome, 150–152
    multivariable assessment of, 20–21
    novel, 19–20
    obesity, 14
    thyroid disease, 18–19
secular trends in, 13–14
stroke after
    incidence of, 69
    prevalence of, 123
stroke prevention in patients with, **125–135,**
    211–212
    apixaban in, 128
    aspirin in, 125–128
    cardioversion in, 128–129
    dabigatran in, 128
    new agents in, 128
    oral anticoagulants in, long-term use issues,
       129–131
    radiofrequency ablation in

Atrial (*continued*)
  long-term anticoagulation after, 127
  overview after, 131–132
  rivaroxaban in, 128
  warfarin in, 124–125
  sustained, patterns of activation at pulmonary vein and pulmonary vein–left atrial junction during, 36–37
  sympathetic activation during, 38
  symptomatic, management of, cardioversion in, 93–94
  symptoms of, 187
  thromboembolism in, historical perspective on, 6–7
  thyroid disease and, 18–19
  unanswered questions about, **201–216**
  vagal, in heart failure, CA$_i$ dynamics and, 40
  Wolff-Parkinson-White syndrome and, management of, 195
Atrial Fibrillation and Congestive Heart Failure (AF-CHF) trial, 83–85
Atrial Fibrillation Clopidogrel Trial with Irbesartan for Prevention of Vascular Events, 116
Atrial Fibrillation Follow-Up Investigation of Rhythm Management (AFFIRM) trial, 5, 83–85, 107–108, 129–130, 161, 188, 190
Atrial flutter
  management of, cardioversion in, 102
  terminology related to, 55
  type 1
    described, 55
    diagnosis of, ECG in, 57
    electrophysiologic mapping of, 57–58
    management of
      medical therapy vs. catheter ablation in, 57
      radiofrequency catheter ablation in, 58–64. See also *Radiofrequency catheter ablation, in type 1 atrial flutter management.*
    pathophysiologic mechanisms of, 257
  type(s) of, 55
  typical, **55–67**
Atrial pacing, in postoperative atrial fibrillation prevention, 72
Atrial repolarization delaying agents, in atrial fibrillation management, 114–115
Atrial Septal Pacing Efficacy Clinical Trial (ASPECT), 144
Atrioventricular junction ablation, in atrial fibrillation management, pacing in, 142–143
Atrioventricular nodal conduction, regulation of, pacing in, 142
Atrioventricular node ablation, 162–164
  of atrial fibrillation
    limitations of, 163–164
    outcomes of, 163–164
    overview of, 162–163
    techniques, 163
Autonomic nervous system, atrial fibrillation and, 39
AVE0118, in atrial fibrillation management, 114
AZD7009, in atrial fibrillation management, 114–115
Azimilide, in atrial fibrillation management, 113–114
Azimilide Postinfarct Survival Evaluation trial, 113
Azimilide Supraventricular Arrhythmia Program, 113
Azimilide Supraventricular Tachyarrhythmia Reduction trial, 114

B

BAFTA study. See *Birmingham Atrial Fibrillation Treatment of the Aged (BAFTA) study.*
Balloon ablation catheters, in atrial fibrillation management, 205–207
Balloon cryoablation, in atrial fibrillation management, 206
Balloon-based high-intensity focused ultrasound ablation, in atrial fibrillation management, 207
Balloon-based pulmonary vein isolation, in atrial fibrillation management, 207
Balloon-based radiofrequency ablation, in atrial fibrillation management, 207
Balloon-based visually guided laser ablation, in atrial fibrillation management, 206–207
Birmingham Atrial Fibrillation Treatment of the Aged (BAFTA) study, 127
Biventricular pacing, in atrial fibrillation management, 144–145
ß-Blockers, in atrial fibrillation management, 108
Brugada syndrome, as factor in atrial fibrillation, 150–152

C

Calcium channel antagonists, in postoperative atrial fibrillation prevention, 71
Calcium channel blockers, in atrial fibrillation management, 108
"Calcium-transient triggering" hypothesis, in atrial fibrillation, 38
Canadian Trial of Atrial Fibrillation, 83, 192
Canadian Trial of Physiologic Pacing (CTOPP), 137, 138
Candesartan in the Prevention of Relapsing Atrial Fibrillation trial, 116
Candidate gene studies, in genetics of atrial fibrillation, 28
Cardiac Arrhythmia Suppression Trial (CAST), 4, 192
Cardiac autonomic innervation, during atrial fibrillation, 37
Cardiac resynchronization therapy, in atrial fibrillation management, 144–145
  in CHF patients, 86–87

Cardiomyopathy, tachycardia-induced, prevention of, in atrial fibrillation management, 188

Cardiovascular Health Study, 69

Cardioversion
in atrial fibrillation management, **95–107**
anticoagulation before, 189–190
described, 96
electrical cardioversion, 96–101. See also *Electrical cardioversion, in atrial fibrillation management.*
for rhythm control, 192
historical perspective on, 5–6
indications for, 93–94
pericardioversion anticoagulation in, 94–96
pharmacologic cardioversion, 101–102
specific uses, 93
successful, rates of, 94
in atrial flutter management, 102
in patients with atrial fibrillation and implantable defibrillators, 156
in stroke prevention in patients with atrial fibrillation, 128–129
pharmacologic, in atrial fibrillation management, 109
transthoracic electrical, described, 93

Carto, in diagnosis and ablation of type 1 atrial flutter, 62–64

CAST. See *Cardiac Arrhythmia Suppression Trial (CAST).*

Catheter(s), balloon ablation, in atrial fibrillation management, 205–207

Catheter ablation
curative, of atrial fibrillation, 164–172. See also *Curative catheter ablation.*
for nonparoxysmal atrial fibrillation, 207–208
for paroxysmal atrial fibrillation, 199–200
in atrial fibrillation management, **163–178.** See also specific types, e.g., *Atrioventricular node ablation.*
atrioventricular node ablation, 162–164
curative catheter ablation, 164–172
in CHF patients, 87–88
in type 1 atrial flutter management, 57–64
alternative energy sources for, 64
radiofrequency catheter ablation, 58–64. See also *Radiofrequency catheter ablation, in type 1 atrial flutter management.*
vs. medical therapy, 57
radiofrequency, fundamentals of, 161–162

Celicarone, in atrial fibrillation management, 113

CFAEs. See *Complex fractionated atrial electrograms (CFAEs).*

CHADS$_2$ score, 5, 81, 188–189

Channelopathy(ies), as factor in atrial fibrillation, 150–152

CHF. See *Congestive heart failure (CHF).*

CHF-STAT study. See *Congestive Heart Failure–Survival Trial of Antiarrhythmic Therapy (CHF-STAT) study.*

Cigarette smoking, as factor in atrial fibrillation, 14

Comparison of Rate Control and Rhythm Control in Patients with Recurrent Persistent Atrial Fibrillation trial, 130

Complex fractionated atrial electrograms (CFAEs), 208

Computerized three-dimensional mapping, in diagnosis and ablation of type 1 atrial flutter, 62–64

Congestive heart failure (CHF), atrial fibrillation in, **79–93**
management of, 80–83
anticoagulation in, 80–82
cardiac resynchronization therapy in, 86–87
catheter ablation in, 87–88
enalapril in, 85
nonantiarrhythmic drugs in, 85–86
rate control in, 82
vs. rhythm control, 83–85
rhythm control–acute conversion in, 82–83
rhythm control–maintenance of sinus rhythm in, 83
mechanisms of, 79–80
sinus rhythm and survival in, 85

Congestive Heart Failure–Survival Trial of Antiarrhythmic Therapy (CHF-STAT) study, 83

Corridor procedure, in atrial fibrillation management, 8

Corticosteroid(s), in postoperative atrial fibrillation prevention, 72

Cox maze III operation, in atrial fibrillation management, 178–179

Cryoablation, balloon, in atrial fibrillation management, 206

CTOPP. See *Canadian Trial of Physiologic Pacing (CTOPP).*

Curative catheter ablation, of atrial fibrillation, 164–172
adjunctive techniques, 167–168
background of, 164
end points in, 168
follow-up, 172
future advances in, 172
limitations of, 168–172
outcomes of, 168–172
overview of, 164
patient selection for, 164–166
technical aspects of, 166–167

D

Dabigatran, in stroke prevention in patients with atrial fibrillation, 128

Danish Investigators of Arrhythmia and Mortality on Dofetilide (DIAMOND)-CHF trial, 83, 110

Diabetes mellitus, as factor in atrial fibrillation, 14–15
DIAMOND-CHF trial. See *Danish Investigators of Arrhythmia and Mortality on Dofetilide (DIAMOND)-CHF trial.*
Digitalis, in postoperative atrial fibrillation prevention, 71–72
Digoxin, in atrial fibrillation management, 108–109
Direct heating, 162
Dofetilide, in atrial fibrillation management
    for rhythm control, 192
    for sinus rhythm maintenance, 110
    historical perspective on, 5
Double Blind Placebo Controlled Dose Ranging Study of the Efficacy and Safety of ssr149744c 300 or 600 mg for the Conversion of Atrial Fibrillation/Flutter trial, 113
Dronedarone, in atrial fibrillation management, 111–112
Dronedarone Atrial Fibrillation Study After Electrical Cardioversion trial, 112
Drug(s)
    in atrial fibrillation management, historical perspective on, 4–5
    in patients with atrial fibrillation and implantable defibrillators, 155–156
    in postoperative atrial fibrillation prevention, 70–72

E

ECG. See *Electrocardiography (ECG).*
Echocardiography, in atrial fibrillation, abnormalities seen on, 16
Efficacy and Safety of Dronedarone for the Control of Ventricular Rate trial, 112
Einthoven, Willem, in ECG development, 2
Electrical cardioversion, in atrial fibrillation management
    anesthesia in, 98–99
    biphasic waveform superior to monophasic waveforms, 96–97
    energy selection in, 98–99
    failed, 100–101
        pharmacologic therapy after, 101
    immediate recurrence of atrial fibrillation after, 99–100
    in patients with implanted devices, 99
    internal by way of intracardiac catheters, 99
    outcomes of, 99
    pad or paddle positioning and size in, 98
    practical considerations for, 97–101
    shock delivery in, 98
Electrocardiography (ECG)
    development of, Einthoven, Willem in, 2
    in atrial fibrillation, historical perspective on, 2–3
    in type 1 atrial flutter diagnosis, 57
Enalapril, in atrial fibrillation management, in CHF patients, 85

Encainide, in atrial fibrillation management, historical perspective on, 4
Ensite system, in diagnosis and ablation of type 1 atrial flutter, 62–64
ESC. See *European Society of Cardiology (ESC).*
European and Australian Multicenter Evaluative Research on Atrial Fibrillation and Dofetilide study, 110
European Rythmol/Rytmonorm Atrial Fibrillation Trial 109
European Society of Cardiology (ESC), Working Group of Arrhythmias of, 55
European Trial in Atrial Fibrillation or Flutter Patients Receiving Dronedarone for the Maintenance of Sinus Rhythm, 112

F

Fatty acids, omega-3, in atrial fibrillation management, 117
FDA. See *Food and Drug Administration (FDA).*
Flecainide, in atrial fibrillation management
    for sinus rhythm maintenance, 110
    historical perspective on, 4
Food and Drug Administration (FDA), 5, 60, 83, 110, 111, 125, 139, 140, 180, 189
Framingham Heart Study, 14–15, 40, 187
Framingham risk score, 123

G

Gender, as factor in atrial fibrillation, 150
Genetics
    as factor in atrial fibrillation, 20
    of atrial fibrillation, **25–33.** See also *Atrial fibrillation, genetics of.*
Grupo de Estudio de la Sobrevida en la Insuficienca Cardica en Argentina Trial, 83
Guidant Heart Rhythm Technologies Linear Ablation System, in atrial fibrillation management, 7

H

Harvey, William, role in atrial fibrillation, 1
Heart, electrophysiology of, vagal influences on, 37–38
Heart failure
    atrial fibrillation and, 150
        management of, 195
    in animal models of atrial fibrillation, 50–51
    vagal atrial fibrillation in, CA_i dynamics and, 40
Heart Outcomes Prevention Evaluation Study, 115
Heating, direct, 162
How to Treat Chronic Atrial Fibrillation trial, 83
Human Genome Project, 26
Hypertension, as factor in atrial fibrillation, 15–16

I

Ibutilide
  after failed electrical cardioversion in atrial
    fibrillation management, 101
  in atrial fibrillation management, historical
    perspective on, 5
Implantable defibrillators, atrial fibrillation in patients
  with, **151–161,** 152–154
  cardioversion and, 156
  drugs and, 155–156
  inappropriate shocks from, 152–154

L

Laser ablation, balloon-based visually guided, in atrial
  fibrillation management, 206–207
Left atrial appendage, in atrial fibrillation
  management, 181
Linkage analysis studies, in genetics of atrial
  fibrillation, 26–28
Long Q syndrome, as factor in atrial fibrillation,
  150–152
Losartan Intervention for Endpoint Reduction in
  Hypertension trial, 116

M

Magnesium, in postoperative atrial fibrillation
  prevention, 72
Maintenance of Sinus Rhythm in Patients with Recent
  Atrial Fibrillation/Flutter trial, 113
Maze procedure, in atrial fibrillation management,
  178–179
Mini-Mental State Examination score, 69
Mode Selection in Sinus-Node Dysfunction Trial
  (MOST), 137, 138
MOST. See Mode Selection in Sinus-Node
  Dysfunction Trial (MOST).

N

National Institutes of Health Stroke Scale score, 69
Neural modulation, in atrial fibrillation, 40–41
Nonparoxysmal atrial fibrillation, management of,
  catheter ablation in, 207–208
North American Azimilide Cardioversion Maintenance
  Trial-I, 113
North American Society of Pacing and
  Electrophysiology, 55

O

Obesity, as factor in atrial fibrillation, 14
Omega-3 fatty acids, in atrial fibrillation management,
  117

P

PAC-ATACH trial. See Pacemaker Atrial Tachycardia
  (PAC-ATACH) trial.
Pacemaker(s)
  diagnostics of, 139–145
  in atrial fibrillation management, **137–150**
    atrial therapies in, 145
    atrioventricular junction ablation, 142–143
    biventricular pacing, 144–145
    chronic vs. permanent atrial fibrillation,
      141–142
    in regulation of atrioventricular nodal
      conduction, 142
    paroxysmal vs. persistent atrial fibrillation,
      143–144
Pacemaker Atrial Tachycardia (PAC-ATACH) trial,
  137, 138
Pacemaker Selection in the Elderly (PASE) trial,
  137, 138
Pacing
  atrial, in postoperative atrial fibrillation prevention,
    72
  biventricular, in atrial fibrillation management,
    144–145
  clinical trials in, 137
  in atrial fibrillation management, **137–150**
  physiologic, described, 136–139
Paroxysmal atrial fibrillation
  animal models of, sympathetic nerve recordings
    in, 39–40
  management of, 194
    catheter ablation in, 199–200
PASE trial. See Pacemaker Selection in the Elderly
  (PASE) trial.
PAVE trial. See Post AV Nodal Ablation Evaluation
  (PAVE) trial.
Pericardioversion anticoagulation, in atrial fibrillation
  management, 94–96
Pericarditis, sterile, in animal models of atrial
  fibrillation, 51
Permanent atrial fibrillation, management of, 194
Persistent atrial fibrillation, management of, 194
Pharmacologic cardioversion, in atrial fibrillation
  management, 101–102
Pharmacologic Intervention in Atrial Fibrillation (PIAF)
  trial, 83
Physiologic pacing, described, 136–139
PIAF trial. See Pharmacologic Intervention in Atrial
  Fibrillation (PIAF) trial.
Polymorphisms, atrial fibrillation–related, 29
Pop, defined, 162
Post AV Nodal Ablation Evaluation (PAVE) trial, 82
Postoperative atrial fibrillation, **69–78**
  management of, 72–74, 195
    anticoagulation in, 73–74
    rate control in, 72

Postoperative (*continued*)
    rhythm control in, 73
    predictors of, 70
    prevention of, 70–73
        ß-adrenergic receptor antagonists in, 70
        amiodarone in, 71
        atrial pacing in, 72
        calcium channel antagonists in, 71
        corticosteroids in, 72
        digitalis in, 71–72
        magnesium in, 72
        pharmacologic agents in, 70–72
        sotalol in, 71
        statins in, 72
Propafenone, in atrial fibrillation management
    for sinus rhythm maintenance, 109–110
    historical perspective on, 4
Pulmonary vein(s)
    anatomic and neural substrates in, during atrial
        fibrillation, 37
    autonomic nerves of, structural anatomy of, 38–39
    neural anatomy of, implications of, 39
    patterns of activation at, during sustained atrial
        fibrillation, 36–37
Pulmonary vein isolation, balloon-based, in atrial
    fibrillation management, 207
Pulmonary vein–left atrial junction, patterns of
    activation at, during sustained atrial fibrillation,
    36–37

Q

Quinidine, in atrial fibrillation management, historical
    perspective on, 4

R

RACE trials. See *Rate Control Versus Electrical
    Cardioversion (RACE) trials.*
Radiofrequency ablation
    balloon-based, in atrial fibrillation management,
        207
    in stroke prevention in patients with atrial
        fibrillation
        long-term anticoagulation after, 127
        overview after, 131–132
Radiofrequency catheter ablation
    fundamentals of, 161–162
    in type 1 atrial flutter management, 58–64
        complications of, 62
        computerized three-dimensional mapping in,
            62–64
        outcomes of, 62
        procedure end points for, 60–62
Rate control
    defined, 190–191

in atrial fibrillation management, 190–193
    agents in, 108–109
    described, 190
    in CHF patients, 82
    strategy for, 190
    therapeutic options for, 191
management of, 72
rhythm control vs., in atrial fibrillation
    management, 107–108
    in CHF patients, 83–85
Rate Control Versus Electrical Cardioversion (RACE)
    trials, 5, 83, 107–108
Recurrent atrial fibrillation, management of, 194
Remote magnetic navigation, in atrial fibrillation
    management, 200–202
Remote navigation technology, in atrial fibrillation
    management, 200–205
    image guidance, 203–205
    remote magnetic navigation, 200–202
    remote robotic navigation, 202–203
Remote robotic navigation, in atrial fibrillation
    management, 202–203
Rhythm control
    in atrial fibrillation management, 109, 190–193
        antiarrhythmic medications for, 191–192
        cardioversion in, 192
        described, 190
        nonpharmacologic, 193
        postoperative, 73
        strategy for, 190
        rate control vs., in atrial fibrillation management,
            107–108
        in CHF patients, 83–85
Rhythm control–acute conversion, in atrial fibrillation
    management, in CHF patients, 82–83
Rhythm control–maintenance of sinus rhythm, in atrial
    fibrillation management, in CHF patients, 83
Rivaroxaban, in stroke prevention in patients with
    atrial fibrillation, 128
Rythmol Atrial Fibrillation Trial, 109

S

SAFE-T trial, 83
Serotonin antagonists, in atrial fibrillation
    management, 115
Shock(s), inappropriate, implantable defibrillators in
    atrial fibrillation patients and, 152–154
Sinus rhythm, maintenance of, in atrial fibrillation
    management, 109–110
Smoking, cigarette, as factor in atrial fibrillation, 14
Sotalol
    in atrial fibrillation management
        for rhythm control, 192
        for sinus rhythm maintenance, 110
        historical perspective on, 4–5
        in postoperative atrial fibrillation prevention, 71

Sotalol Amiodarone Atrial Fibrillation Efficacy Trial, 109
Spiral wave model, of atrial fibrillation, 45–46
STAF trial. See *Strategies of Treatment of Atrial Fibrillation (STAF) trial.*
Statin(s)
  in atrial fibrillation management, 116
  in postoperative atrial fibrillation prevention, 72
Sterile pericarditis, in animal models of atrial fibrillation, 51
Steroid(s), in atrial fibrillation management, 116
Strategies of Treatment of Atrial Fibrillation (STAF) trial, 83
Stroke, in patients with atrial fibrillation
  incidence of, 69
  prevalence of, 123
  prevention of, **125–135,** 211–212. See also *Atrial fibrillation, stroke prevention in patients with.*
  risk factors for
    epidemiology of, 123
    stratification schemes for, 123
    Surgical ablation, for atrial fibrillation, **179–188.** See also *Atrial fibrillation, management of, surgical approaches to.*
Sympathetic activation, during atrial fibrillation, 38
Symptomatic Atrial Fibrillation Investigative Research on Dofetilide trial, 110

T

Tachycardia(s), cardiomyopathy due to, prevention of, in atrial fibrillation management, 188
Tachycardia-bradycardia syndrome, management of, 194
Tedisamil, in atrial fibrillation management, 114
Thromboembolism
  atrial fibrillation and, historical perspective on, 6–7
  prevention of, in atrial fibrillation management, 187–188
Thyroid disease, as factor in atrial fibrillation, 18–19
Trandolapril Cardiac Evaluation trial, 115
Transthoracic electrical cardioversion, described, 93

2006 Guidelines for the Management of Patients with Atrial Fibrillation (revised), of ACC/AHA/ESC, 123
  risk factors for stroke in, 128

U

UKPACE trial. See *United Kingdom Pacing and Cardiovascular Events (UKPACE) trial.*
Ultrasound ablation, balloon-based high-intensity focused, in atrial fibrillation management, 207
United Kingdom Pacing and Cardiovascular Events (UKPACE) trial, 137, 138
University College of London, 1
US Food and Drug Administration. See *Food and Drug Administration (FDA).*

V

Vagal atrial fibrillation, in heart failure, CA_i dynamics and, 40
Vagal influences, on cardiac electrophysiology, 37–38
Valsartan Heart Failure Trial, 116
Vernakalant, in atrial fibrillation management, 114
Veterans Affairs Congestive Heart Failure: Survival Trial of Antiarrhythmic Therapy, 109

W

Warfarin
  in atrial fibrillation management, 189
  in stroke prevention in patients with atrial fibrillation, 124–125
Watchman device, 211
Wolff-Parkinson-White syndrome, atrial fibrillation and, management of, 195
Working Group of Arrhythmias, of European Society of Cardiology, 55

Y

Yellow Emperor's Classic of Internal Medicine, 1

Moving?

Make sure your subscription moves with you!

To notify us of your new address, find your **Clinics Account Number** (located on your mailing label above your name), and contact customer service at:

E-mail: elspcs@elsevier.com

800-654-2452 (subscribers in the U.S. & Canada)
314-453-7041 (subscribers outside of the U.S. & Canada)

Fax number: 314-523-5170

Elsevier Periodicals Customer Service
11830 Westline Industrial Drive
St. Louis, MO 63146

*To ensure uninterrupted delivery of your subscription, please notify us at least 4 weeks in advance of move.

Printed and bound by CPI Group (UK) Ltd, Croydon, CR0 4YY

03/10/2024

01040348-0004